Welcome

Gluten. It's a word that has become very familiar from supermarket shelves, product packaging, bakery displays and restaurant menus. But what is it, where does it come from and why does it cause a problem for so many people?

This publication aims to answer all those questions and to provide a guide to living your best life gluten-free. Whether you are someone who has to avoid it, or you have a friend or family member you want to support, there are pointers on day-to-day shopping for food and beauty products – what to look for and what to avoid – as well as on eating out and travelling.

You will also find chapters on identifying the many different conditions that can arise from eating gluten, and how to get a diagnosis if you are one of the people who suspect their symptoms are diet-related but don't know for sure. It's estimated that more than 60% of people with a gluten condition have not been clinically diagnosed.

We highlight the helpful organisations to seek out and useful books, websites and apps to explore – there is a lot of information and some great gluten-free recipes to be found on internet blogger sites, and many self-help and cookery books you can order online, and we cover some of those too.

We also include a few simple and delicious recipes for savoury dishes and desserts for you to try, and, as a bonus, you will find a handy conversion chart for US cups, metric and imperial measures on the inside back cover. If you cut this out and keep it on the fridge it will be a handy reference for following any gluten-free recipes you come across.

The world of gluten-free living is a complex one and can be daunting, whether it affects you directly or someone you love. Hopefully you will find our handbook an invaluable help in navigating that world.

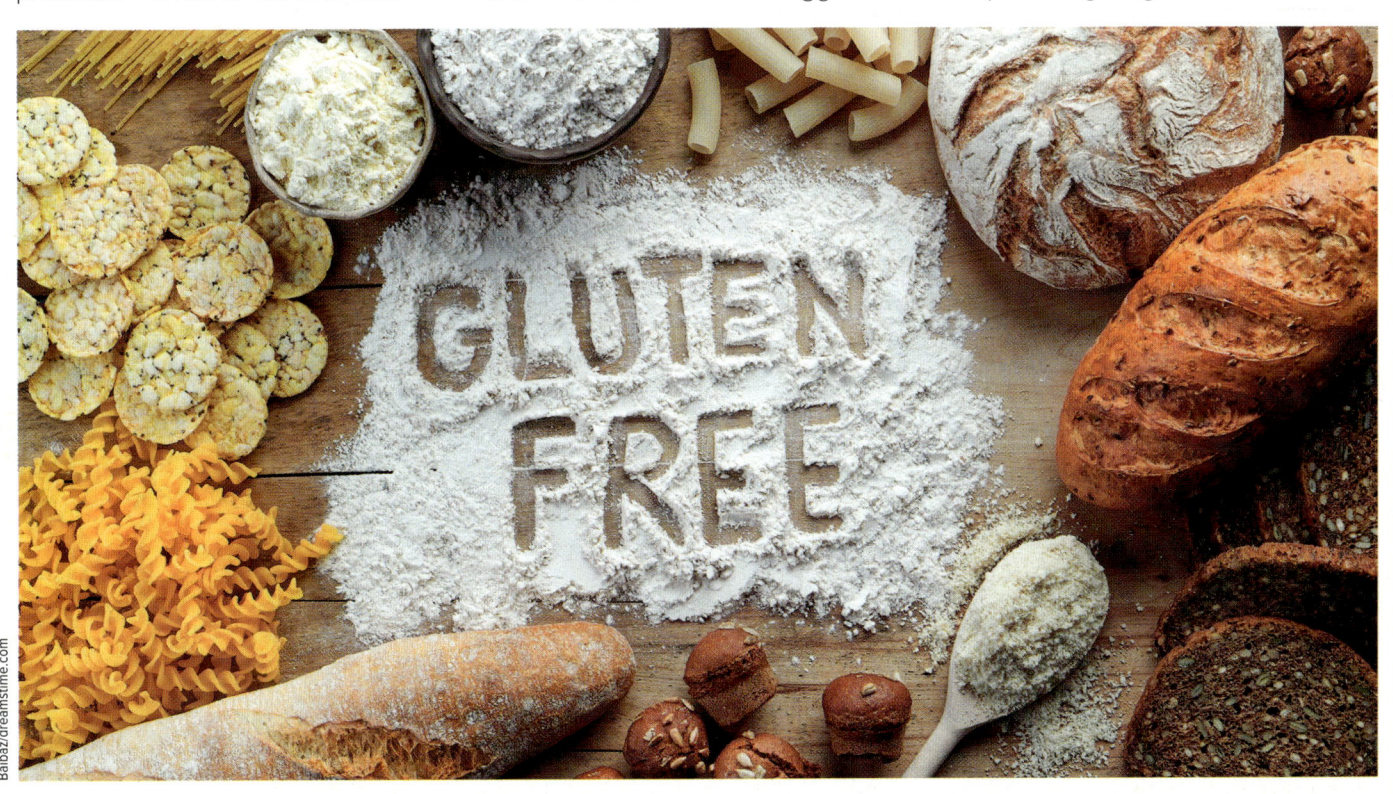

ISBN: 978 1 83632 085 2
Editor: Sheena Harvey
Senior editor, specials: Roger Mortimer
Email: roger.mortimer@keypublishing.com
Cover Design: Steve Donovan
Design: SJmagic DESIGN SERVICES, India.
Advertising Sales Manager: Sam Clark
Email: sam.clark@keypublishing.com
Tel: 01780 755131
Advertising Production: Becky Antoniades
Email: Rebecca.antoniades@keypublishing.com

SUBSCRIPTION/MAIL ORDER
Key Publishing Ltd, PO Box 300,
Stamford, Lincs, PE9 1NA
Tel: 01780 480404

Subscriptions email: subs@keypublishing.com
Mail Order email: orders@keypublishing.com
Website: www.keypublishing.com/shop

PUBLISHING
Group CEO and Publisher: Adrian Cox

Published by
Key Publishing Ltd,
PO Box 100, Stamford, Lincs, PE9 1XQ
Tel: 01780 755131
Website: www.keypublishing.com

PRINTING
Precision Colour Printing Ltd, Haldane,
Halesfield 1, Telford, Shropshire. TF7 4QQ

DISTRIBUTION
Seymour Distribution Ltd, 2 Poultry Avenue, London, EC1A 9PU
Enquiries Line: 02074 294000.

We are unable to guarantee the bona fides of any of our advertisers. Readers are strongly recommended to take their own precautions before parting with any information or item of value, including, but not limited to money, manuscripts, photographs, or personal information in response to any advertisements within this publication.

© Key Publishing Ltd 2025. All rights reserved. No part of this magazine may be reproduced or transmitted in any form by any means, electronic or mechanical, including photocopying, recording or by any information storage and retrieval system, without prior permission in writing from the copyright owner. Multiple copying of the contents of the magazine without prior written approval is not permitted.

THE GLUTEN-FREE HANDBOOK

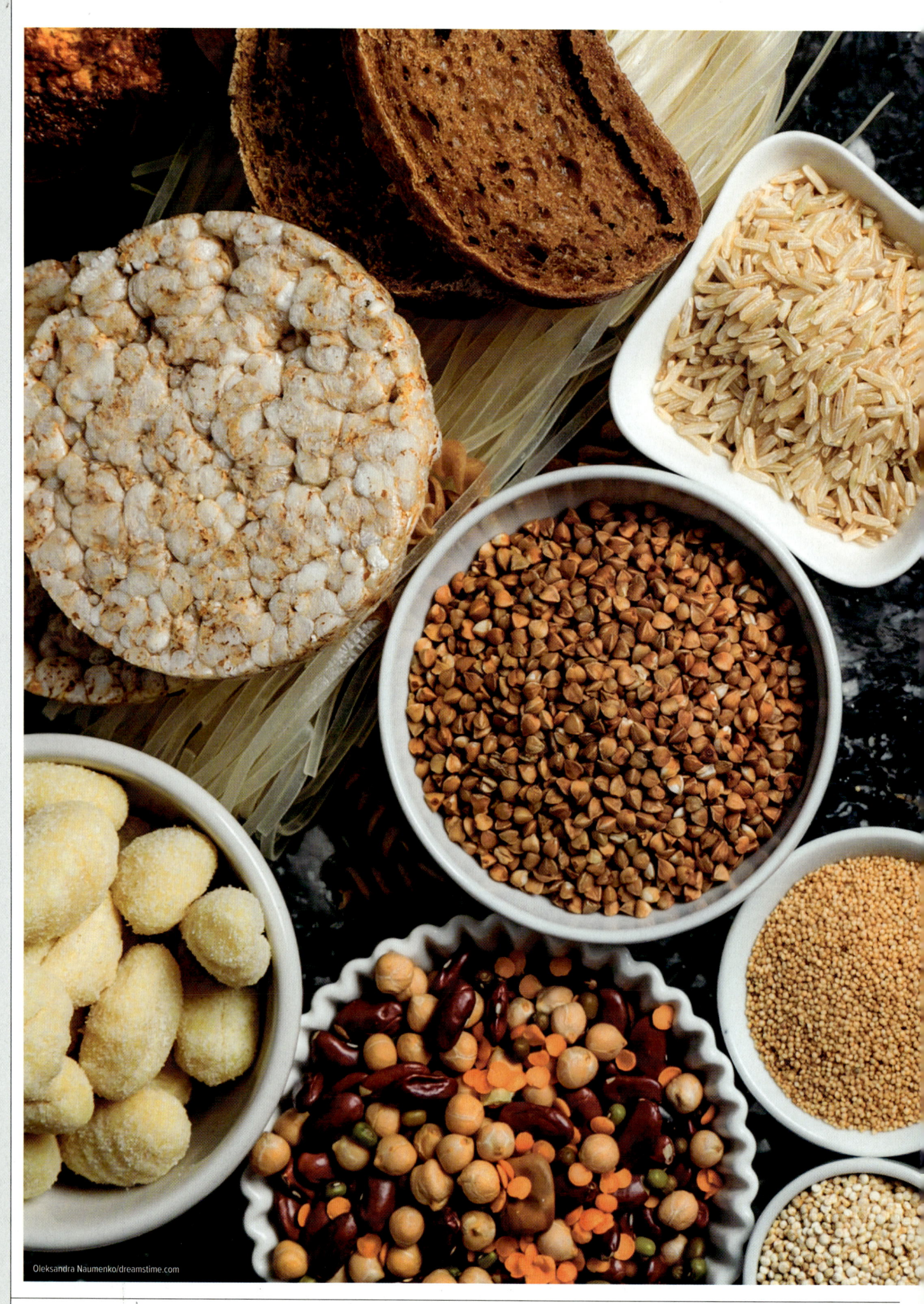

CONTENTS

Oleksandra Naumenko/dreamstime.com

GLUTEN FREE

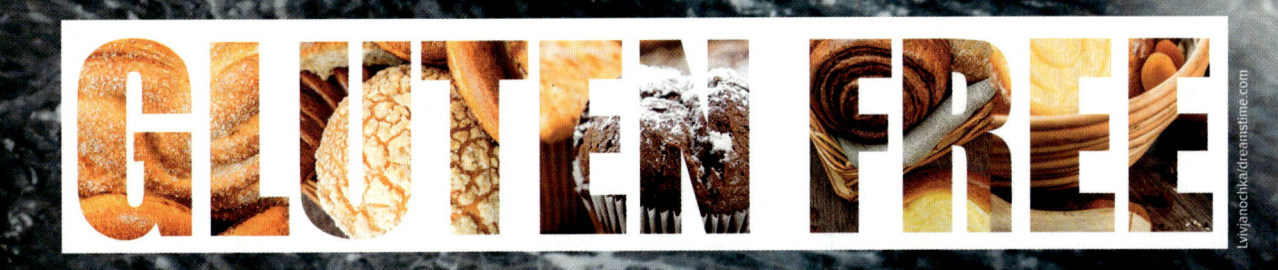

CONTENTS

6   **What is gluten?**
The discovery of gluten, where it comes from and how it affects the body.

16   **Where do you find gluten?**
A rundown of all the products that contain gluten – some of them hidden – and what ingredients to look out for.

28   **Coeliac Disease**
One of the most dangerous conditions caused by gluten, how it is diagnosed, how it has been treated in the past, plus celebrity champions for coeliac awareness.

38   **Non-coeliac Gluten Sensitivity**
How to tell this from other digestive issues, what else can lead on from having the condition and famous people who live gluten-free.

46   **Wheat allergy**
How and why wheat allergy differs from Coeliac Disease, together with the conditions that spring from it – Baker's Asthma, and Wheat-dependent Exercise-induced Anaphylactic Reaction.

54   **Gluten Ataxia**
An attack on the body's nervous system that can damage parts of the brain.

58   **Dermatitis Herpetiformis**
What happens when gluten causes skin eruptions and irritations.

62   **Coeliac Awareness Month**
Promoting knowledge of the condition and how to get a diagnosis, as well as fundraising events around the world.

64   **How to live gluten-free**
Shopping and food swaps, labelling laws and guidelines, plus gluten-free manufacturers and products.

74   **Gluten-free recipes**
Fourteen savoury and sweet dishes that are easy to make and delicious for all the family, not just gluten avoiders.

102   **Eating out gluten-free**
Planning your trip to a restaurant and which country's foods provide the most choice.

106   **Travel gluten-free**
Choosing a holiday, navigating the transport hazards, finding the right hotel and things to consider when travelling in a foreign country.

110   **Books, apps, and websites**
Sources of information and inspiration as well as practical help.

114   **Helpful organisations**
Coeliac societies in the UK, United States, Canada, and Australia.

115   **Conversion chart**
A handy guide for adapting recipes in US cups, metric, and Imperial to your preferred measures.

What is gluten?

It has become such a familiar word in recent years, on food packaging and restaurant menus, although many people don't know what it is and why it causes problems.

The science

Gluten is an example of what are termed 'structural proteins'. These give support and shape to the cells in all living things. In the case of gluten, it is found in the seeds of many cereal plants and its function within the seeds, or grains, is to hold together two individual proteins, Prolamin and Glutelin, that nourish the developing plant. When water is added to crushed grains, the gluten protein molecules form into sticky and elastic chains which provide the binding properties that make bread and other doughs flexible.

As this flour and water mix is kneaded, it stays stretchy and doesn't tear. Air pockets are formed within the gluten strands, and they help the dough rise. This is what makes bread, in particular, light, and airy.

Gluten also contributes to trapping water molecules in the dough, so the baked goods remain moist. It gives a chewy texture to bread, pasta, pastry, and biscuits, stopping them becoming excessively dry and crumbly.

Because it gives this desirable consistency and mouth-appeal to food, it is often extracted from the raw grains by manufacturers to add to a wide range of products, beyond just baked ones. It is concentrated and added to food as a binding agent to hold processed ingredients together and give them shape.

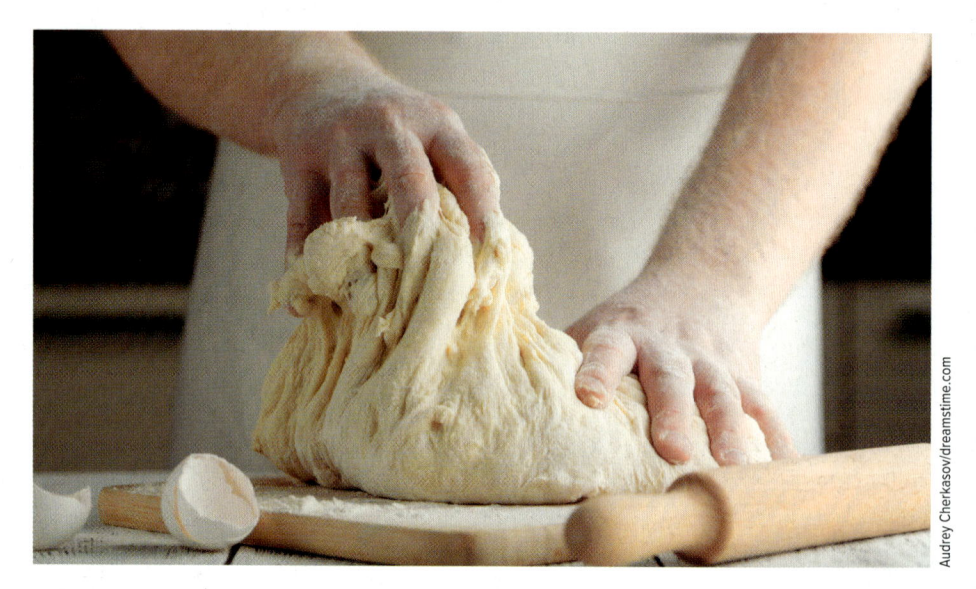

How does gluten affect your body?

Digestive enzymes in our stomach and small intestine break down the food we eat into much smaller particles called amino acids. These can then be absorbed into the bloodstream and be carried to all the cells around the body.

However, the enzymes are not strong enough to completely break down the gluten mixture of proteins found in bread, pastry, pasta, and the like, so an amount passes down the small intestine in its raw state. It is this that triggers a variety of unpleasant reactions.

The effects of eating gluten are very personal to the individual. For a majority of people, it passes through the digestive system with little or no bad effects, just helping to deliver nutritious grain protein to the body's cells to nourish and grow them.

For anyone who has Coeliac Disease, though, the gluten acts directly on the lining of the small intestine, fooling the immune system into attacking its own body

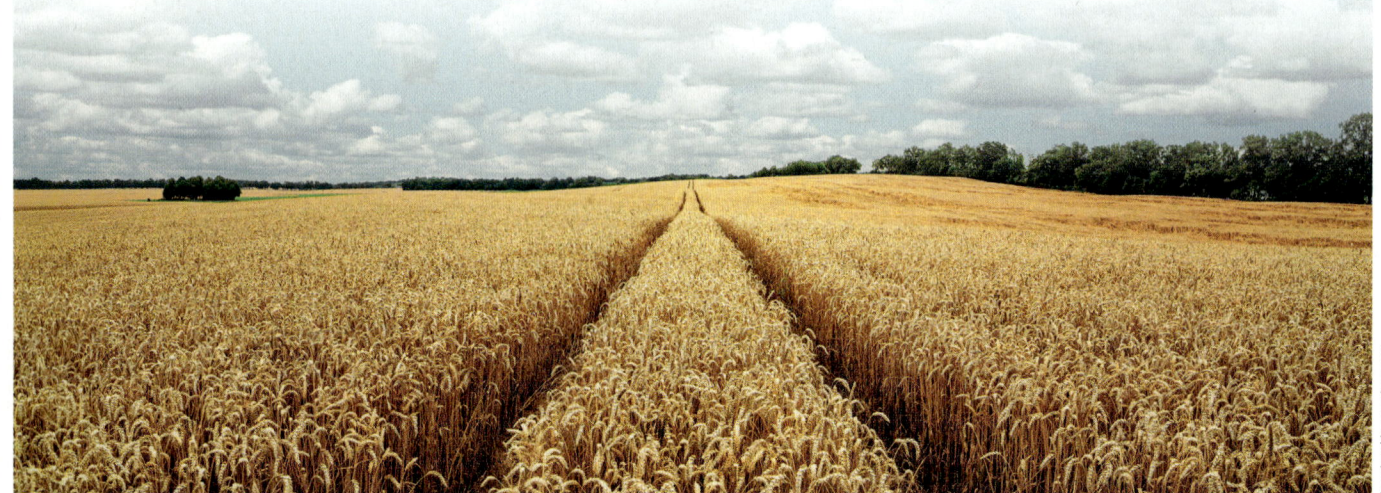

WHAT IS GLUTEN?

IT STARTED WITH A SORE MOUTH
Liz from Cheshire

"In 2003 I went to see my GP as I had this annoying crack on the side of my mouth that wouldn't heal. On bad days, my lips also shed their skin, and no amount of lip balm/Vaseline solved the problem.

After my GP tried out medicated cream with no success, he ran some blood tests. The results showed my iron levels were a little low and I was prescribed an iron supplement. Unfortunately, this didn't fix things, so more bloods were taken. A week or so later my GP gave me a call to let me know that a blood test for Coeliac Disease had come back positive (neither I nor my husband had heard of coeliac). He stressed at this stage it was important to remain on a normal diet, as I would require an endoscopy to confirm Coeliac Disease. Removing gluten before an endoscopy test for coeliac will start the healing process and will prevent you from getting an accurate test result.

It was a couple of months before I had the endoscopy and I did as my GP instructed and maintained my normal diet, making the most of eating whatever I wanted without any boundaries – doughnuts, Chinese banquets, etc – it was great! If gluten had to remain for now, I was not going to do it by halves. I was extremely lucky that I did not have upset tummy symptoms at this time. I appreciate it's a much harder process when you feel unwell.

I remember walking out of the hospital thinking 'I've got this covered', I'm a trained chef with lots of catering experience and love my food. I shouldn't have a problem managing my new gluten-free diet. But a few days later reality hit, and I realised it was going to be harder than I first thought. Luckily for me, a family friend who had been diagnosed for a long time came around laden with gluten-free recipes.

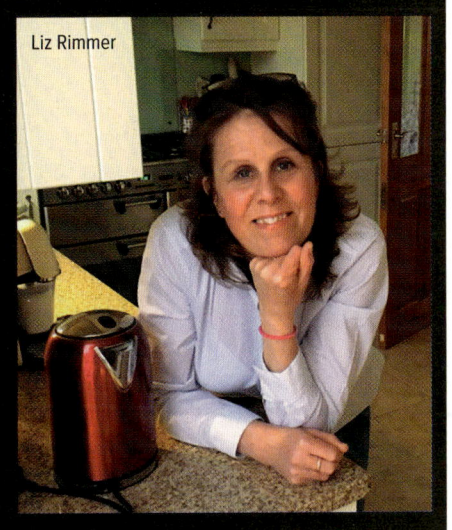

I think the realisation of the importance of my gluten-free diet was at my first appointment with a dietician. Until then I was under the impression it was occasionally OK to eat gluten – I was completely wrong about this. The dietician stressed, for my gluten-free diet to be effective it had to followed for life. She also explained that as I did not react with tummy upsets, etc, I had to be extra careful to make sure I was not unknowingly still eating gluten."

Liz's website www.coeliacbydesign.com and YouTube channel offer practical help for people with Coeliac Disease and lots of easy-to-follow recipes.

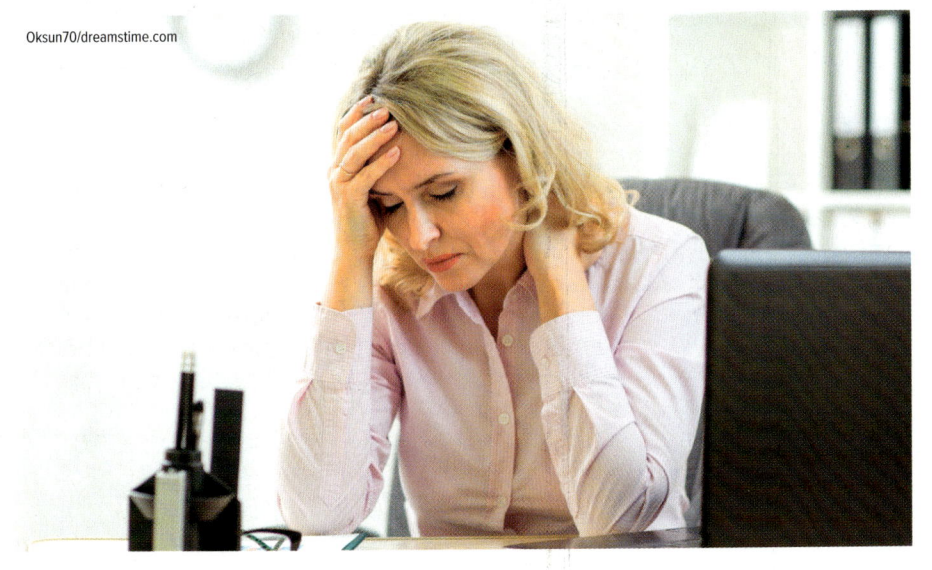

---

as if repelling an invader from outside.

Others, who do not experience such a strong autoimmune response, may nevertheless have a pronounced allergic reaction as gluten passes through the walls of the small intestine and is absorbed into the system.

Possible symptoms
Digestion
Nausea, diarrhoea, vomiting, bloating, flatulence, constipation, stomach pain.

Skin
Numbness and tingling, rashes, itchy or burning blisters and raised red patches.

Body overall
Breathlessness, wheezing, mouth ulcers, damage to dental enamel, fatigue, brain fog, dizziness, loss of coordination and balance, weight loss, infertility, osteoporosis, malnutrition, throat swelling and difficulty swallowing.

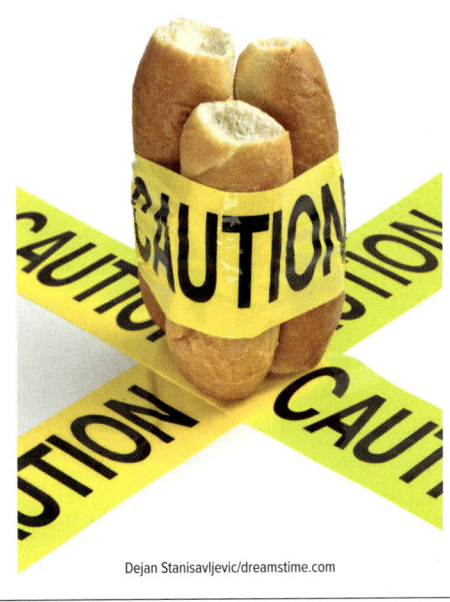

THE GLUTEN-FREE HANDBOOK

WHAT IS GLUTEN?

The different reactions to gluten

People who are sensitive to gluten react in different ways – some simply inconvenient and embarrassing, some more disabling, and even life-threatening.

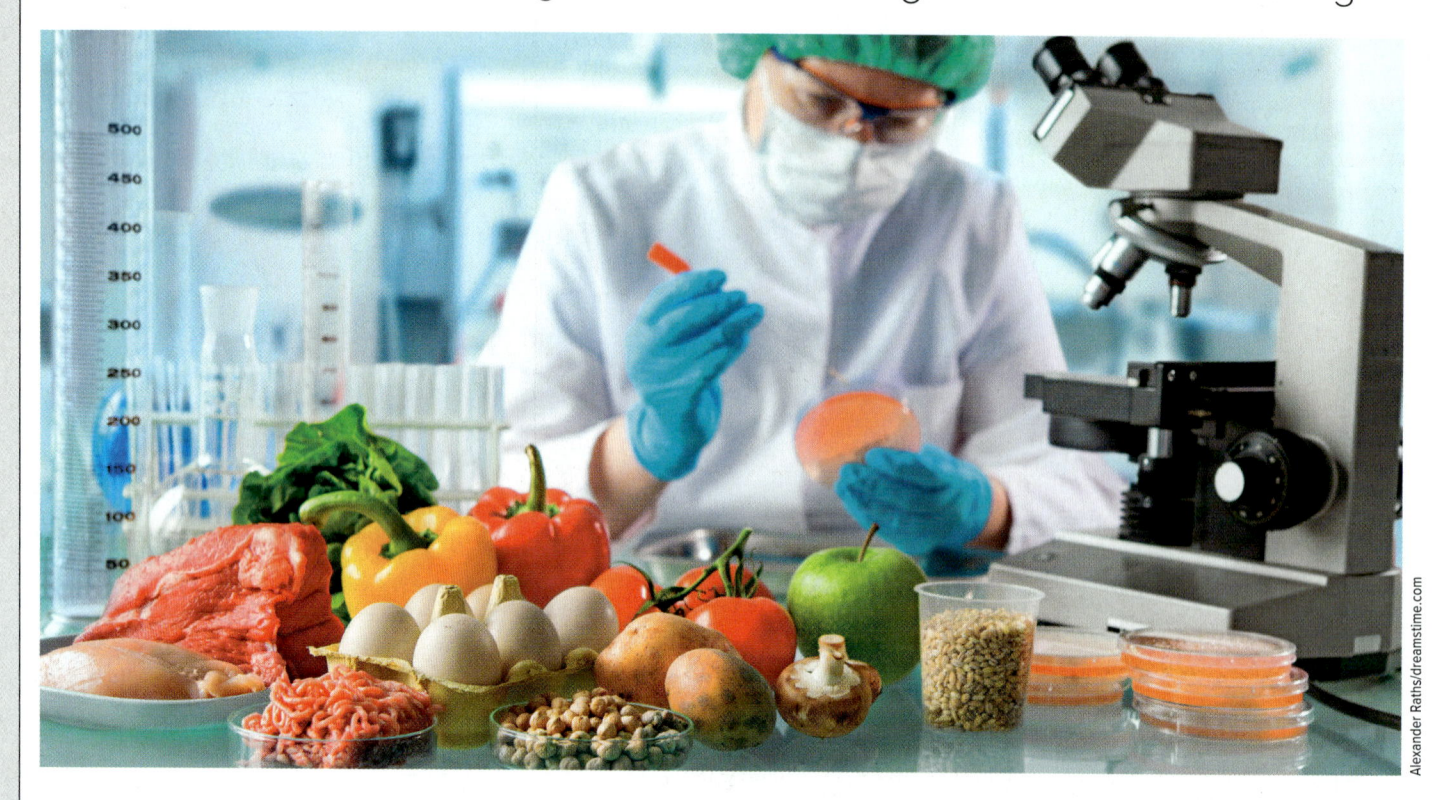

The ways gluten affects people can be classed into five broad categories:

Coeliac Disease
Also spelt Celiac and pronounced SEE-lee-ak, this is the most severe of reactions to the gluten protein. In people with this condition, eating gluten can cause what is often irreparable damage to the lower intestine if left undiagnosed. It leads to painful abdominal discomfort, extreme fatigue, skin complaints and bad mouth ulcers.

Non-coeliac Gluten Sensitivity
A complex and hard-to-diagnose condition that mimics Coeliac in large part but does not cause long-term or permanent damage to the digestive system.

Wheat Allergy
A reaction that occurs only in response to wheat proteins and not other grains. But unlike Coeliac and Non-coeliac, it can be activated by inhaling wheat flour dust, which causes a condition known as Baker's Asthma. On rare occasions, eating wheat products followed by exercise can also trigger a life-threatening anaphylaxis shock.

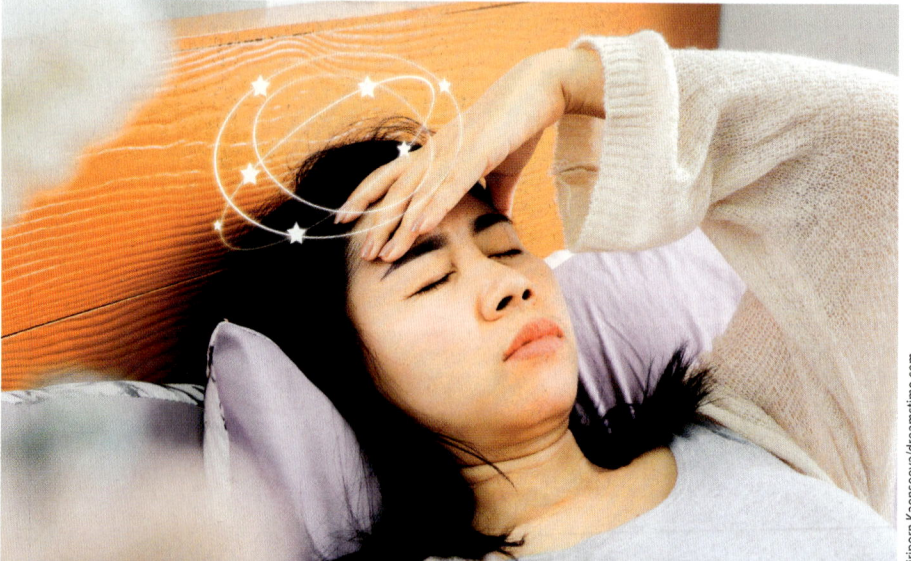

Gluten Ataxia
Antibodies produced by the body in an immune response to gluten attack the nervous system as well as the digestive one. This is relatively rare but can damage the cerebellum area of the brain if left untreated.

Dermatitis Herpetiformis
Antibodies triggered by gluten gather under the skin and cause itchy blisters that can burst and become infected.

Each of these conditions will be covered in more detail in following chapters.

8

www.keypublishing.com

WHAT IS GLUTEN?

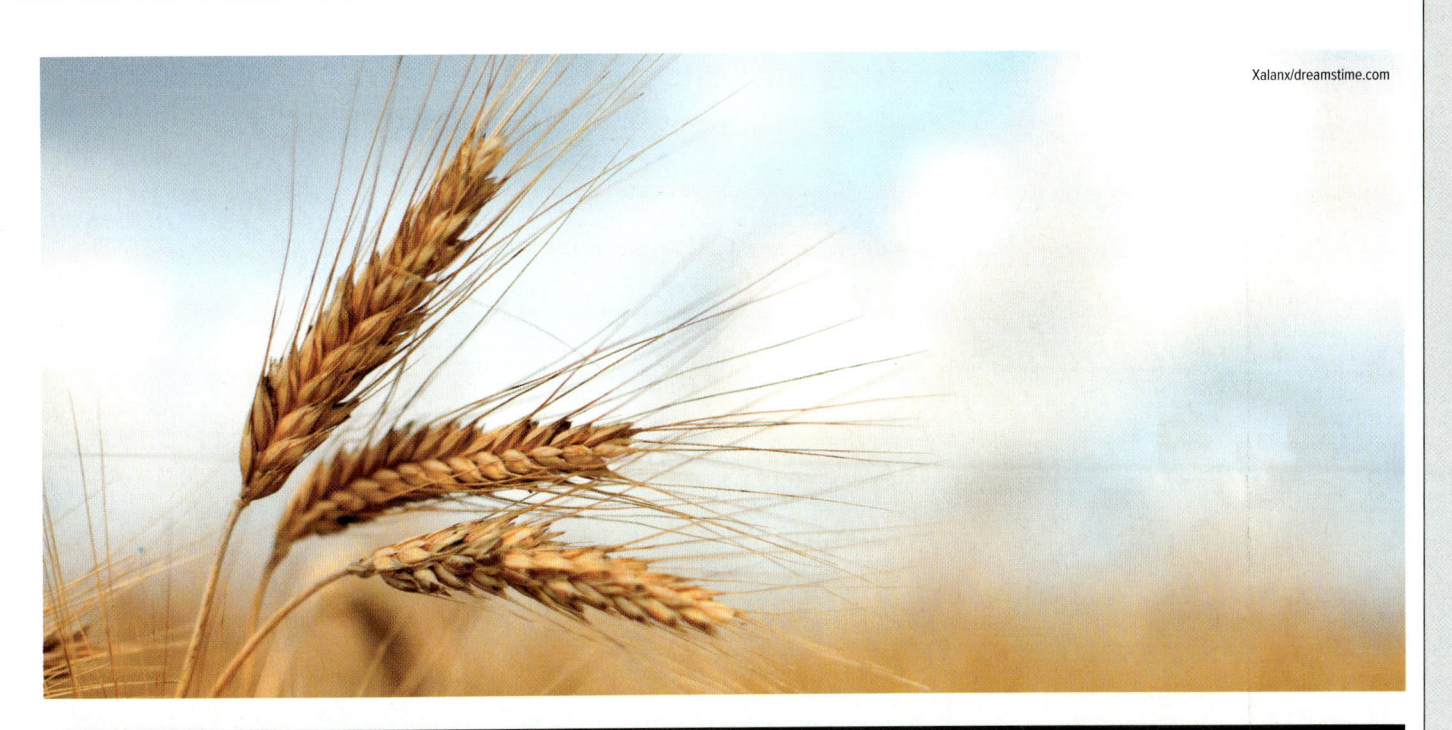

Xalanx/dreamstime.com

TWENTY-FIVE YEARS OF EXPERIENCE
Laura from the UK

Laura Strange

"I thrived as a baby, so when I started to get poorly at around seven years old, no one suspected that it could be Coeliac Disease. Our GP wrote it off as anxiety and growing pains, despite my parents knowing that it wasn't the cause. They were frustrated that the doctor wouldn't even go down the route of testing me.

As the years passed, I became severely underweight, in regular pain, completely exhausted and really struggled to function. I remember sitting at school, trying to gather up the strength to go to my next lesson. Everyday tasks were a struggle. Many people assumed I was seriously ill or had an eating disorder (by the time I was 14 I only weighed six stone) and I remember being so frustrated at not knowing what was wrong.

Then one day we had a lucky break. My regular GP was on holiday, and we were seen by another doctor. She decided to get my bloods done, which revealed severe anaemia. Some more tests and one painless upper GI endoscopy later I finally received a concrete diagnosis of Coeliac Disease.

I had never really heard of a gluten-free diet before, let alone Coeliac Disease, but an NHS dietician talked us through it all and off we went. I quickly gained a stone, then another stone until I was finally a healthy weight for my age and height. I now had boundless energy and truly felt like a new person. It took a few months for my gut to repair itself, but everything was soon back in full working order.

Coeliac Disease, of course, has its struggles, and 25 years on I think I have come up against pretty much every awkward social situation, accidental 'glutening' and rookie gluten-free error in the book. Pizza parties at university, welcome lunches at new jobs, kind colleagues making me a gluten-free birthday cake then unwittingly topping it with (gluten-containing) Smarties, me not realising that soy sauce contained gluten, etc. These days I consider myself to be a gluten-free pro, but it has certainly been a journey of (often painful) discovery getting to this point."

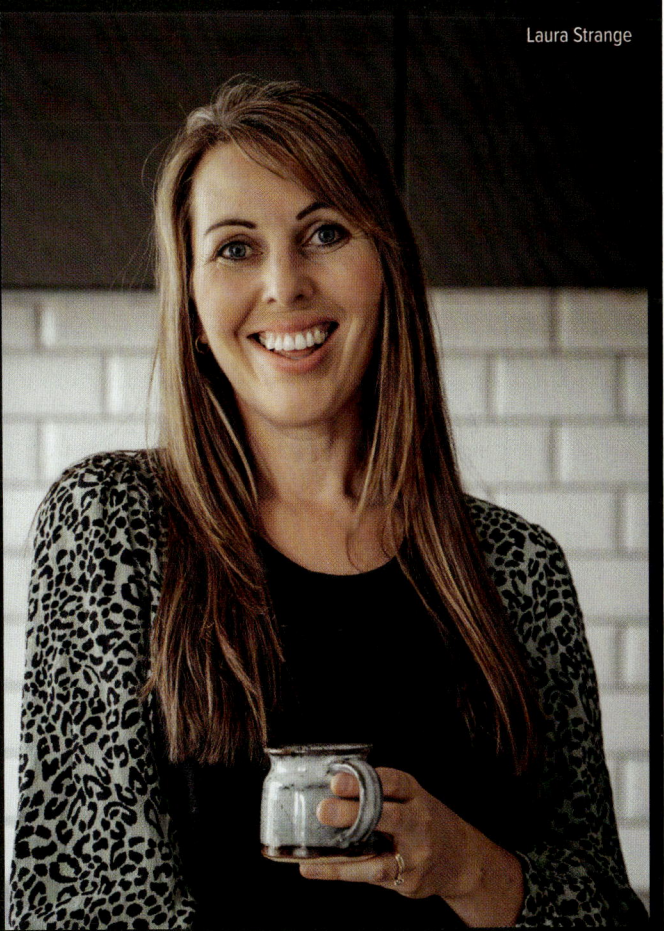

Laura Strange has written cookbooks and meal planners for gluten-free living, including at Christmas, as well as travel guides to many countries. She also gives cookery demonstrations. www.mygfguide.com

THE GLUTEN-FREE HANDBOOK

WHAT IS GLUTEN?

The discovery of gluten

Long-term digestive problems have been known about for as long as people have been eating wheat and other grains, but pinning down the cause to those foods has taken a long time.

In the 2nd century AD/CE, in the Cappadocia region of Greece that was then under Roman control, there was a physician called Aretaeus. He has been celebrated as one of the most important earliest recorders of medical matters. He wrote eight books with in-depth descriptions of different diseases and conditions and his treatment of them, including asthma, diabetes, and tetanus, many of which conform to modern-day medical thinking.

Included in his writings is the first known account of symptoms that can now be identified as stemming from an allergic reaction to gluten. He named it the disease of the abdomen – κοιλιακός (pronounced see-lee-a-KOS) from the word for abdominal in his Greek dialect.

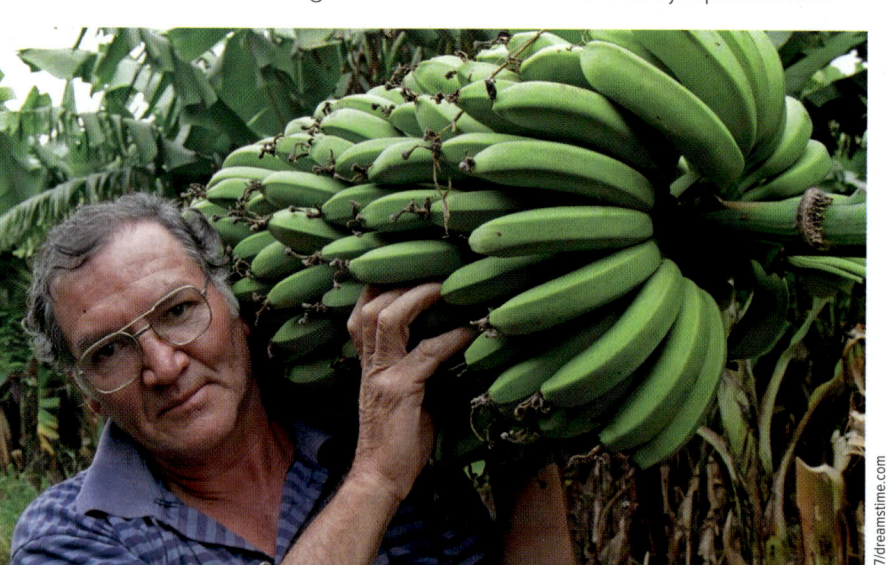

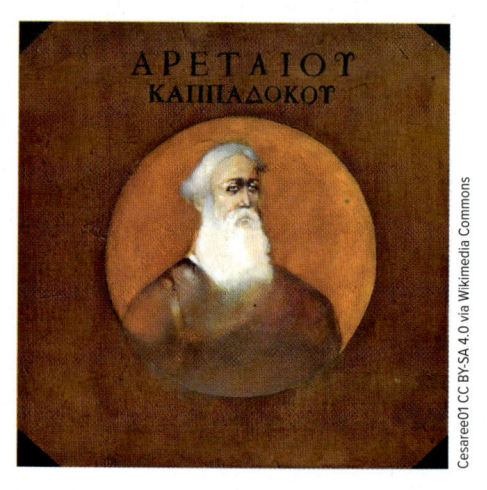

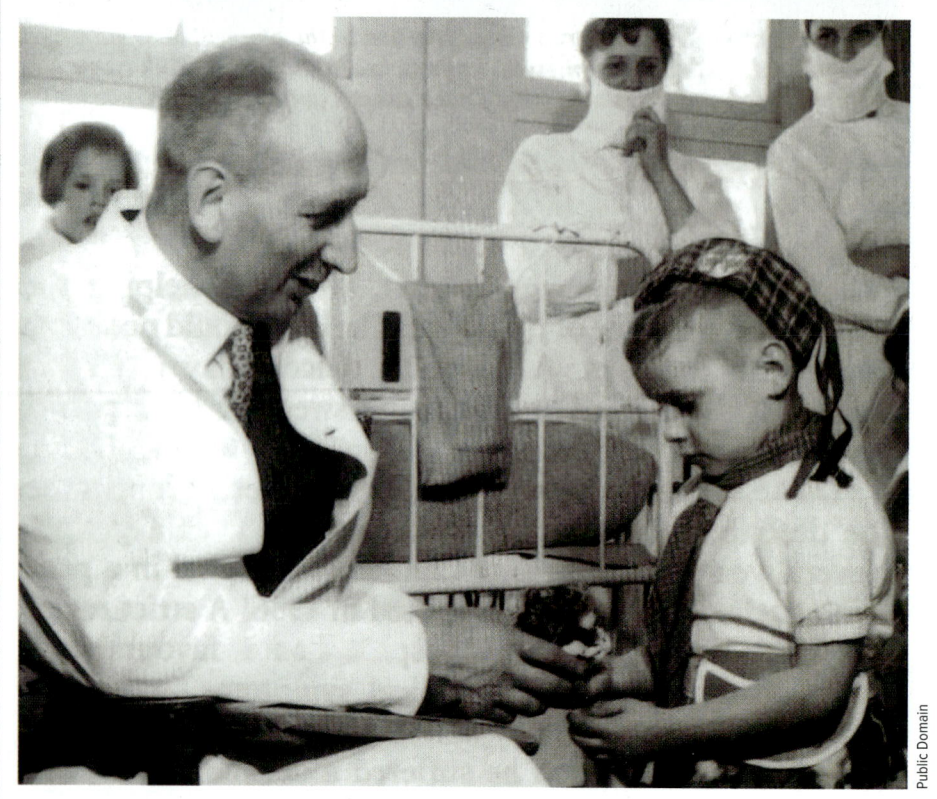

In 1852 in Venice, Aretaeus' work was reproduced for the first time in Latin. Shortly after, in 1856, UK medical writer Francis Adams edited and translated the volume for the Sydenham Society, a London institution that aimed to improve the sharing of medical texts. This was when the word coeliac, taken from κοιλιακός, first came to prominence as the name for the autoimmune condition we know today.

Looking to diet

In 1888, Dr Samuel Gee, working at The Hospital for Sick Children on Great Ormond Street in London, put forward a theory based on his observations of some of his patients that a 'coeliac affliction' could be improved by a change of diet. But he was unable to put his finger on just what foodstuff made them ill.

Nearly 40 years later an American paediatrician, Dr Sidney Valentine Haas, improved the lives of many children by putting them on a high-calorie banana diet that did not contain any starchy food but did include daily bananas, milk, cottage cheese, meat, and vegetables.

WHAT IS GLUTEN?

IT SHAPES YOUR EVERYDAY LIFE
Arabella from London

"I discovered my gluten intolerance when I was around 18, just as I was starting my undergraduate studies. The journey to a diagnosis was surprisingly long, even though the test itself is relatively straightforward. I experienced a range of gut-related symptoms, including severe bloating and persistent stomach issues, and I was quite unwell for a significant period before receiving a proper diagnosis.

It wasn't until I went on a summer holiday that the extent of my symptoms became undeniable – I was constantly bloated, and it began to affect not just my digestion but also my joints, skin, and overall mood. It felt like the condition was taking over every aspect of my life. Eventually, I was fortunate to meet a compassionate consultant who conducted thorough testing and finally identified the root cause. Since then, with their help, I've been able to manage my condition effectively and regain control over my health.

Living with gluten intolerance does somewhat shape your daily life. Every meal requires careful consideration, as ingredients in common products often change, and even menus at your favourite restaurants can be altered without notice. At home, I'm fortunate that cooking gluten-free is relatively easy and stress-free, especially since I enjoy it. My household tends to eat the same meals as me, though I spare them from my gluten-free bread and cakes – poor things! Thankfully, they don't mind gluten-free soy sauce.

When it comes to social occasions, things are improving. Awareness of gluten intolerance has grown significantly, and gluten-free options are becoming more widely available. However, travel remains my biggest challenge. Airports often lack decent gluten-free options, and the limited choices are rarely nutritionally balanced, which can leave you feeling frustrated – and often 'hangry'. I'll never forget a 15-hour flight where the gluten-free meal option consisted of melon for all three meals! I've learned to carry snacks with me now, but it's not ideal – they're often repetitive and not what you really want.

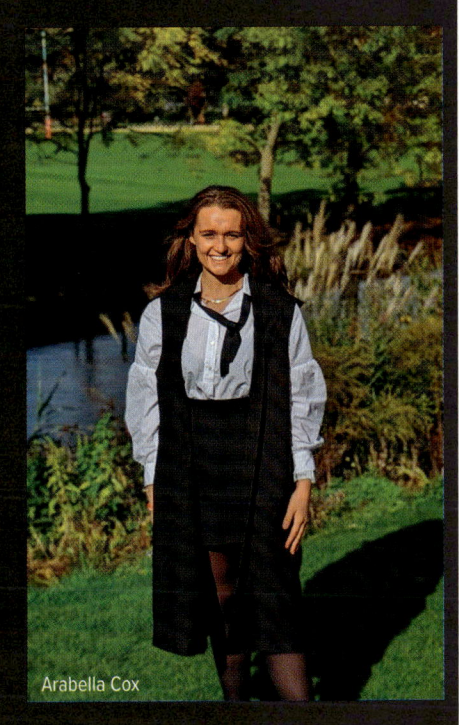

Overall, managing a gluten-free lifestyle day-to-day is doable, but in situations where access to safe food is limited, it can feel isolating and lonely. It's those moments that remind you how much of a challenge it can be.

One unexpected joy of my gluten-free journey has been becoming much more adventurous in the kitchen, particularly with baking, which feels like an art form just to make things edible! My partner and I have a weekend ritual where we visit different bakeries in search of gluten-free treats, which we then rate out of 10. It's been an emotional rollercoaster! My favourite so far is Libby's in Belsize Park, London; they make incredible gluten-free croissants (though I probably shouldn't mention that to anyone from Paris)."

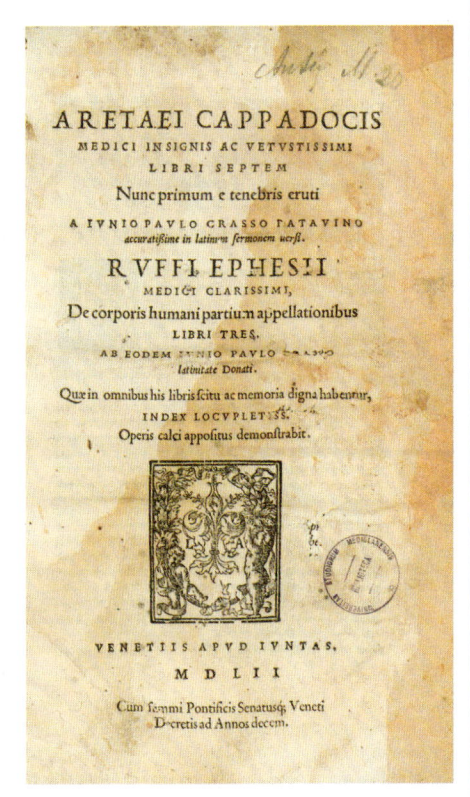

Arabella Cox

Public Domain

He had formulated the diet having visited a town in Puerto Rico where the inhabitants ate a lot of bread and suffered widely from Sprue – a condition where food is not properly absorbed into the body. On the other hand, he found that poor farmers living outside the town who lived mostly on bananas as their staple carbohydrate foodstuff had no such digestive problems. By advocating his banana diet with his patients back home, he successfully eliminated gluten from their systems without knowing that that was the root cause of their issues.

From the 1920s to the early 1950s this was the recommended 'cure' but, unfortunately, once cured, many children returned to the normal family diet and suffered further dangerous long-term damage to their digestive systems.

Finally, in the 1940s a Dutch doctor, Willem Karel Dicke (pic far left), made the connection between wheat and a coeliac condition when he noted that as bread became unavailable in the Netherlands during the World War, so the patients presenting to him with the disease dropped dramatically.

This was followed up in the early 1950s by a study conducted by a British medical team that pinpointed the gluten protein in wheat, barley, and rye as being the trigger for digestive illness.

WHAT IS GLUTEN?

The Gluten TIMELINE
The Early Days

200 BCE — Aretaeus of Cappadocia writes about an abdominal disease he names κοιλιακός.

1 CE — Bread made from wheat becomes popular in ancient Rome and bakers wear masks when preparing bread as they recognise the condition of Baker's Asthma.

1662 — French mathematician and philosopher Blaise Pascal dies of extreme long-term stomach problems, headaches, and depression. An autopsy reveals much damage to his intestines and other internal organs that has since been thought to be caused by Coeliac Disease.

1800 — British physician and pathologist Matthew Baillie describes a condition of patients suffering chronic diarrhoea and malnutrition that improves if they are put on an exclusively rice-based diet.

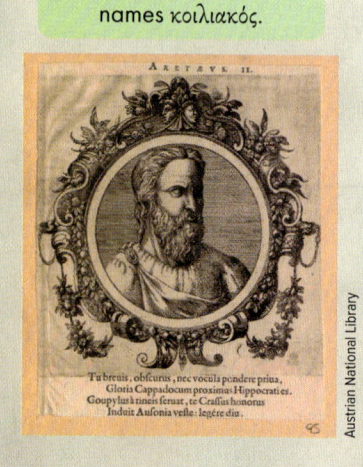

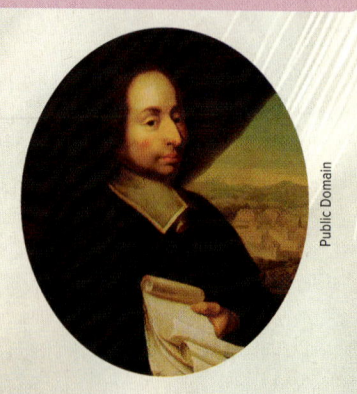

1856 — Medical writer Francis Adams highlights the works of Aretaeus of Cappadocia concerning Coeliac Disease.

1888

www.keypublishing.com

WHAT IS GLUTEN?

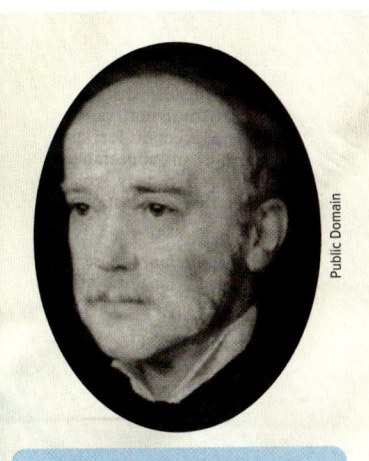

English physician Dr Samuel Gee gives the first modern description of Coeliac Disease and advocates diet as a cause, but he cannot isolate which foodstuff is the culprit.

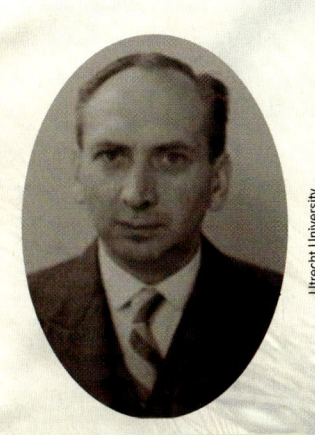

Dutch paediatrician Willem Karel Dicke first isolates wheat as the root cause of Coeliac Disease and creates the first gluten-free diet.

Consultant physician John Paulley in the UK identifies the causes of coeliac symptoms after examining surgical specimens and seeing the damage to the villi in the gut.

1924

1940s

1952

1954

1956

American paediatrician Dr Sidney Valentine Haas successfully treats Coeliac children with his banana diet. For more on this, see page 32.

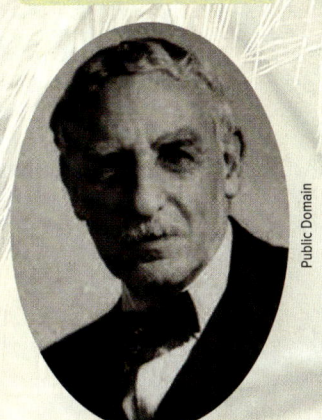

A British team of scientists pinpoint the gluten component of wheat, rye, barley, and oats as the disease trigger. Dietary advice is to look for alternative sources of carbohydrate proteins, such as corn.

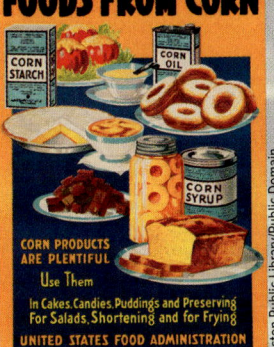

German/English gastroenterologist Margot Shiner develops the Shiner mucosal biopsy tube which enables her to take small samples of tissue from the intestine to test for coeliac markers.

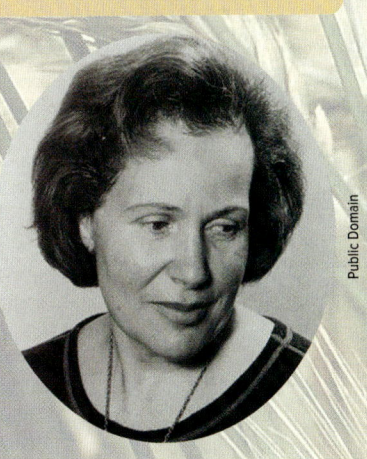

THE GLUTEN-FREE HANDBOOK

WHAT IS GLUTEN?

Into the swinging sixties

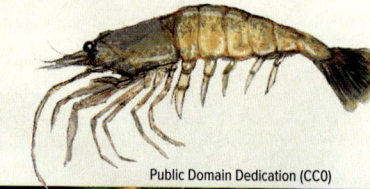

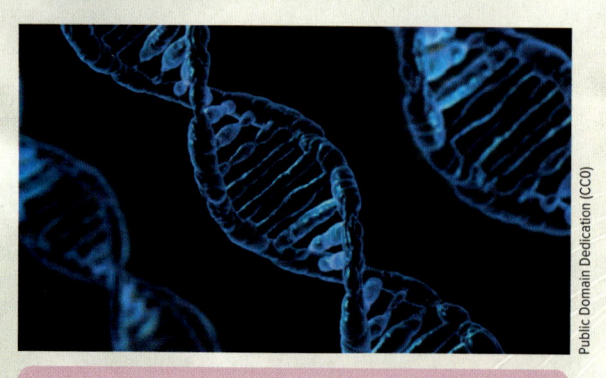

The HLA-DQ2 gene is discovered, associated with Coeliac Disease and Dermatitis Herpetiformis.

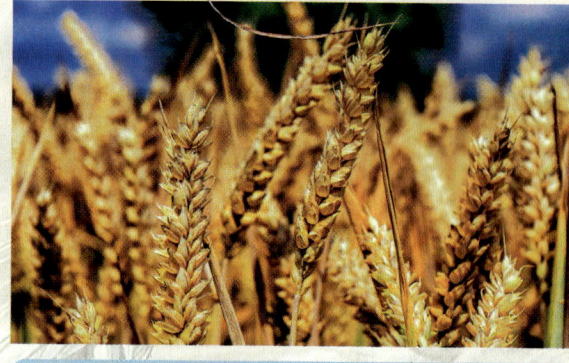

The condition of Food-dependent Exercise-induced Anaphylaxis is first described in relation to shellfish. Wheat is later found to be an important trigger and the most widespread.

1960

1970s

1978

1979

1980s

Australian scientist Dr Charlotte Anderson irrefutably links damage to the intestinal villi with gluten by testing patients before and after they eliminate it from their diets.

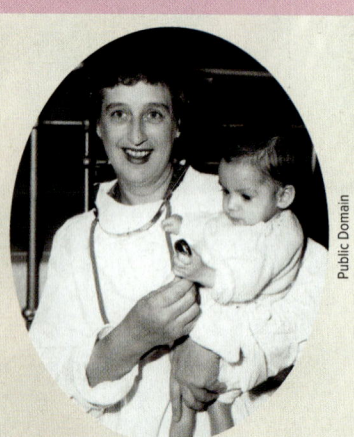

The condition of Non-Coeliac Gluten Sensitivity is identified, prompted by a rise in the general public themselves choosing to alleviate their undiagnosed symptoms by eliminating gluten products.

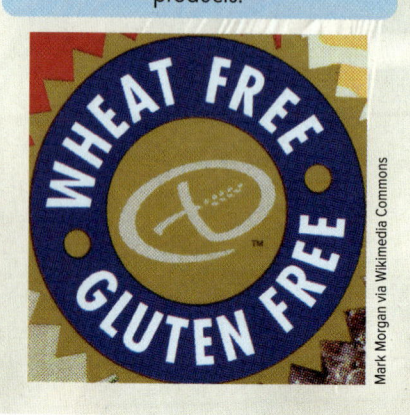

Coeliac Disease is accepted by the medical community as an autoimmune condition.

WHAT IS GLUTEN?

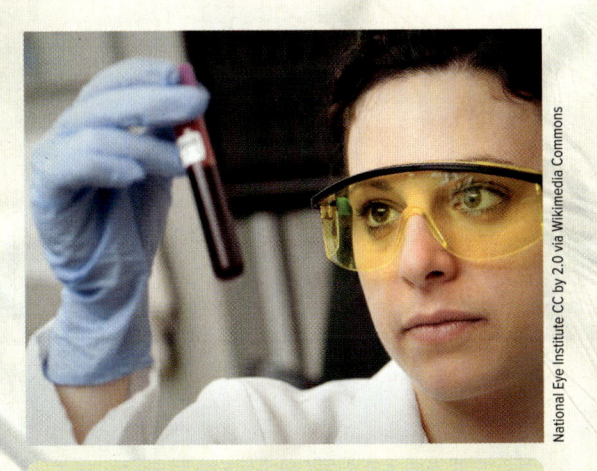

IgA anti-tissue transglutaminase antibodies are discovered to be linked to Coeliac Disease, which greatly improves diagnosis when they are found in a blood test.

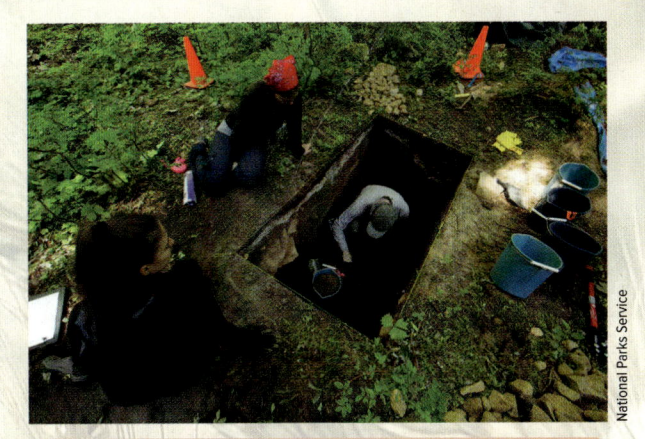

An archaeological dig in Italy finds the body of a young woman from the 1st century CE showing signs of extreme malnutrition. A test of her DNA reveals the presence of the coeliac gene HLA-DQ2.

1997

2006

2008

2012

Research and clinical trials of drugs that could be used to treat Coeliac Disease begin and are ongoing around the world.

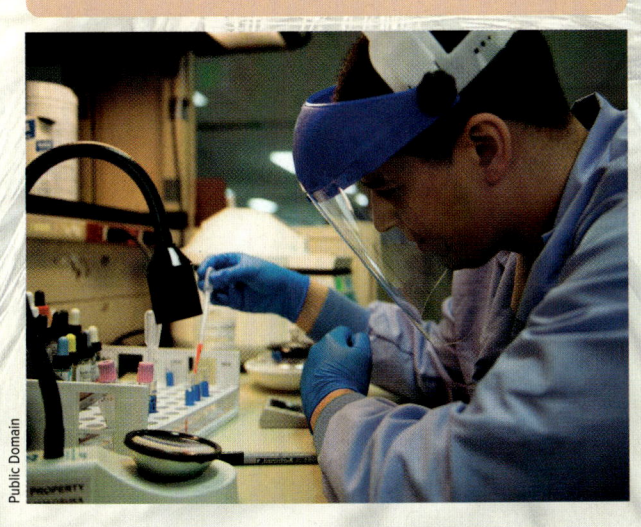

An article in the *British Medical Journal* formally describes the spectrum of gluten-related disorders and states the medical community's consensus on naming such as Non-Coeliac Gluten Sensitivity and Wheat-dependent Exercise-induced Anaphylaxis.

THE GLUTEN-FREE HANDBOOK

Where do you find gluten?

The main direct derivations of gluten are the grains of a number of grass plants, commonly known as cereals, but these can be turned into many different products and some of them are not so obvious.

Cereals
Wheat
This is the principal cereal associated in most people's minds with gluten. Rather than being the name of one single plant, wheat is a collective term for a number of domesticated grasses that are cultivated in order to harvest their grains for food. They are an important source of the starch carbohydrate that we need for energy, to fuel the muscles and keep our organs in good working order.

Different types of wheat include:

Common, or bread, wheat – the most widely cultivated type that forms 95% of the wheat eaten globally. In the UK, the wheat grains are classified as Winter and Spring, Hard and Soft. In the US they are divided into Hard Red Spring and Winter, Soft Red Winter, Hard and Soft White. In Australia there are Prime Hard, Hard, Premium, Standard and Soft grains.

Spelt, or Dinkel wheat – an historic grain that was cultivated widely in Europe from 5,000 BCE, and America from the 1890s, until the 20th century when Common wheat became more popular. Nowadays it is most often used in artisan bread and pasta, as well as breakfast cereal.

Durum, or Pasta wheat – a grain that originated in the eastern Mediterranean and northern Africa. It is the hardest wheat to mill and has a high gluten content, which means it is very stretchy when formed into dough. This makes it particularly useful for pasta and it is also often made into couscous and semolina.

Emmer, or Farro, and Einkorn wheats – very ancient species of wild wheats that produce grains with a nutty flavour.

Khorasan, or Kamut wheat – an ancient species that produces very large grains, also with a nutty flavour. It is grown in Afghanistan and Iran.

Barley
This is another member of the grass family that was one of the first

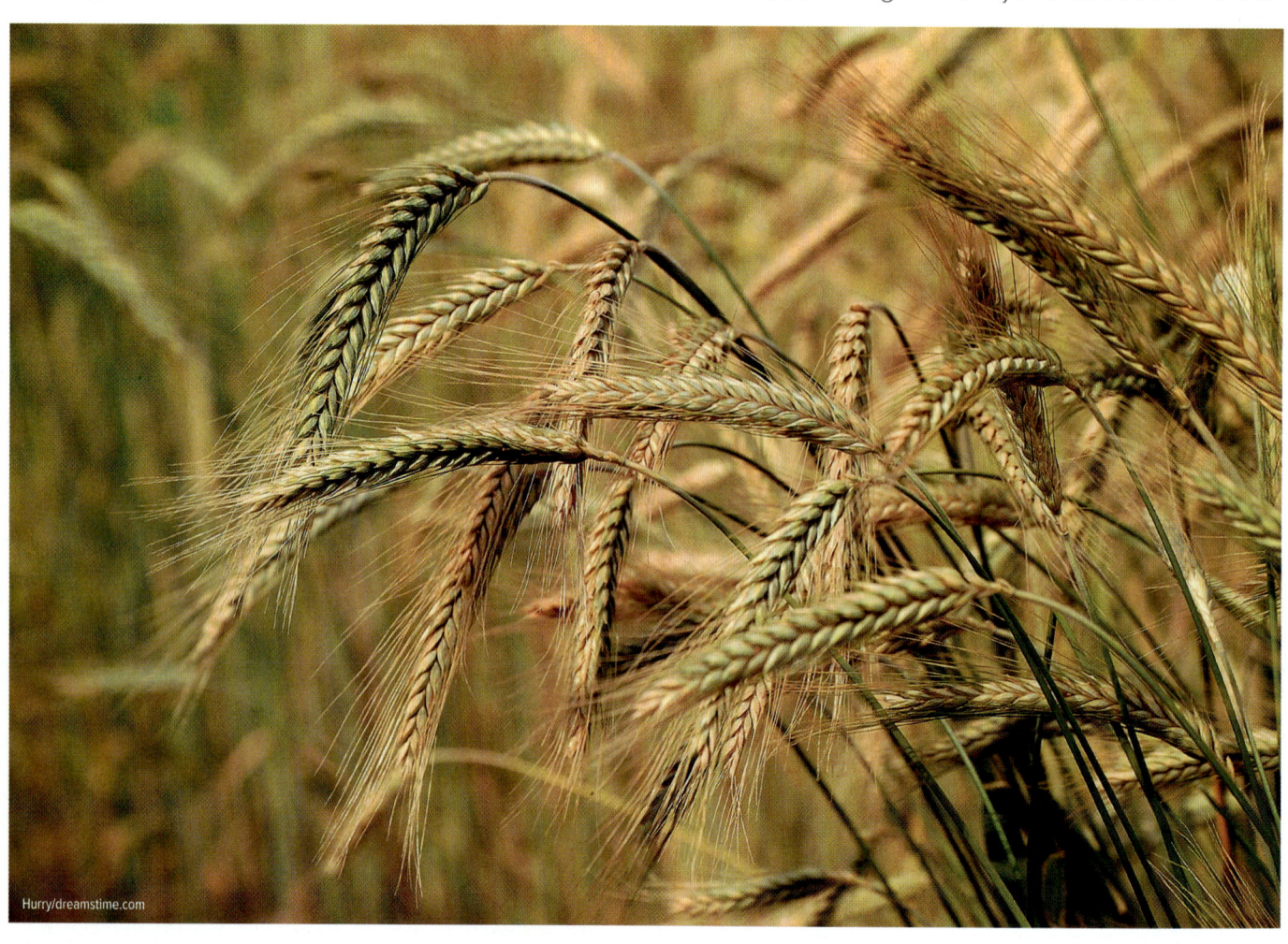

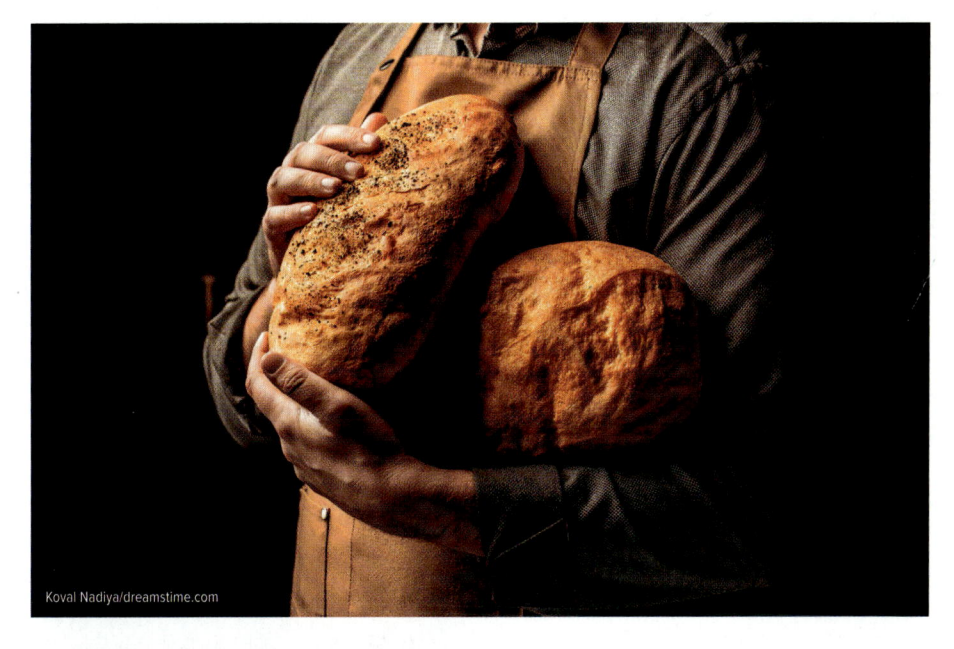

WHERE DO YOU FIND GLUTEN?

It is also added to milk to make drinks such as Horlicks, Ovaltine, and Milo, and to sweets, bagels, and biscuits.

Rye

A grass from Eastern and Northern Europe and Russia that is now grown in the Americas, Oceania, and China, and used extensively as animal fodder.

For human consumption, rye grain is used to make whiskey and beer, and a low-alcohol drink known as kvass. Rye grain is also refined into flour to make bread such as pumpernickel and Scandinavian crispbreads.

Triticale

This is a 19th century laboratory-bred plant that is a hybrid of wheat and rye. The grains are more nutritious than wheat because they have a higher protein content, but they still contain gluten.

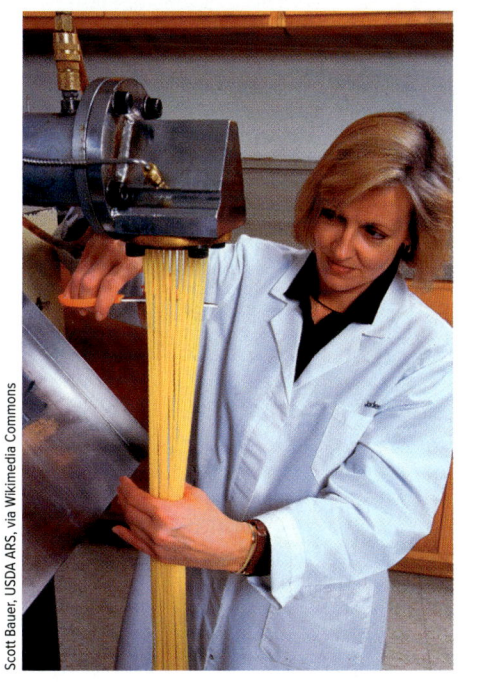

Malt – barley is soaked in water until it germinates and then it is dried out with hot air. The end product is used in beer making and malt vinegar, soft drinks and squashes, and barley wine.

of these to be domesticated in the Middle East around 9,000 BCE.

Different types of barley include:

Scotch, or Pot barley – a version that has the grain's outer husk removed and is used for soups and stews.

Pearl barley – is also de-husked, but the outer layer – the bran – is removed as well. It is the main ingredient in dishes such as Italian orzotto where it takes the place of rice in a risotto-style recipe.

Barley meal – is ground barley that is made into bread and biscuits.

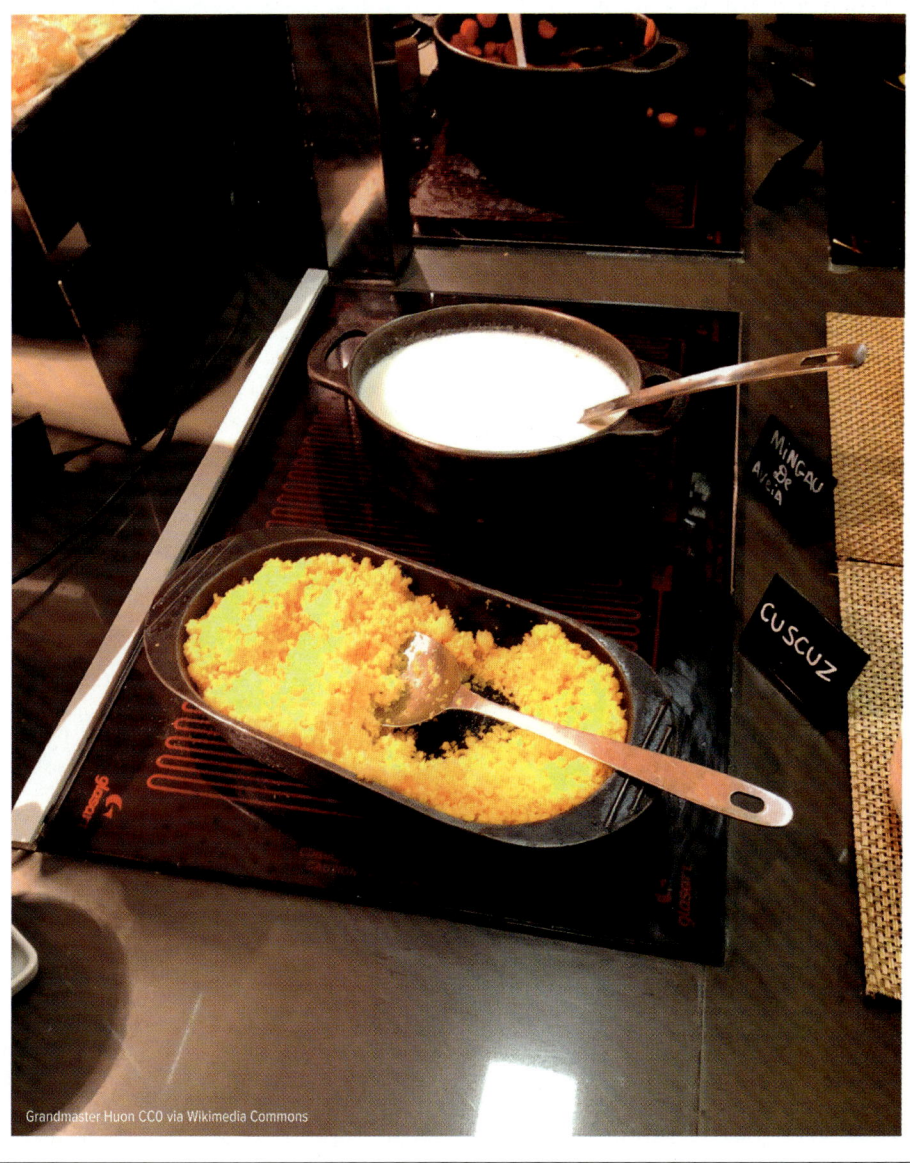

THE GLUTEN-FREE HANDBOOK

17

WHERE DO YOU FIND GLUTEN?

What not to eat

This looks like a long and quite depressing list. But these days a lot of these products are made without gluten, or there are gluten-free versions, so this is just a matter of drawing your attention to the potential so you can check the labels.

Carbs
Pastas, raviolis, dumplings, couscous, and gnocchi.

Noodles – ramen, udon, soba (those made with only a percentage of buckwheat flour), chow mein, egg noodles (rice noodles and mung bean noodles are gluten-free).

Breads and pastries – croissants, pittas, naan, bagels, flatbreads, cornbread, potato pancakes, muffins, doughnuts.

Crackers, oatcakes.

Flour tortillas.

Snacks
Flavoured crisps and popcorn – may use gluten in the flavourings.

Flavoured rice cakes – plain ones should be OK but check the labels.

Tortilla chips that are not entirely corn based.

Dry roast nuts – often coated in wheat flour.

Pretzels.

Sauces and condiments
Malt vinegar.

Soy sauce – Japanese tamari can be used as a substitute.

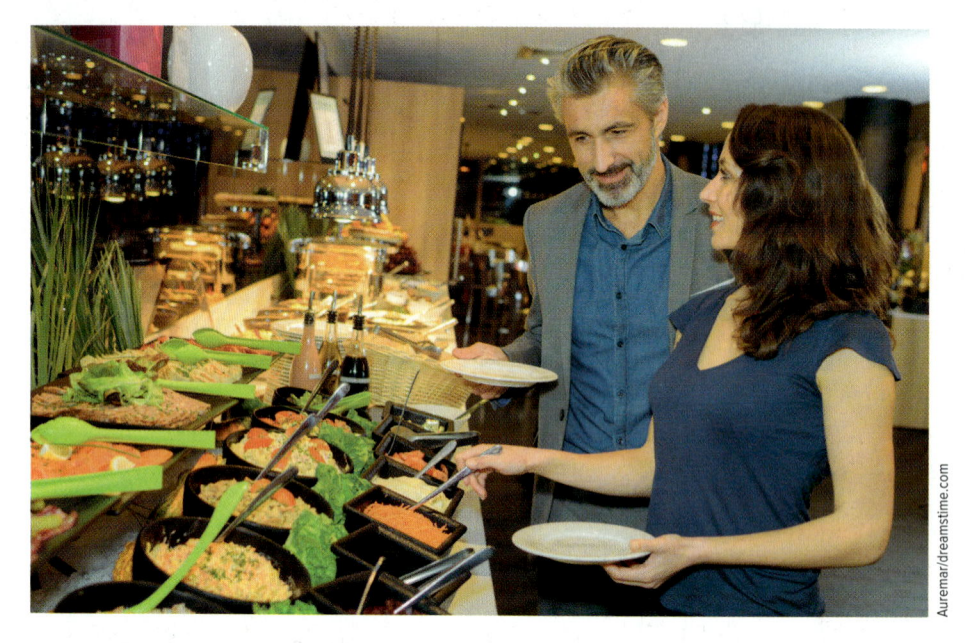

Curry powder – check that wheat flour hasn't been used to stop the ground spices from clumping.

Sauces such as Worcestershire (Lea & Perrins is gluten-free in the US, but not in the UK where it's made with malt vinegar), Tartare, BBQ Sauce.

Stock cubes – some brands contain wheat.

Salad dressings and marinades – may contain malt vinegar, soy sauce and flour.

Mustards that contain wheat flour and malt vinegar.

Breakfast foods
Pancakes, waffles, French toast.

Corn flakes, rice puffs and other breakfast cereals – may contain barley malt extract.

Energy/granola bars – some bars may contain wheat as an ingredient, and most use oats that are not gluten-free.

Yeast spreads such as Marmite and Vegemite.

Peanut butter.

Sweets
Cakes, biscuits, cookies, brownies, eclairs, Danish pastries.

Crêpes.

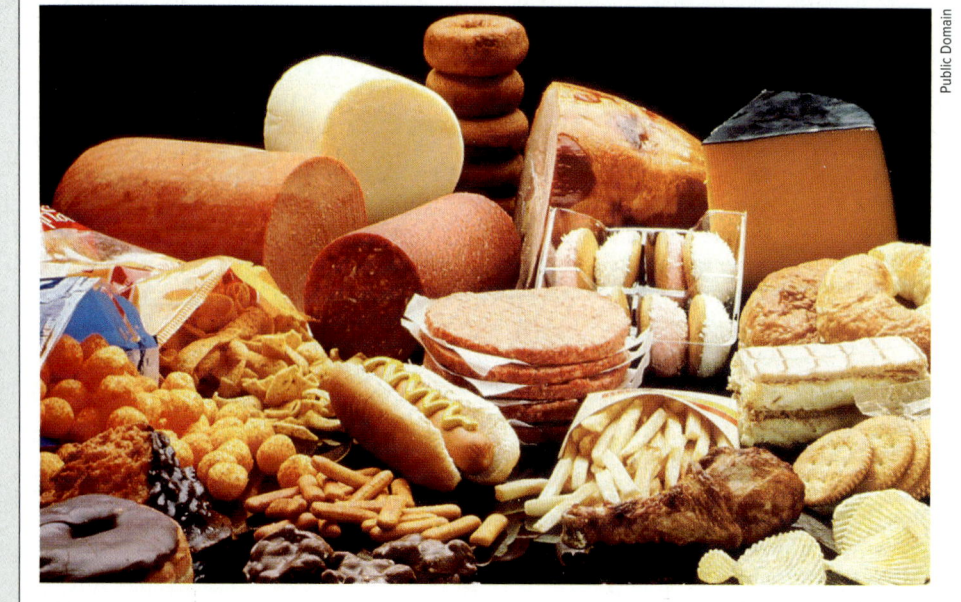

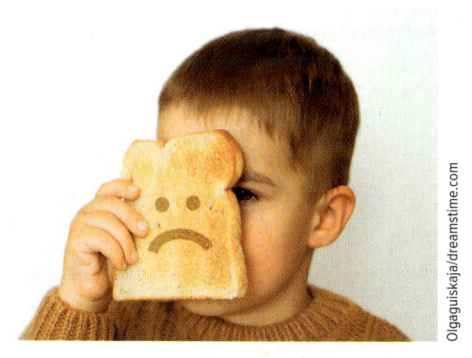

WHERE DO YOU FIND GLUTEN?

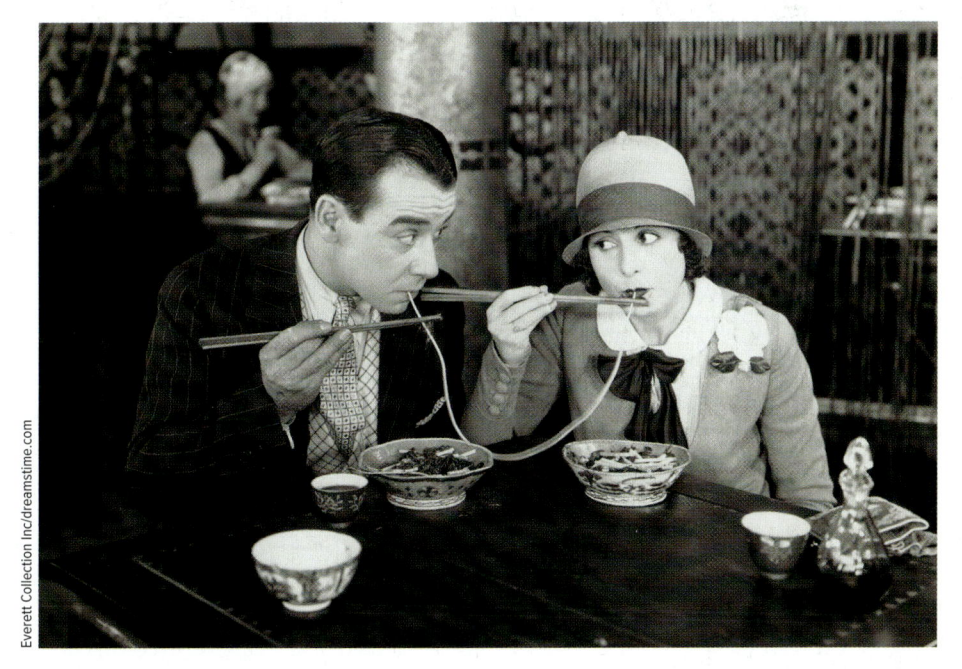

Trifles, fruit pies and strudels.

Chocolate and other treats that contain malt or biscuit pieces.

Fruit gums and other sweets that may contain wheat thickeners and glucose syrup made from wheat.

Cooking ingredients
Breadcrumbs and ready-made coating mixes.

Baking powder if it is made from wheat starch rather than corn or rice starch.

Croutons.

Brown rice syrup – may be made with barley enzymes.

Suet – may be coated in flour to extend its life.

Pre-packed grated cheese – if wheat flour has been used to stop it clumping.

Non-alcoholic drinks
Zero alcohol beer.

Soft drinks containing barley malt extract.

Tomato juice if it contains Worcestershire Sauce.

Malted hot drinks.

Drinking chocolate – may contain wheat.

Fruit barley squashes.

Processed food
Ready-made stuffing.

Frozen potato products – chips, hash browns, potato wedges, potato waffles may all contain a wheat-based flavouring or coating.

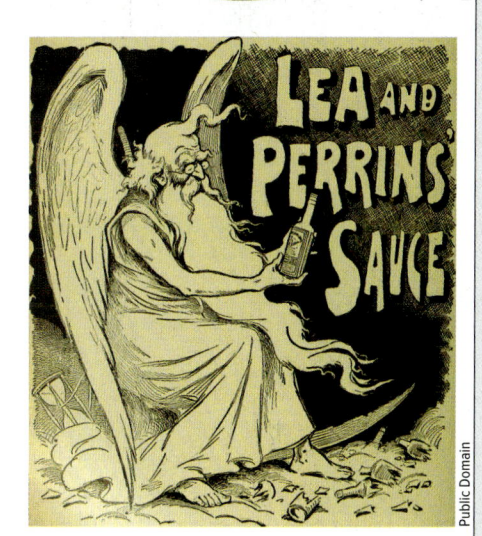

Sausages – these may contain rusk and wheat flour.

Processed meats – salamis, hot dogs, pepperoni, liver sausage, pâté, all potentially contain grains.

Taramasalata – may contain bread.

Spreadable cheese and cheese products – may contain modified food starch.

Ready-made and tinned soups – especially creamy ones that may have flour as a thickener and broths that may contain barley.

The other hazard for anyone trying to avoid gluten products is potential cross-contamination of anything that is produced or served in a gluten environment. This is covered in detail on page 22.

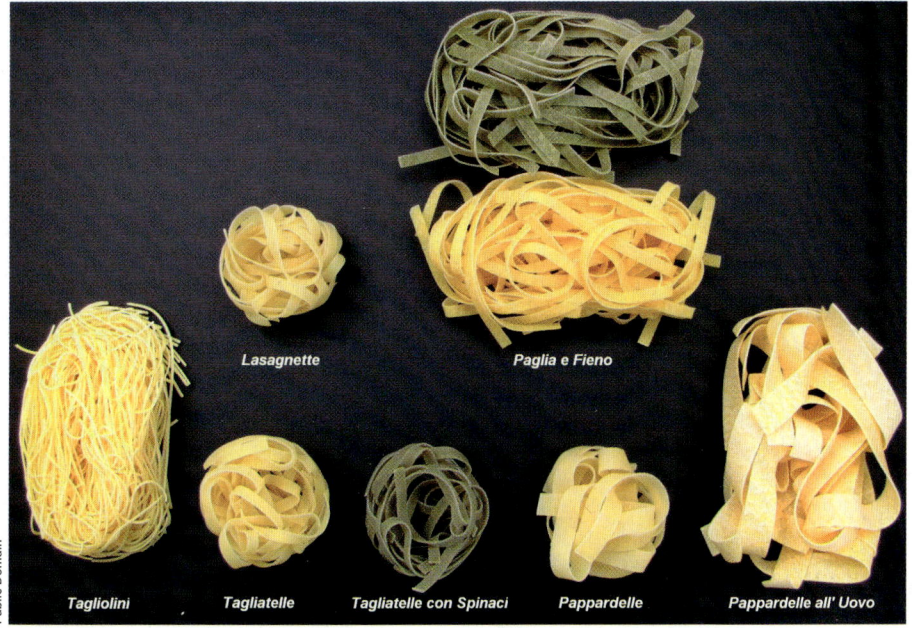

THE GLUTEN-FREE HANDBOOK

WHERE DO YOU FIND GLUTEN?

Alcohol

Most alcoholic beverages, such as wine, sherry, champagne, gin, whisky, brandy, rum, and vodka are gluten-free but there are some to look out for.

Grains are used to make distilled alcohol, such as whisky, but the process of producing them does not heat the plant liquid to a high enough degree to vaporise the gluten, so it is left behind in the distillation process.

However, there are some alcohol products that must be avoided or the labels checked to make sure that they don't contain any traces of gluten. Unfortunately, drink labels don't always list all the ingredients, but there should be an allergy warning if it is applicable.

Beer, ale, lager, and stout
These are traditionally made from barley and wheat, and the brewing process does not remove the gluten. Some brewers are now making gluten-free beers using an enzyme to break down the gluten proteins, but traces can remain so coeliacs need to be wary.

There are also now beers made from non-gluten grains and pseudocereals, such as maize, millet, amaranth and quinoa.

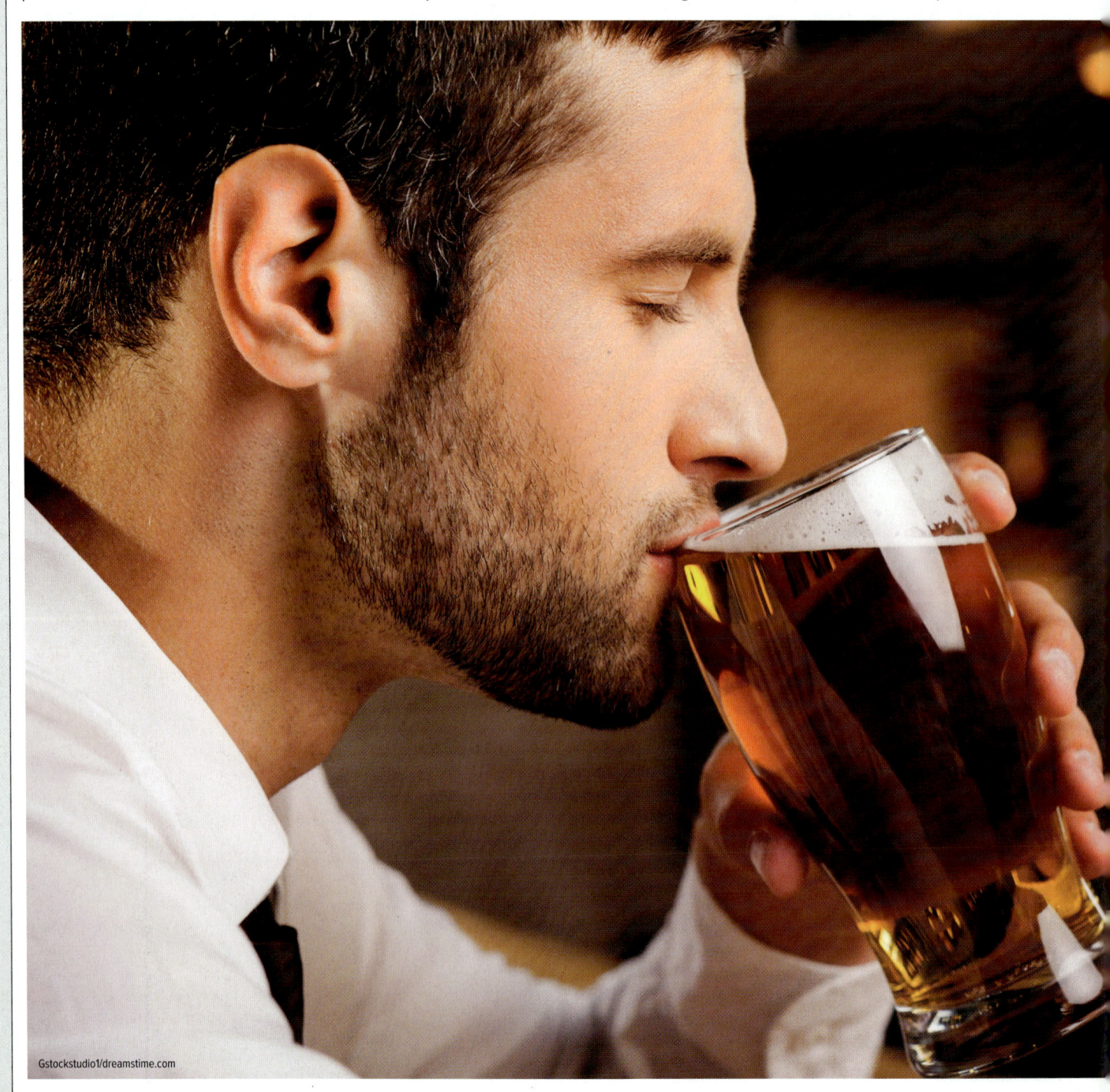

WHERE DO YOU FIND GLUTEN?

Dessert wines
Extra flavourings can be added to some dessert wines, so it is best to avoid unless it's possible to check what flavourings have been used.

Ciders
Most are fine for anyone avoiding gluten, but some manufacturers add flavourings to their cider that can contain gluten, so go for the pure apple or pear varieties.

Liqueurs
Drinks such as amaretto, schnapps, and brand names such as Tia Maria, Cointreau and Grand Marnier are made from distilled alcohol to which sugar and flavouring have been added. In some cases, the flavourings may contain gluten so avoid unless you can see the ingredients or check the manufacturers' websites.

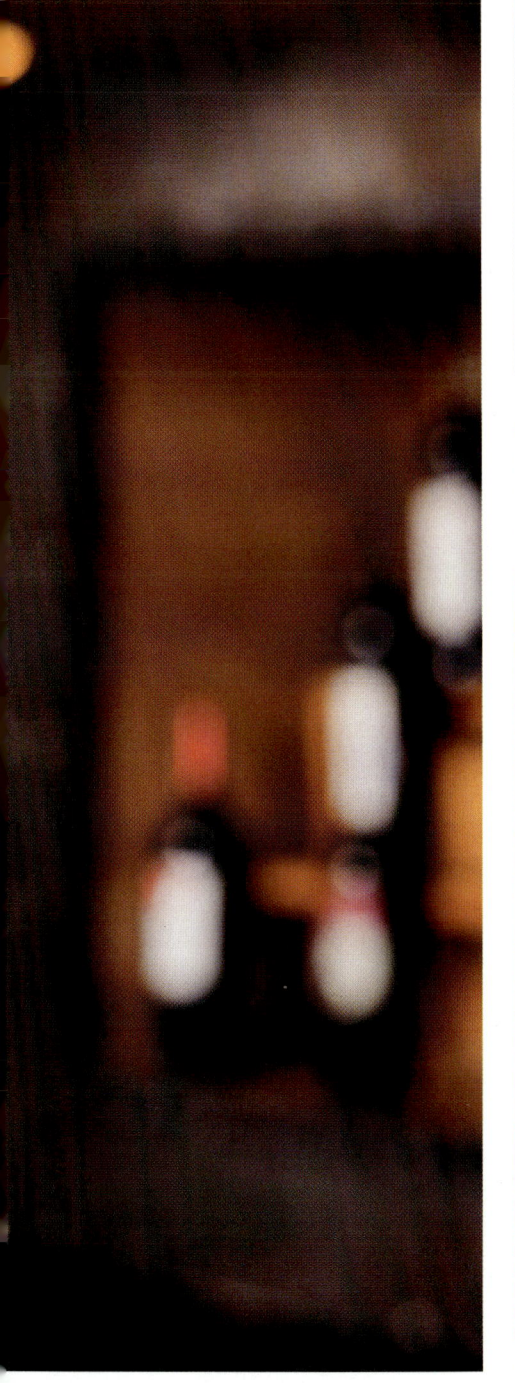

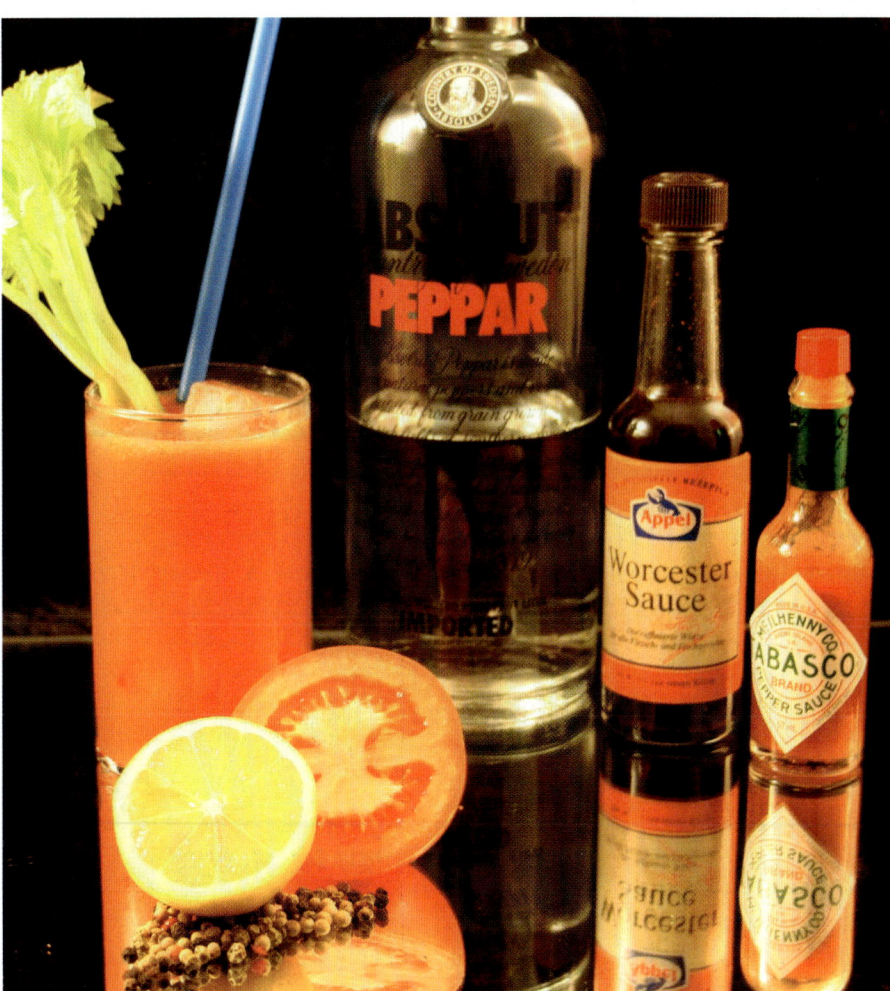

Cocktails
To be properly safe, quiz the bartender on all the ingredients. Most will be fine if they use distilled alcohol and fruit juices, but a Bloody Mary, for instance, will have a dash of Worcestershire Sauce.

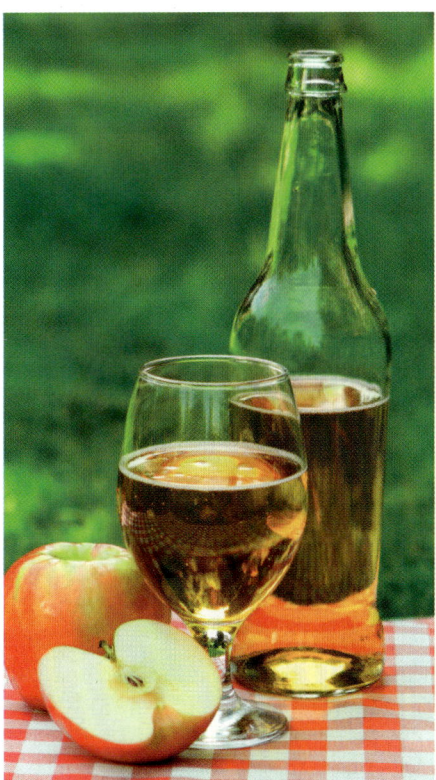

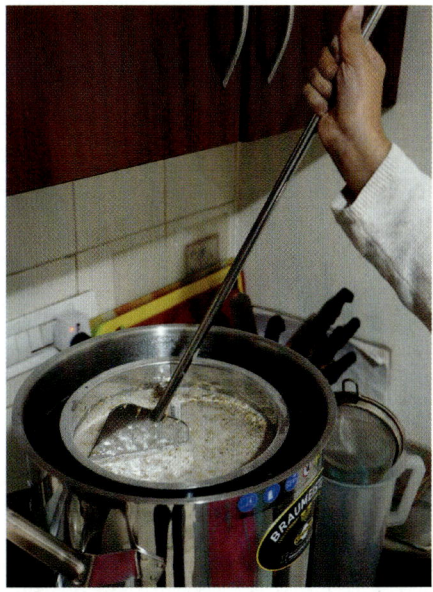

Darya Petrenko/dreamstime.com

Mike Prince via Wikimedia Commons

THE GLUTEN-FREE HANDBOOK

A note on cross-contamination

This is one important hidden source of gluten that anyone who is in any way sensitive to the protein or, indeed, to any wheat product, needs to know about.

The typical farming practice of crop rotation, as well as the shared use of harvesting and transport equipment and storage silos, often results in gluten-containing grains coming into contact with other grains, legumes and seeds that are naturally free of gluten.

Food processing factories and bakeries that use shared production equipment to produce foods both with and without gluten can also result in gluten cross-contact.

In the past few years, we have become used to seeing specific notices on food labels, in shops and restaurants warning us that what we are about to eat or buy has been made or packaged in an establishment where nuts are present. These enable those who are highly sensitive to make a judgement on the risks of continuing with the purchase.

Much less in use are warnings about wheat and gluten – although certification is becoming more widespread – so there just has to be an awareness, especially in the very sensitive, that contamination is possible.

If in doubt, contact the manufacturer or take advice from one of the recognised support organisations – Coeliac UK, Celiac Disease Foundation in the US, Coeliac Australia, and Celiac Canada, all of whom operate a helpline service. See page 114 for more details.

Things to be aware of at home

Utensils, pots and pans, strainers, and colanders with fine holes.

Kitchen equipment such as food processors, blenders, grill pans, toasters, air fryers, barbecues and pizza ovens that are hard to clean thoroughly enough to remove traces of gluten.

Fan ovens that recirculate the air – keep gluten-free food well covered in these, throughout the cooking process.

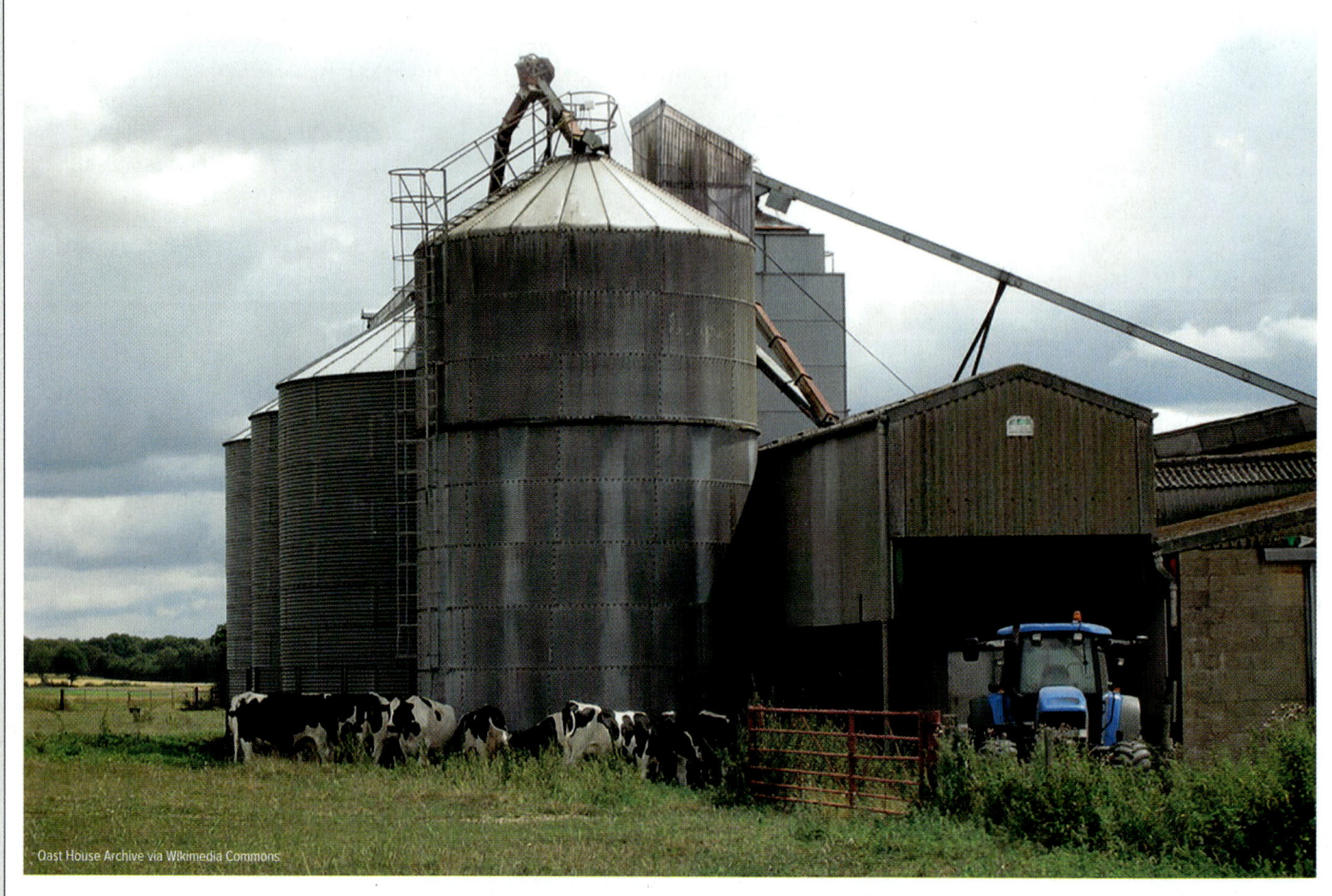

WHERE DO YOU FIND GLUTEN?

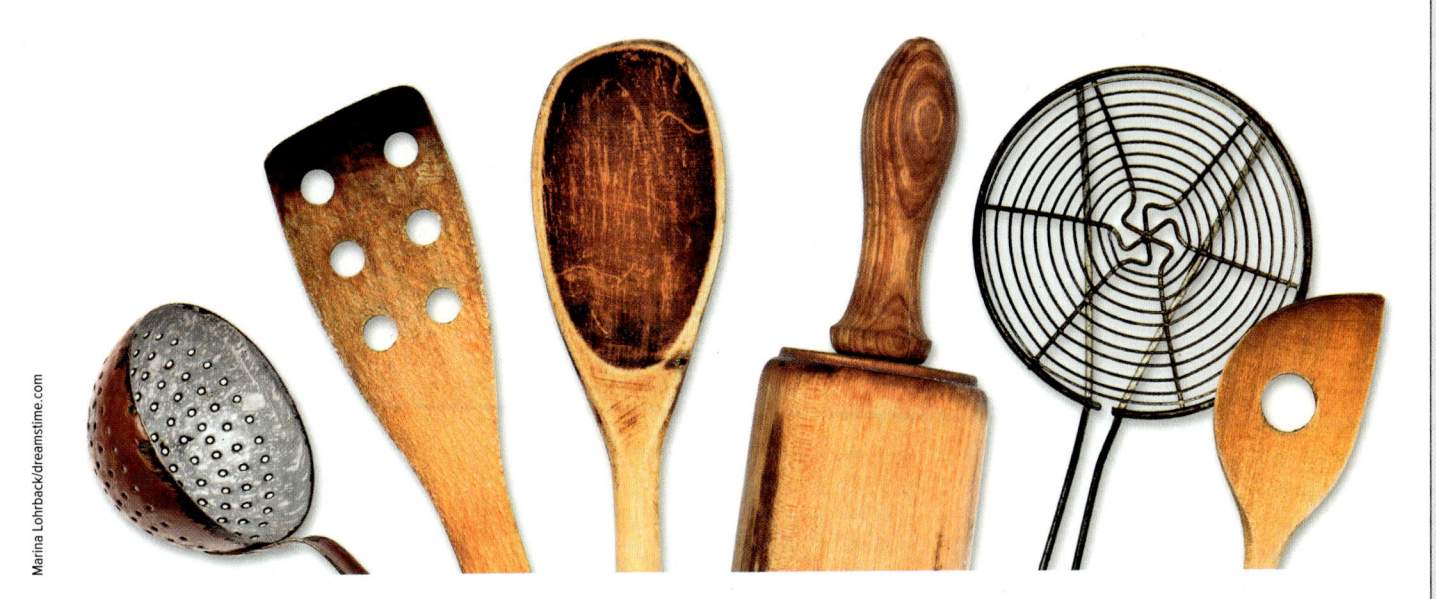

Bread boards that can be shared between gluten and gluten-free foods.

Storage containers with multiple uses, such as biscuit tins and cake boxes.

Pantry shelves – store gluten-free products above gluten ones and make sure non-gluten-free flour bags don't spill any of their contents.

Oven gloves that you use to handle both gluten and gluten-free dishes.

Drying towels that can often be used to transfer food out of an oven in place of oven gloves.

Cooking oil that is reused for deep fat frying.

Chopping and serving surfaces have not been thoroughly cleaned after they have been used in the preparation of a gluten product.

Ingredients coming into contact with flour or other ground grains in a fridge or on a worktop while they are waiting to be used.

Butter knives and jam spoons becoming contaminated with non-gluten-free bread and cake crumbs.

How to minimise cross-contamination

If you live in a mixed Coeliac, non-Coeliac household you don't have to go to the expense of having double of absolutely everything! Simple washing of most kitchen equipment and work surfaces with soap and hot water will remove traces of gluten. For toasting you can buy a number of different brands of reusable toaster bags. And covering food up in clingfilm or foil or using wax wrappers and plastic boxes that can be washed, will help keep stored items away from each other.

What do you need two of?

A separate bread board might be a worthwhile purchase, but if you have a dishwasher or the washer-upper is careful, you shouldn't have to buy extra chopping boards.

Two pairs of readily identifiable oven gloves are also a good idea if a mixture of foods is being prepared in the kitchen every day. Otherwise, if it's only occasionally that food has to be prepared for either a gluten or a gluten-free eater, then you just need to make sure the gloves are washed in between.

Wooden utensils and bowls are harder to wash and more porous so they can absorb particles of gluten. A separate set of these could be important for coeliacs and others who are very sensitive.

Another duplicate to consider is a separate oil pan if the pan used for deep frying isn't routinely emptied and washed out.

And if pans are very pitted and scratched, they can harbour contaminants in the grooves, so replacing them or having a couple of extras that are exclusively gluten-free would be safest.

All-in-all, you should use the same approach to the matter as you would with a smelly food – fish, garlic, onion, for instance – and cover effectively, keep well away from everything else and make sure equipment is washed up after use.

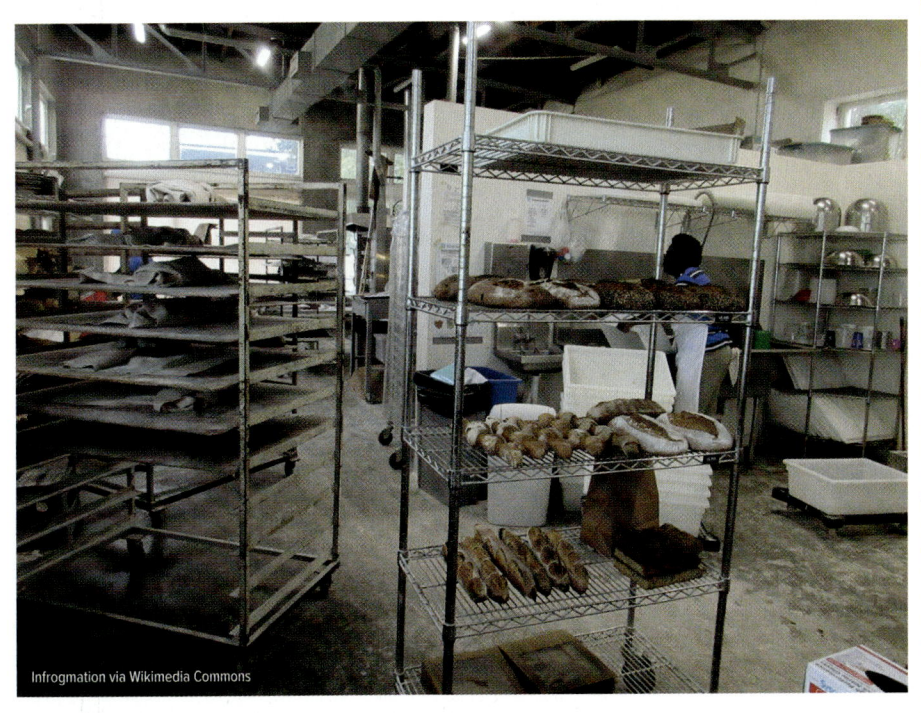

THE GLUTEN-FREE HANDBOOK

WHERE DO YOU FIND GLUTEN?

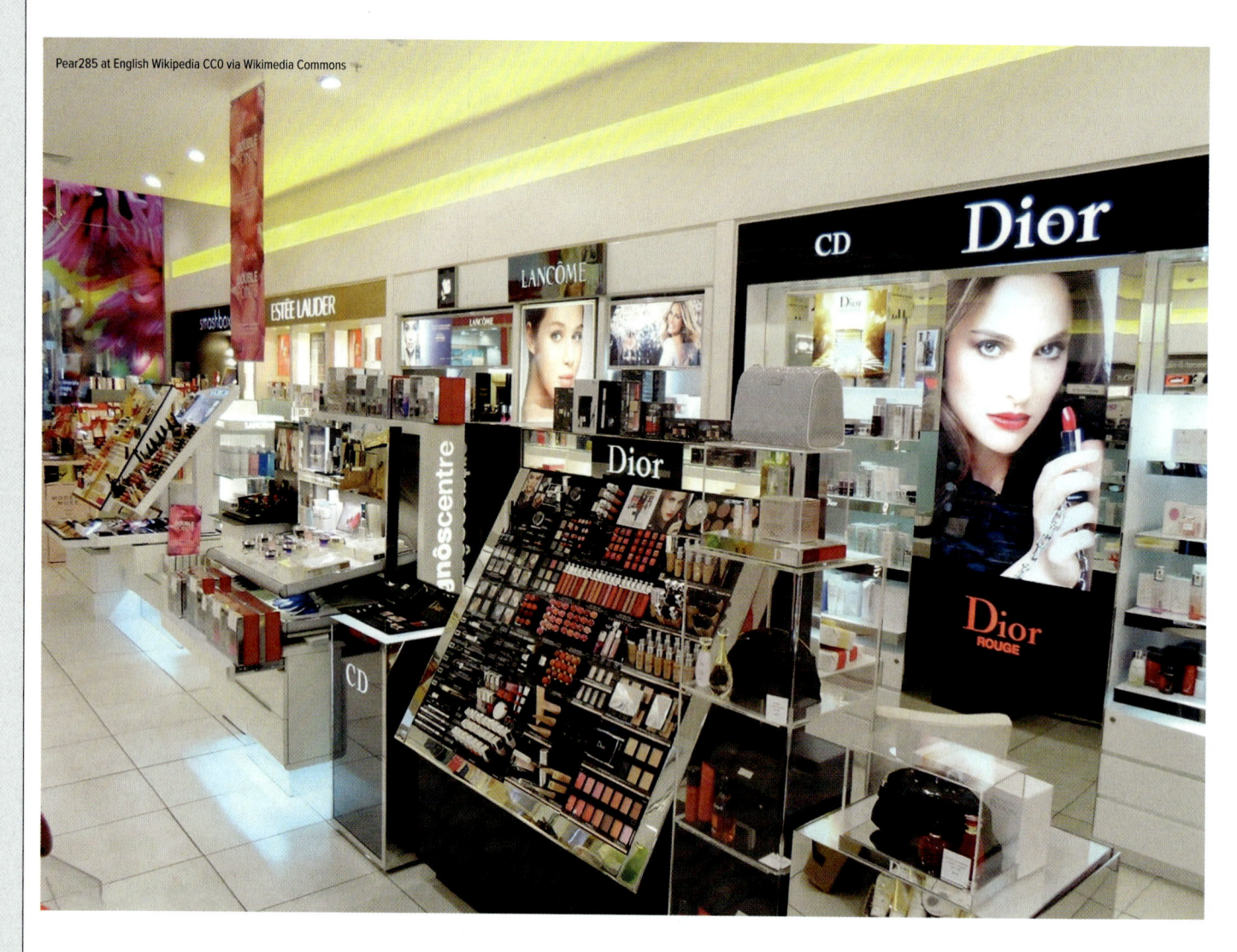

Pear285 at English Wikipedia CC0 via Wikimedia Commons

The hidden gluten

Lots of products use binding agents for texture and to hold ingredients together, and these may have been extracted from wheat and other grains.

Some of the less obvious foodstuffs can be an unforeseen source of harmful gluten, but there are also other products, unrelated to what we eat, that can also be a hidden hazard. When in doubt, consult the label, contact the manufacturer, or take advice from one of the Coeliac support organisations outlined on page 114.

Foods that look harmless… but aren't!

Cereal and granola – corn flakes and puffed rice often contain malt extract and granola is often made with regular oats, not gluten-free ones

Ready-made sauces and gravies – it's the thickening agent used in these that's likely to be suspect

Dried and brewer's yeast – fresh yeast is usually gluten-free but other versions need checking

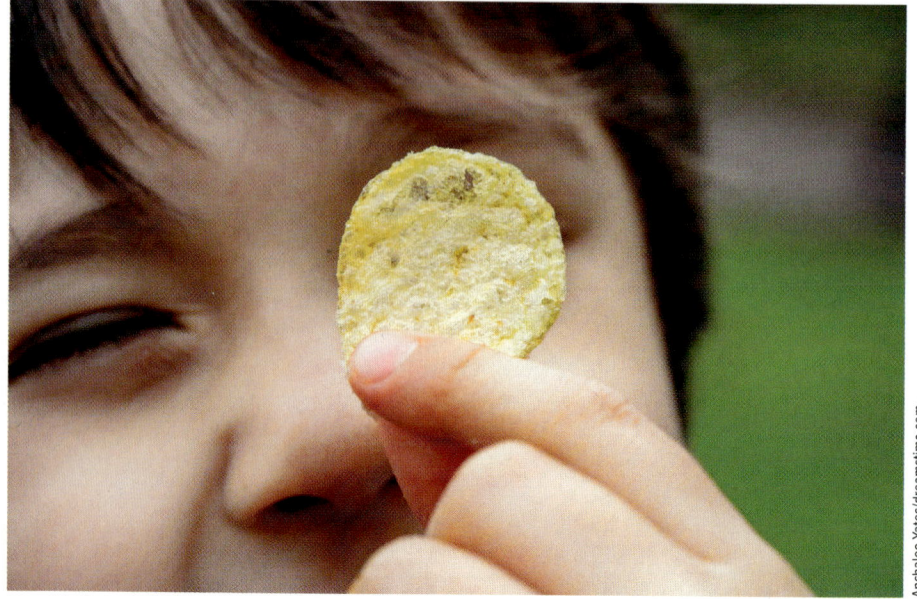

Anchalee Yates/dreamstime.com

WHERE DO YOU FIND GLUTEN?

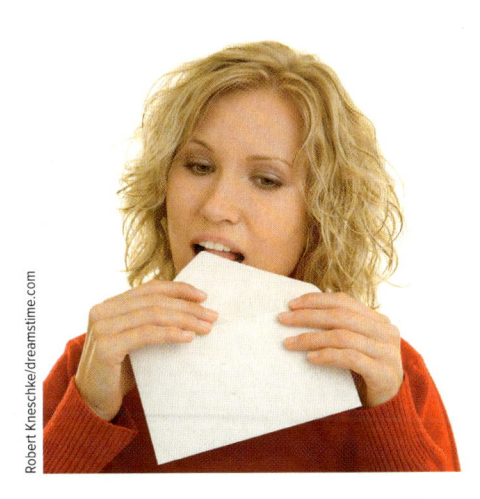

Traditional soy sauce – Tamari is a gluten-free version

Blue cheese – the mould spores can be grown on a gluten product

Stock cubes – wheat flour can be used as a thickener

Jam – gluten can be used as a thickener

Icing sugar – may have wheat starch added to stop it clumping

French fries/chips – if fried with fish these may be cross-contaminated from the batter or may themselves be coated in wheat flour to keep them separate

Meat substitutes such as veggie burgers and vegetarian sausages that may contain bread or have bread-based coatings

Chewing gum – can contain glucose syrup made from wheat

Ready meals unless they specifically say they are gluten-free

Crisps/potato chips – some potato chip flavours may contain malt vinegar or wheat starch

Chocolate – some varieties are not gluten free so the ingredient list should be checked

Burgers and sausages – sometimes contain wheat rusk

Ice cream – most single flavour ice creams are gluten-free, however certain flavours and toppings may contain ingredients that are not

Beauty products

Although gluten cannot be absorbed through the skin, many of the cleansing, moisturising and beauty products we use contain gluten that can be ingested accidentally if we lick our lips or fingers, or if we have a habit of absentmindedly sucking our hair or biting our nails.

These include:

- Dry shampoo
- Face cream
- Face powder and blusher
- Foundation
- Hair products – mousse, gel, hair spray
- Lipstick and lip balm
- Nail polish
- Shampoo and conditioner
- Soap (some contain bran)
- Sunscreen
- Tanning products
- Toothpaste

There are gluten-free versions of all these products, so check the labels for the magic words 'gluten-free' or check the packaging for any problematic ingredients (see the list on page 26).

Unexpected gluten

Then there are products that, even more than beauty products, no one would imagine contain gluten. For example:

The glue used on lickable envelopes, stamps, and address labels

Paper paste, finger paints and play-dough – while adults are unlikely to ingest these, children of play school age almost certainly will

Communion wafers.

Some medicinal products and vitamins – all oral medicine and supplements should be checked for gluten and starches as they are often used as one of the inactive ingredients, for instance as a binder to hold tablets together. Also be aware that generic versions of drugs may differ from branded ones, depending on the practices of the different manufacturers.

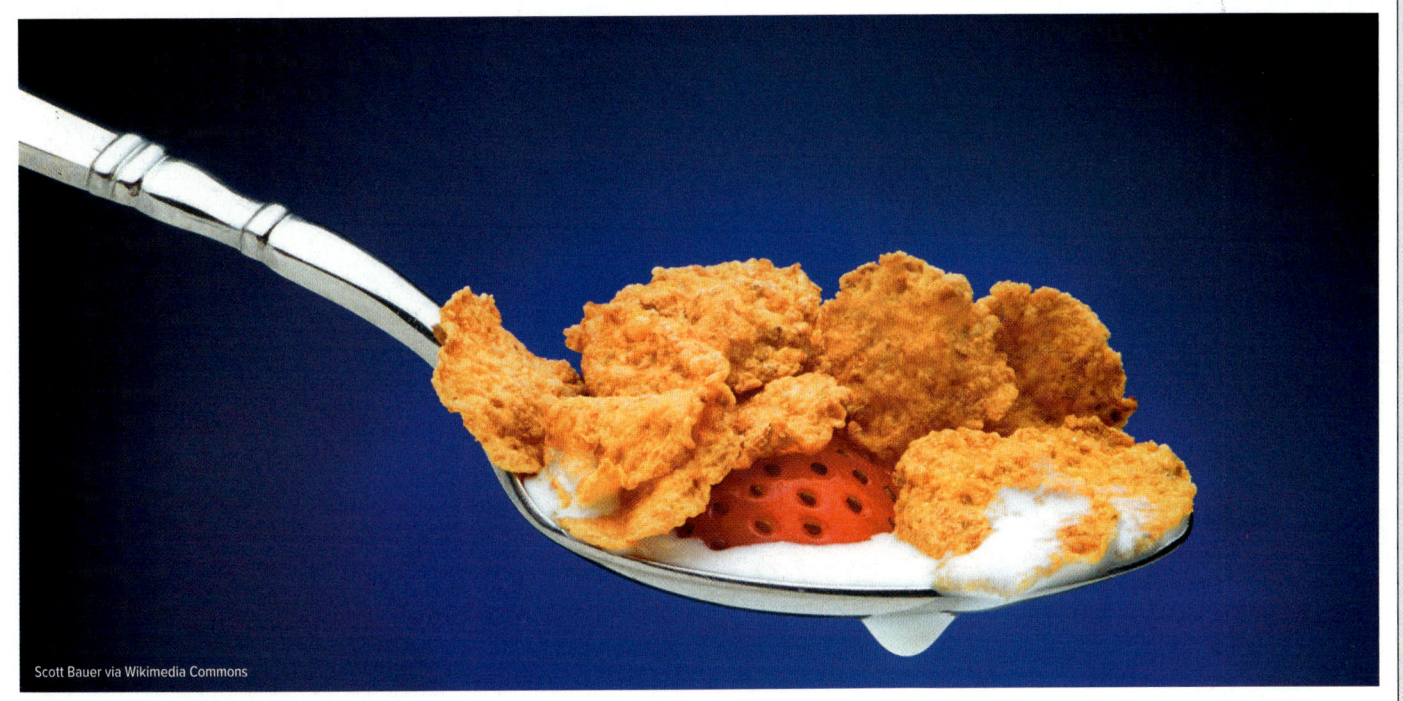

THE GLUTEN-FREE HANDBOOK

WHERE DO YOU FIND GLUTEN?

What on the labels says gluten beware?

One thing everyone who cannot eat gluten has to get into the habit of doing is carefully reading product labels.

Sometimes there's a helping hand for consumers in the form of the words 'Gluten Free' on packaging. Manufacturers can only apply these words to their labels if they can guarantee that no more than 20 parts per million of gluten is present in their product.

There's additional help if the products have been given the right to use a certification logo from one of the recognised authorities. This means that the products have been thoroughly tested and found to be truly gluten-free. See the *How to live gluten-free* chapter starting on page 64 for more information on these.

Ingredients to look out for

If the following appear on product labels for both food and beauty products then it's not safe to buy them. In alphabetical order:

Avena sativa (oats)
Barley
Barley malt extract
Barley meal
Beta-glucan (frequently derived from wheat)
Brewer's yeast
Brown rice syrup
Colloidal oatmeal
Contains Gluten – pretty obvious one this!
Cyclodextrin
Dextrin
Dextrin palmitate (starch, possibly gluten-based)
Dinkel
Durum
Einkorn
Emmer
Farina
Faro/Farro
Graham
Hordeum vulgare (barley)
Hydrolysed wheat protein
Hydrolysed vegetable protein (may contain wheat)
Kamut
Khorasan
Laurdimonium hydroxypropyl (hydrolysed wheat protein)
Malt
Malt extract
Modified food starch
Modified corn starch
Modified wheat starch
MSG (Monosodium Glutamate)

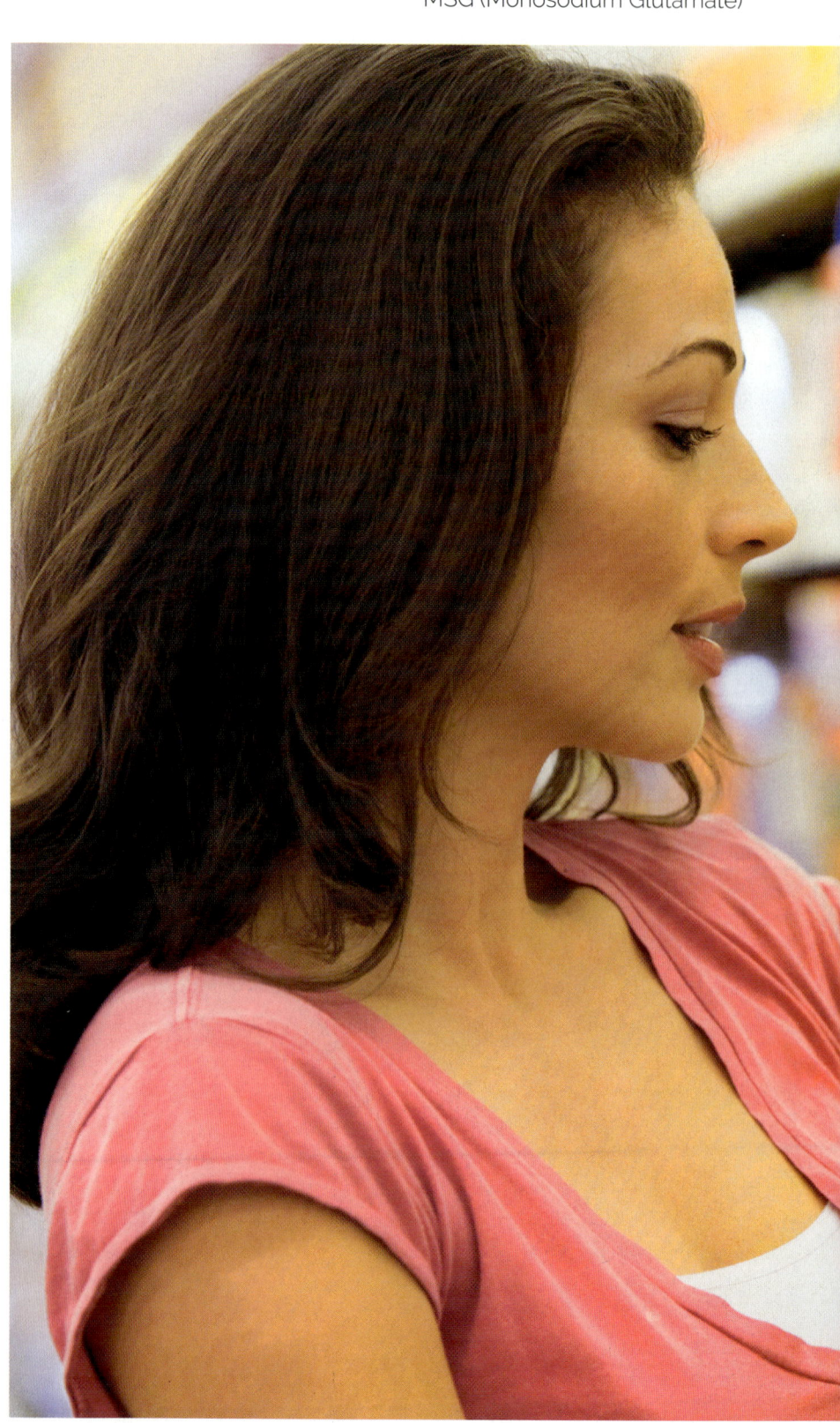

WHERE DO YOU FIND GLUTEN?

- Oats (unless specifically stated to be gluten-free)
- Pearl barley
- Pot barley
- Rye
- Scotch barley
- Secale cereale (rye)
- Semolina
- Smoke flavouring (sometimes uses barley malt flour to capture the smoke)
- Soy sauce
- Spelt
- Starch (this can be derived from wheat; to be safe look for specific types of starch – corn, rice, or potato)
- Stearyl dimonium hydroxypropyl (hydrolysed wheat protein)
- Triticale
- Tricalcium phosphate
- Triticum amino acids
- Triticum lipids
- Triticum vulgare (wheat)
- Udon (wheat pasta)
- Vegetable protein (may contain wheat, barley, rye, and/or oats)
- Vitamin E (can be derived from wheat germ oil)
- Wheat
- Wheat berries
- Wheat bran
- Wheat germ
- Wheat germ oil
- Wheat starch
- Yeast extract

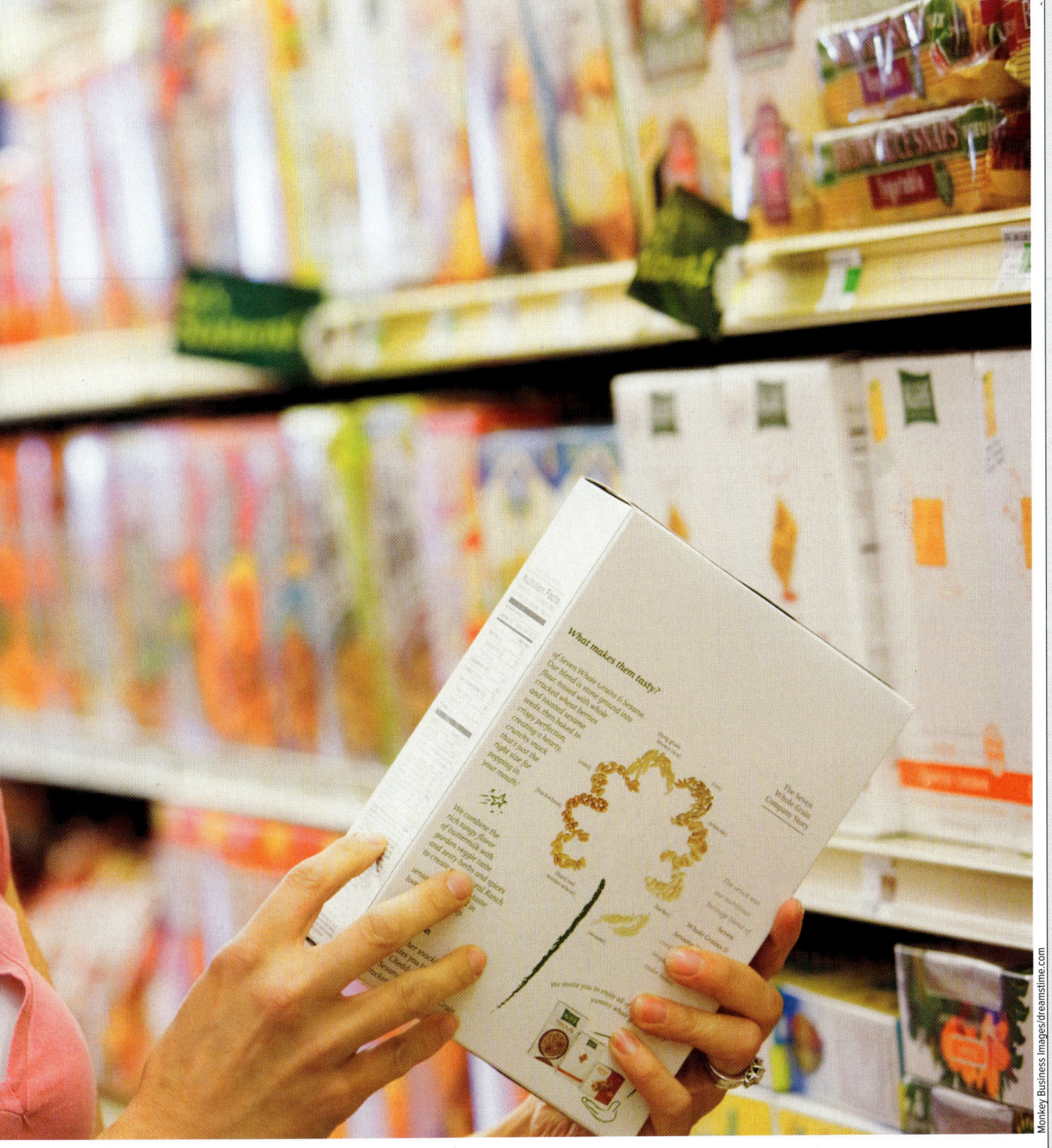

THE GLUTEN-FREE HANDBOOK

Coeliac Disease

This is the most dangerous of human reactions to ingesting gluten as it can be life-threatening if untreated.

Coeliac Disease is not simply an allergic reaction, it is an autoimmune condition that is activated by eating gluten. A person's body misidentifies a harmless substance absorbed into the digestive system as something dangerous to the body's survival. In defence it triggers the immune system to mistakenly attack its own tissues.

When this happens in the gut it leads to inflammation of the small intestine, the section of the digestive tract immediately after the stomach.

It is known that some people are born with a gene – one of either HLA DQ2.5 (commonest), HLA DQ8 (less common) or HLA DQ2.2 (least common) – that make them susceptible to developing Coeliac Disease. That means the condition can run in families, although this isn't inevitable. On the other hand, there

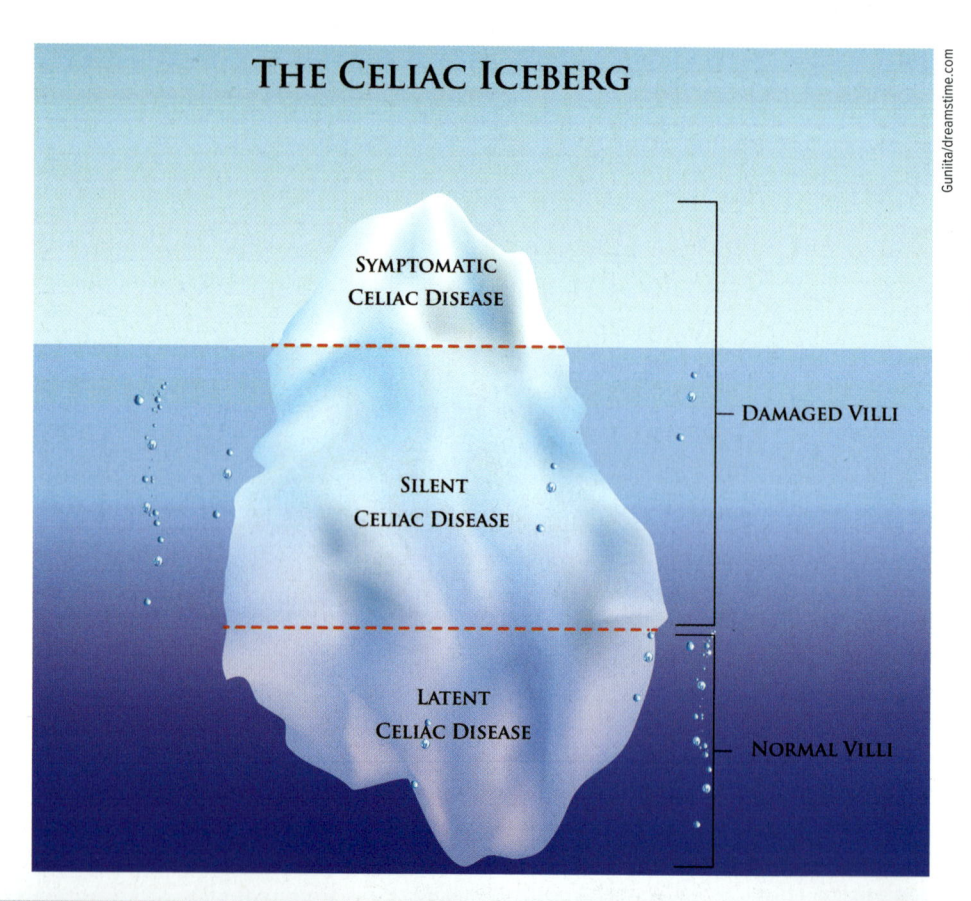

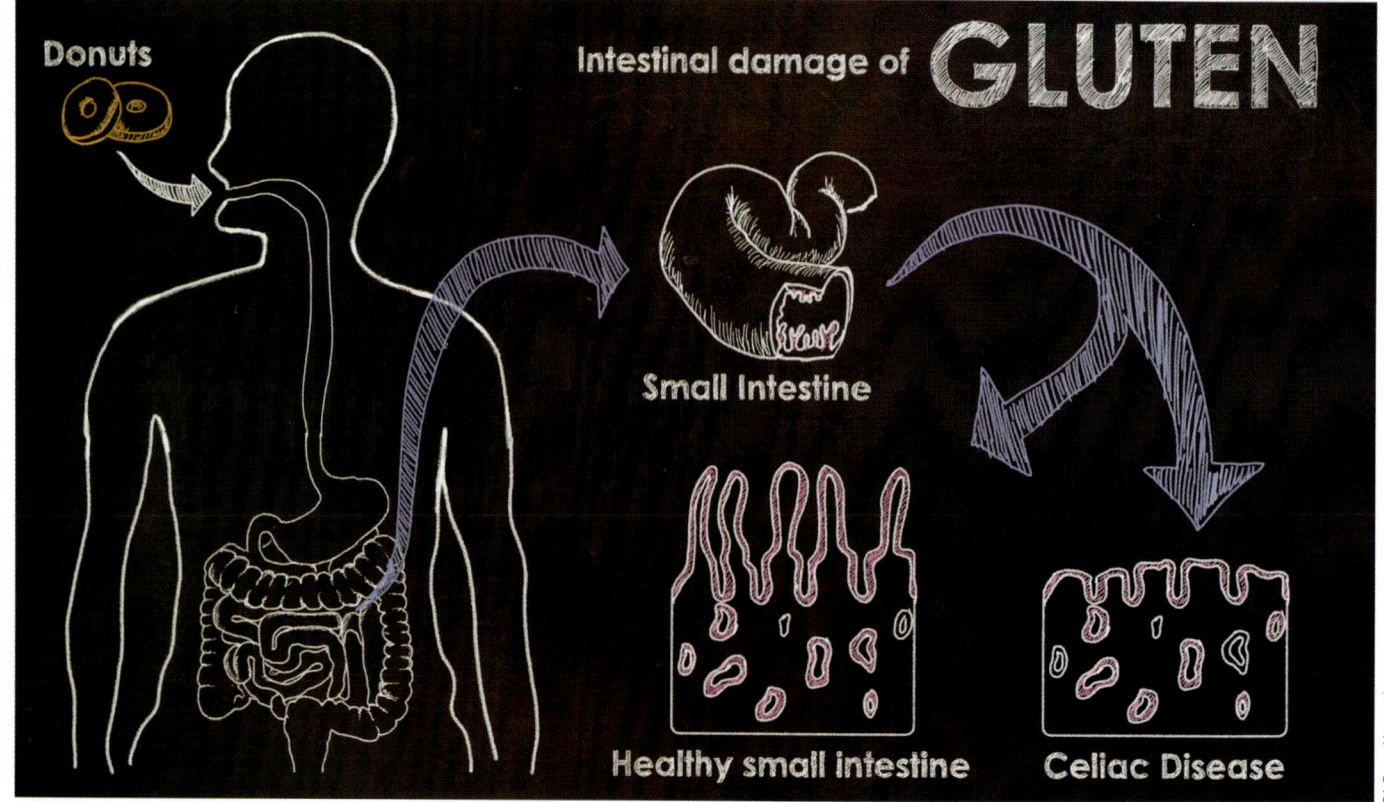

COELIAC DISEASE

A FEELING OF COMMUNITY
MasterChef winner, Jane Devonshire's son Ben was born with Coeliac Disease

"When he was two years old Ben screamed all the time," Jane Devonshire said in an interview with the *Belfast Telegraph* in 2020. He looked unwell and could not be taken to toddler clubs because he would bite people. Devonshire knew instinctively that something was wrong, but visits to the doctor proved futile. She recalled feeling as if the GP presumed her child was fractious because she was not coping. Then they moved home and got a new GP.

"He sat and he listened," she said. "He referred us and within about three months we had a diagnosis. It turned out it was Coeliac Disease. Within weeks, the difference in Ben [who is now 22] was profound and now he is probably the most chilled of all my children. He's so laid back, he's so kind, he's completely different to the child you would have seen."

Since 2019 Devonshire has been an ambassador for Coeliac UK. She knows how important a feeling of togetherness with the coeliac community can be.

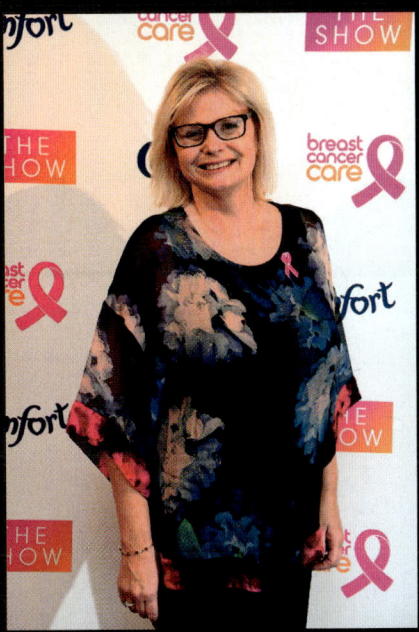

Eamonn M McCormack/Getty Images for Breast Cancer Care

"We survived on our own," she said. "That feeling of community is really overwhelming. I've been close to tears at times at coeliac shows because I didn't know that [community] existed when I had Ben. If I'd have known I could've accessed so much help, so much advice, and not thought I was on my own with this."

---

diarrhoea and weight loss, but Coeliac has been called an 'iceberg disease' because it can often be present with fewer, or less obvious, symptoms affecting other areas of the body apart from the gut.

Official advice for assessing whether to test for Coeliac Disease suggests being suspicious of unexplained abdominal complaints, constant fatigue, unexpected weight loss, severe mouth ulcers, unexplained vitamin and iron deficiencies, unexplained numbness and muscle weakness and a range of other seemingly unrelated symptoms, either together or in isolation.

To be certain, a doctor will order blood tests to find if antibodies are present when the person is following a diet that contains gluten-rich products. These tests are relatively inexpensive and are available on the NHS in the UK and covered by Australian and Canadian Medicare and most insurance companies in the US. Follow-up biopsies are similarly covered.

If antibodies are found, the next step is generally a biopsy of the lining of the small intestine, although this is often not needed when assessing children.

are many other people who are not born with the gene but can still be afflicted at any stage in their life.

Around one in every 100 people in the UK has been diagnosed with the condition, according to Coeliac UK. For the United States, the known figure is around one in 141 as estimated by John Hopkins Medicine, and Coeliac Australia says that in its country it's one in 70 people.

Globally, the estimate based on known coeliacs is around 1% of the total population, and while the percentage may seem small, the number it represents is not – around 80 million worldwide. And the likelihood is that there will be many more, as yet undiagnosed.

Diagnosing the disease
The classic complaints seen by medical practitioners are

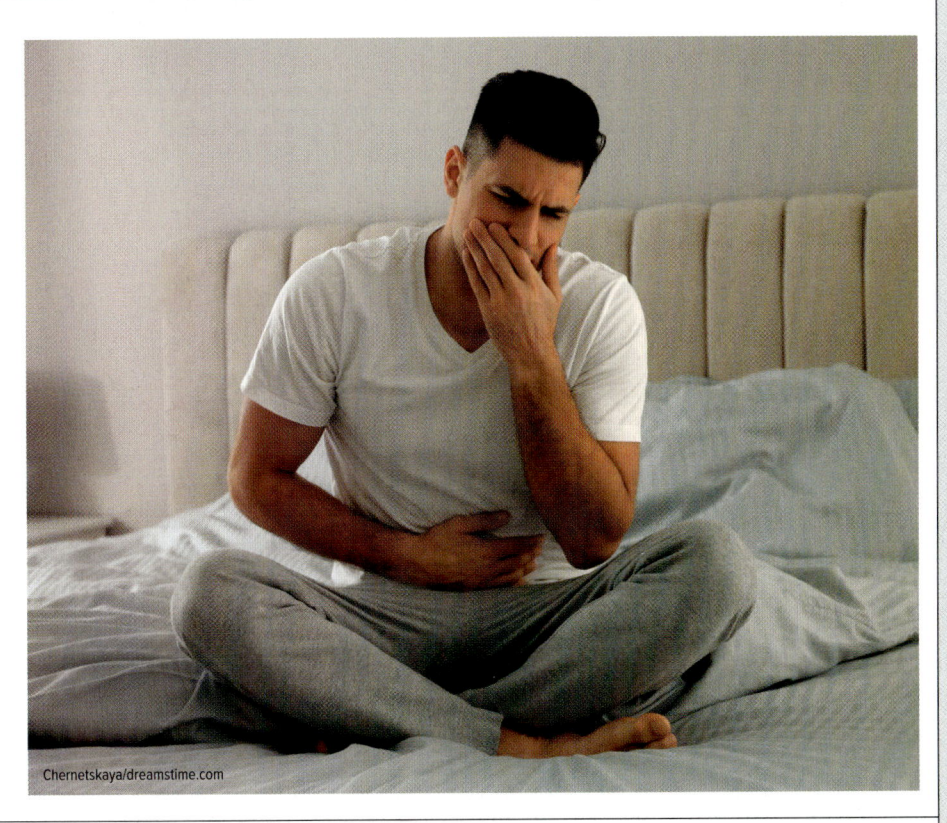

Chernetskaya/dreamstime.com

THE GLUTEN-FREE HANDBOOK

COELIAC DISEASE

What happens if Coeliac Disease is not diagnosed

The consequences of continually subjecting the body to a heightened immune reaction can be life-threatening. The attacks by the immune system damage the finger-like projections called villi in the wall of the small intestine that greatly expand the surface area of the gut. This increases its ability to absorb sugars, fats, proteins, vitamins, and minerals into the bloodstream.

When they are attacked, the villi flatten and stop properly absorbing nutrients from the food passing through them, which leads to severe malnutrition, no matter how much food the person eats. The lack of nutrients inhibits the ability of the body's muscles and organs to function well. There is also a greater chance of the coeliac individual developing bowel cancer, diabetes, asthma, infertility, and epilepsy.

A coeliac patient may also find that they are lactose intolerant because of the damage that has been done to their lower intestine.

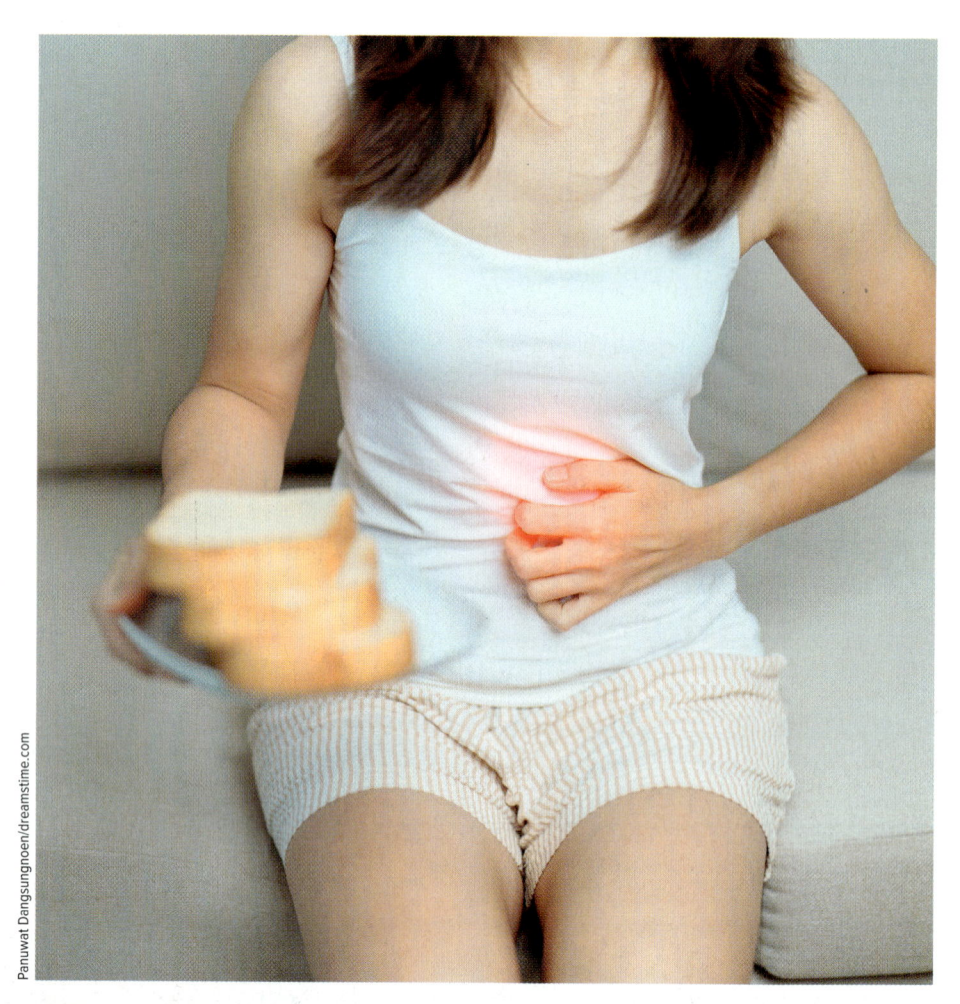

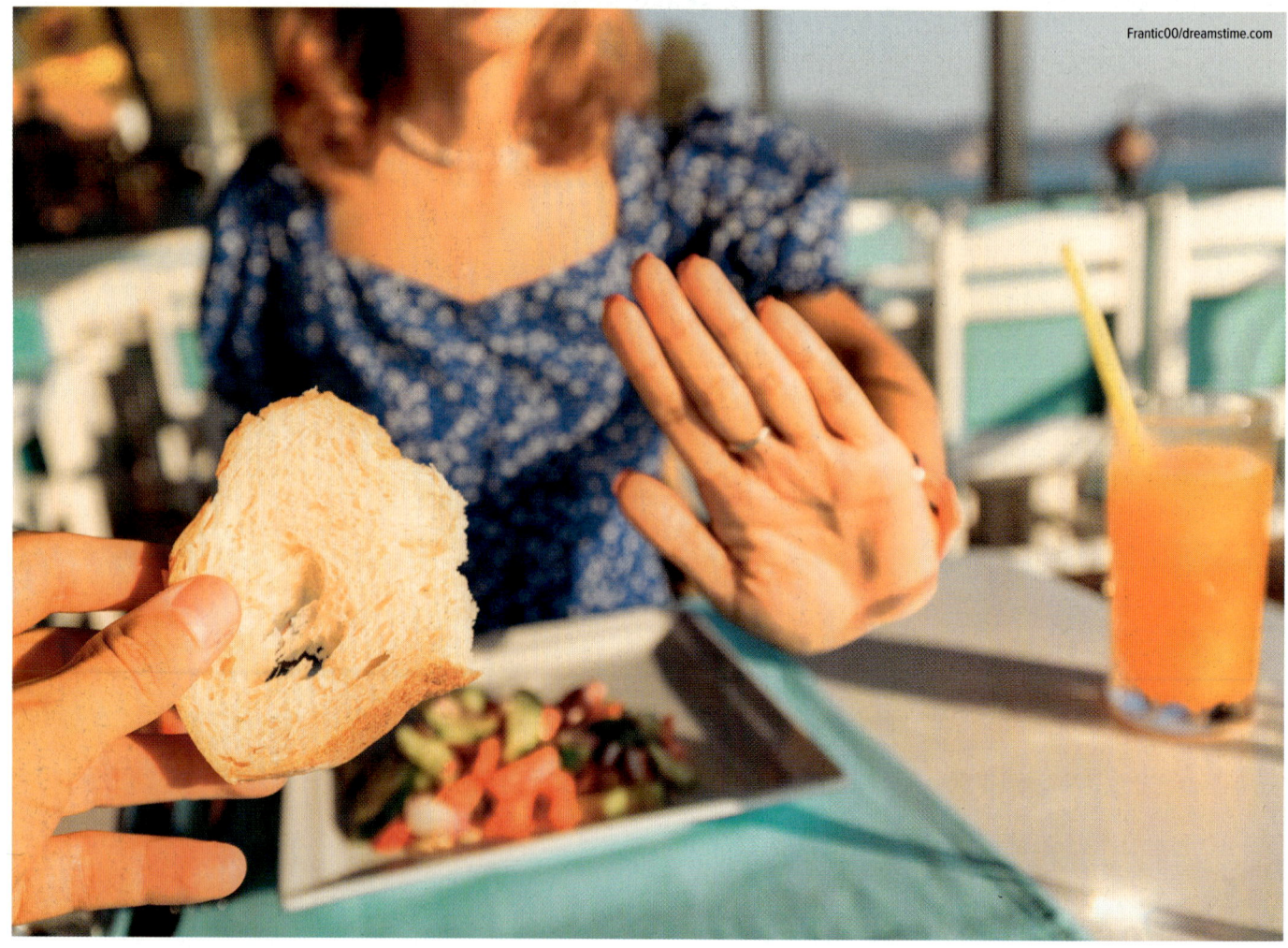

COELIAC DISEASE

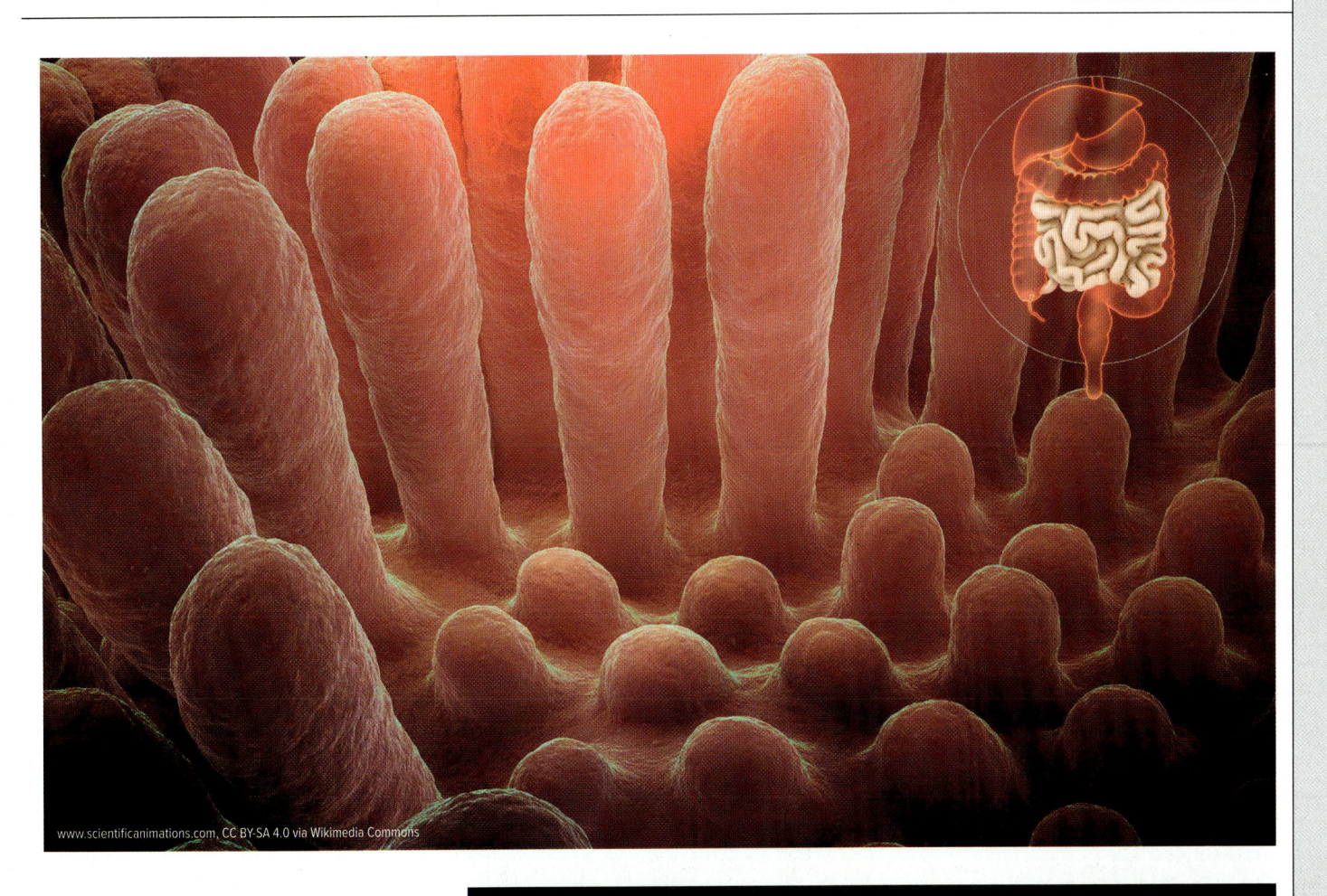

www.scientificanimations.com, CC BY-SA 4.0 via Wikimedia Commons

Many find that once they have eliminated gluten and the gut has recovered, they are able to enjoy dairy products again.

How is it treated?

There is currently no cure for Coeliac Disease, nor can you 'grow out of it'. The only effective treatment is for the person to switch to a strictly gluten-free diet. Even a small amount of gluten in coeliac patients can set off the damaging chain reaction.

The good news is that the controlled-diet treatment is highly effective, and people generally start to feel better in as short a space of time as the first few weeks after changing what they eat. It is true that for anyone who has had long-term damage to their small intestine, full recovery can take years, but the body does start the process of regeneration relatively quickly in most cases.

A few people can find that a gluten-free diet alone does not alleviate all their symptoms. If that is the case, they should consult a nutritionist about the possibility of also having an intolerance to FODMAPs. These are explained in the chapter on Non-Coeliac Gluten Sensitivity starting on page 38.

TAKE A SELF-ASSESSMENT
Derek Roberts from Coeliac UK

"My symptoms started back in 2013 with calcium, vitamin D and iron deficiency anaemia, alongside extreme fatigue. After struggling to find answers for years, I finally had a blood test in early 2016 after a brief period where I began to experience the more recognised symptoms of Coeliac Disease (diarrhoea, excessive wind, and bloating – I compared it to feeling seasick), which indicated I might have the disease. I had to continue eating gluten until my biopsy a few months later, which confirmed the diagnosis.

It was a long and difficult journey, especially adapting to the gluten-free diet and learning about cross-contamination. One of the biggest shocks was discovering the higher cost of gluten-free food, particularly bread. Social situations such as dining out and having a beer with friends also became a challenge, but Coeliac UK's resources, including their app and social media, were invaluable during this time. I would encourage everyone to check out the self-assessment tool at isitcoeliacdisease.org.uk, which can help people determine if they should be tested for Coeliac Disease."

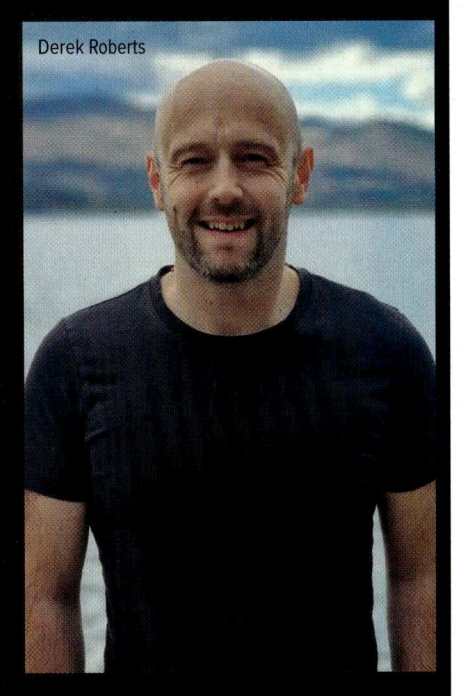

THE GLUTEN-FREE HANDBOOK

COELIAC DISEASE

The Banana Diet

What seemed like a breakthrough in the successful treatment of Coeliac Disease came in 1924. But while it was effective, it did not work in the way it was thought to.

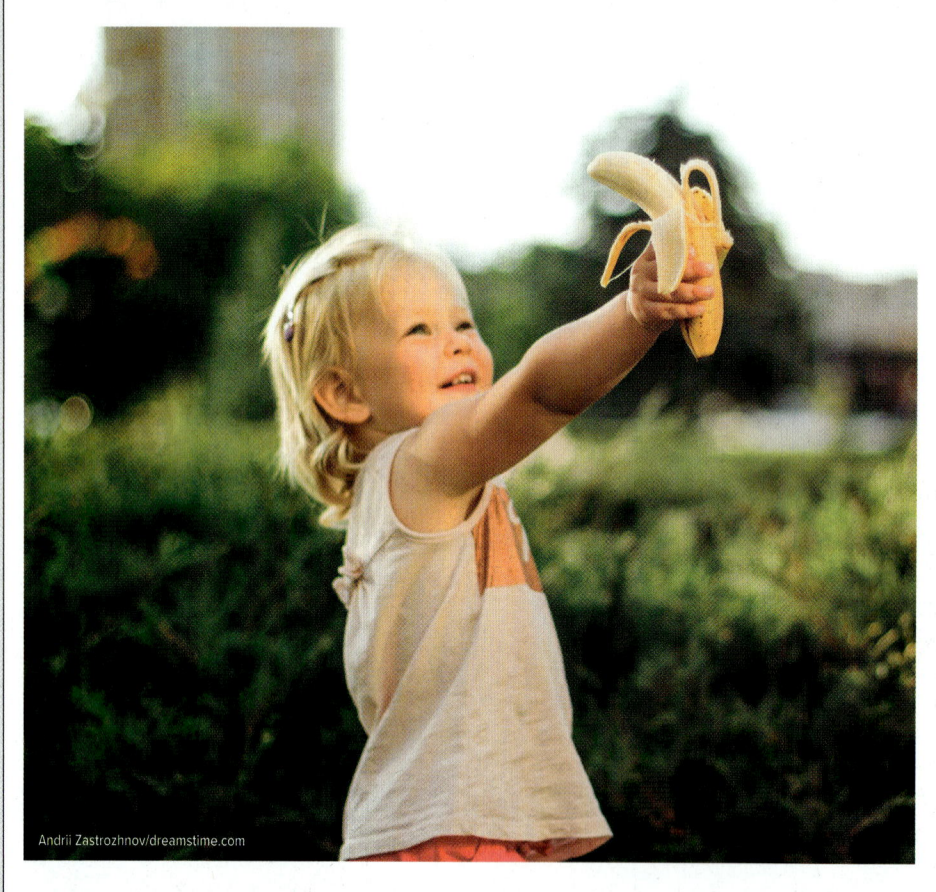

The miracle of the ripe banana

Haas was working with the information available at the time, which had not yet made the connection between Coeliac Disease and gluten. It had been noted that carbohydrate appeared to trigger symptoms, and he noted that in one town in Puerto Rico, where the

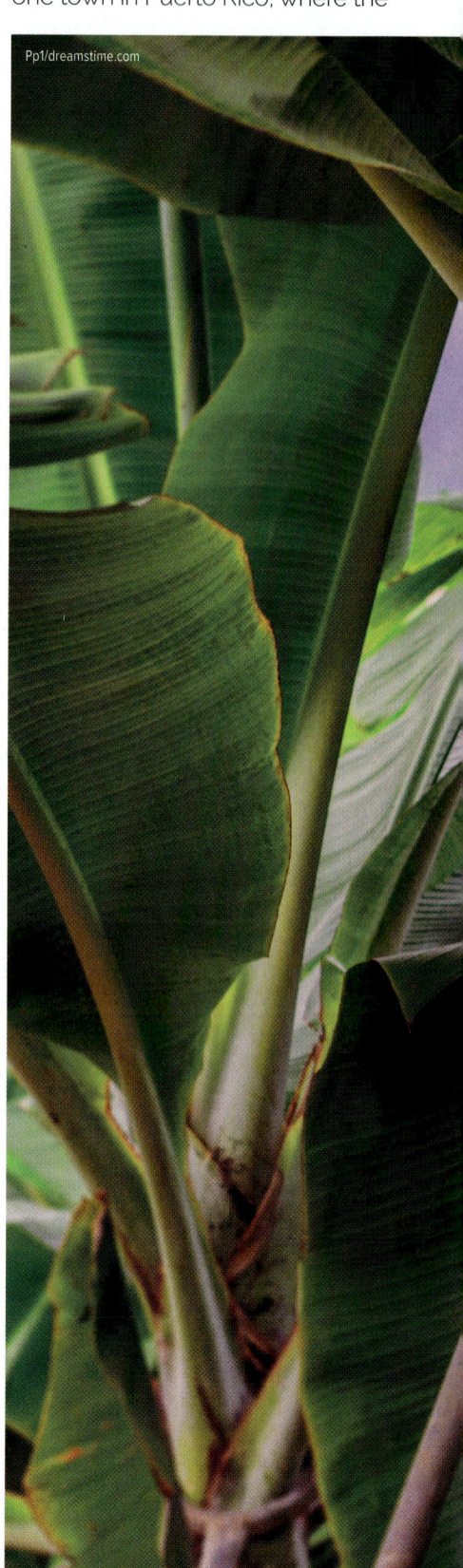

A young doctor called Sidney Valentine Haas specialised in paediatrics in 1920s New York. Following a visit to the islands of Puerto Rico and work with a young anorexic patient, he published a medical paper, *The Value of the Banana in the Treatment of Celiac Disease,* in *The Journal of Diseases of Children*. His theory introduced a whole new treatment for the disease that went on to save many lives, albeit not for the reasons he thought.

In the paper he stated: "Some years ago I treated a child, aged three years, who suffered from a severe case of anorexia nervosa. She had reached a serious state of depletion and weakness from her self-imposed starvation, refusing all food, and regurgitating that fed to her by gavage [tube into the stomach]. She finally accepted a banana, with the result that other food was taken in a more or less normal amount within 48 hours. There was a complete relapse when the banana was withheld, and food was taken normally only with bananas.

This experiment was repeated to test the validity of the observation, always with the same result, until a time came when her appetite was normal whether bananas were included in the diet or not… It was natural, therefore, to test bananas in a case of Celiac Disease where anorexia was a prominent symptom.

Celiac Disease is probably the most troublesome disturbance of nutrition of late infancy and early childhood. The consensus of opinion is that it is a functional disease characterised by inability to utilise properly carbohydrates and fats."

COELIAC DISEASE

inhabitants ate a lot of bread, there was a high incidence of 'Sprue', another term for Coeliac Disease. Farmers in the countryside around the town, on the other hand, ate bananas rather than bread and suffered far less from intestinal problems.

Haas put his young patients on a diet of ripe bananas – noting that under-ripe fruits were starchy whereas in over-ripe ones most of the starch had turned to sugar – milk, cottage cheese, vegetables, oranges, and a small amount of meat. As the diet was gluten-free (although Haas didn't realise that was what was making the difference) and high in calories, it gave the children's intestinal villi the chance to heal, and their lives were saved.

Parents from all over the United States brought their children with Coeliac Disease to Haas and he eventually successfully treated over 600 people. This was at a time when around 30% of children with coeliac died in their infancy.

The banana diet continued to be used to treat some children until the early 1950s. But as it was not addressing the root cause of the disease in the first place, only its symptoms temporarily, it had a downside. When parents thought their children were cured, they allowed them to return to the family's normal eating habits, which meant that their intestines continued to be damaged into adulthood. This damage would eventually catch up with them unless they subscribed, 20 or 30 years later, to the newly recommended gluten-free diets.

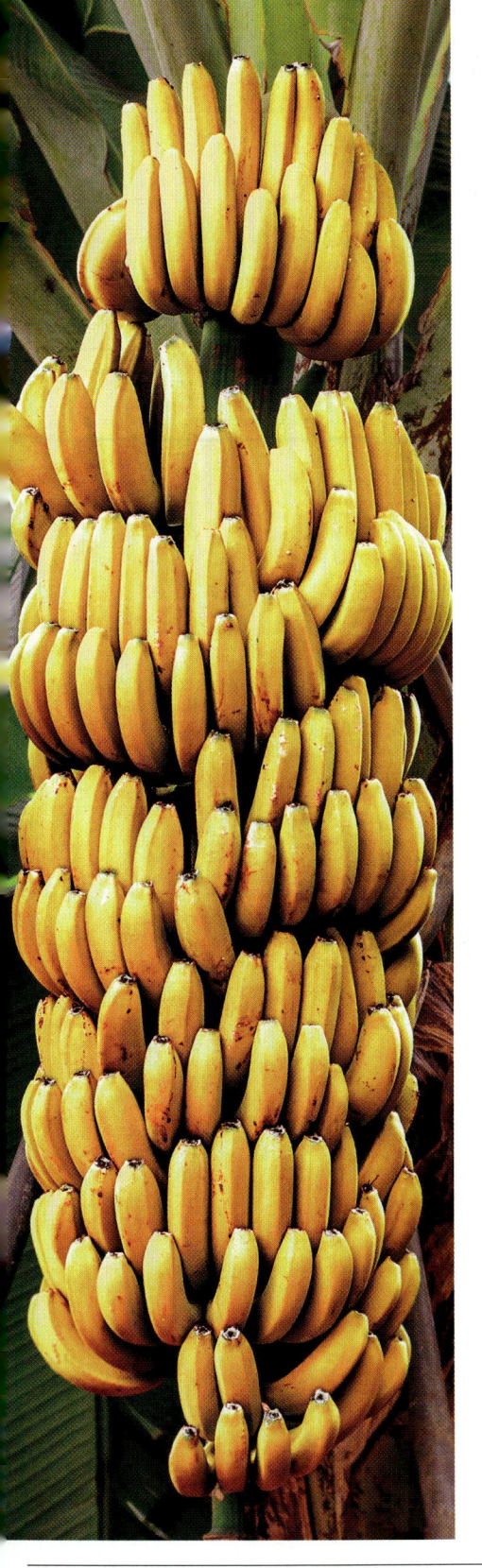

THE STORY OF A BANANA BABY
Tricia Thompson MS, RD

A former patient of Dr Sidney Haas shared her story with Tricia Thompson, founder of the Gluten Free Watchdog (www.glutenfreewatchdog.org) in 2008.

"I was born with coeliac 77 years ago. I was a year old, and my brother was three when it was discovered we both had celiac. I was told many years later that my brother had been close to death... My mother had to prepare a formula with bananas that took hours to complete. My parents would have to buy 'trees' of bananas because that is the way they were sold.

Every time a new food was added to our diet, Dr Haas had us take castor oil to clean out our stomach. This was terrible for me because my father had to chase me around the house.

By the time I was 12 years old, I was able to eat 'everything'. I was brought up to believe that sugars and starches were what a celiac was not able to digest. I was also told that I was 'cured'."

[The woman then went on to have two children, both of whom exhibited signs of Coeliac Disease. She put them on Dr Haas's diet, and they recovered, but the intestinal issues did not fully resolve.]

"I have always had problems with my stomach. Around the age of 30-something, I found that I could not eat lettuce or even fresh vegetables or fruits. Everything had to be cooked. When I reached 50, I became lactose intolerant.

From then until now, I've had periods of sudden upset stomachs (I thought for no reason), and it would take over a month-and-a-half to get better.

This past year I have had terrible pains of gas in my chest... After going through test after test at the cardiologist to test my heart and finding my heart very healthy, I discussed with my gastroenterologist about going on a celiac diet, which he agreed that I should do.

I only knew it to be a diet free of sugars and starches. I certainly have been shocked to find out, since Dr Haas was honoured worldwide by physicians, that the word 'starches' has been replaced by the word 'gluten'. For the past three months now, being on a gluten-free diet has certainly helped with all the terrible gas pains. I can now, suddenly, eat a moderate amount of fresh fruit and vegetables.

Thank goodness for all the research that was done in finally discovering that gluten was the 'culprit'. If Dr Haas was alive today, I would again give him a big hug for saving my brother, my children, and my life."

THE GLUTEN-FREE HANDBOOK

Celebrity Coeliacs

In the world of entertainment there are many high-profile people who have been diagnosed with the condition.

Caroline Quentin
UK actor

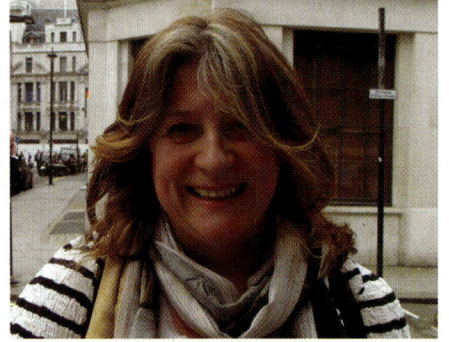

Eimaiegw CC BY-SA 4.0 via Wikimedia Commons

"I struggled for years with stomach pains, vomiting, bloating, headaches, and total exhaustion. But I didn't know they were symptoms of Coeliac Disease. I was really busy, and I honestly thought it was stress. I'd have a bowl of pasta or a slice of toast and soon afterwards I would be sick.

The good news is that once you're properly diagnosed, although there isn't a cure, you don't need medicine. All you have to do is avoid gluten and you won't have any issues. The earlier you are diagnosed the lower the risk of health problems."

Caroline wanted to get the message out to other people who might have her condition, and she is now an ambassador for Coeliac UK.

Katherine, Duchess of Kent
The duchess, who is now 92 years old and the oldest living member of the British Royal family, has had a long history of illness, being diagnosed with several disorders to explain her failing health, including chronic fatigue syndrome and Coeliac Disease, which could also account for her exhaustion as she was not properly absorbing food. When asked about her illness, she once simply said: "None of us goes through life unscathed."

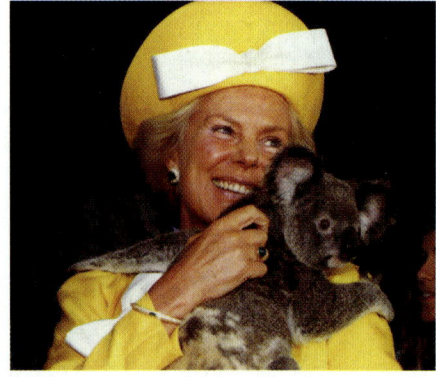

Queensland State Archives CC BY 3.0 AU via Wikimedia Commons

Zooey Deschanel
US actor and singer/songwriter Zooey has said she had been feeling unwell most of her adult life and guesstimates it was at least 13 years before she realised how sick she really was and got her Coeliac Disease diagnosis. Many of her symptoms she misinterpreted as irritable bowel syndrome, or the strains of a busy life. She now knows that she can't eat dairy, eggs, wheat, or gluten.

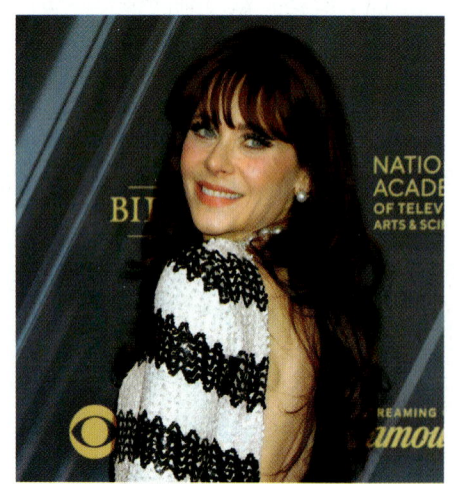

Hutchinsphoto/dreamstime.com

Bob Holness
Former television presenter on *Call My Bluff* and *Blockbusters*, who died in 2012

In 2002, after he suffered a stroke that left him temporarily paralysed down his left side, brain scans revealed he had suffered 'multiple minor strokes' or TIAs (transient ischaemic attacks) over the previous decade. Within nine months he was "amazingly better", said his wife, Mary.

"He was back doing voice-overs and public appearances for charities. He'd had trouble going downstairs, but this improved. Best of all, his speech became clear, and he began to sound like the old Bob."

However, about a year after the stroke, Bob went into an unexpected decline. He began falling over when out for a walk. He also fell downstairs carrying a tray of tea and scalded himself. Then in 2005, he was found to be anaemic and needed an emergency blood transfusion. The cause of the anaemia was not identified until a biopsy was taken of his gut. It revealed that he had Coeliac Disease.

Jennifer Esposito
US TV Actress from *NCIS* and *Blue Bloods*

The 51-year-old told *People* magazine she grew up seeing someone close to her struggle with illnesses, stress anxiety, panic disorder, bipolar disorder and more – all of which she believed was normal. So, when she began to experience panic attacks and stomach issues, she didn't raise it with anyone.

"I thought having panic disorder and having panic attacks all the time was normal," she said. "I thought my stomach being sick all the time was normal. I thought that sleeping all through lunch was normal. I thought highs, lows, and rage; I thought it was normal."

Esposito was often dealing with fatigue, hair loss, difficulty walking, vomiting, sinus infections and more. Her health continued to decline until she was in "really bad shape".

She saw a number of doctors to try to find solutions to her health

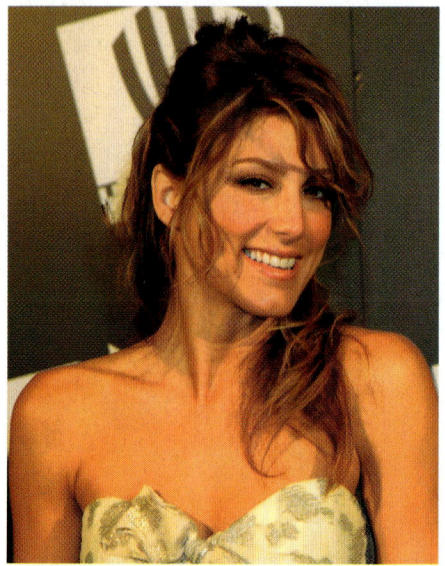

Carrienelson1/dreamstime.com

problems, but she didn't receive a diagnosis until her ear, nose and throat specialist recommended her to yet another doctor.

"I went to this woman. I told her everything. She said to me, 'I'm gonna test you for everything. I'm gonna get this, give me a few days.' She called me two days later and said, 'You have the worst case of Coeliac Disease I think I've ever seen. I don't know how you're alive.'

Esposito said that following her diagnosis she was able to stabilise her gut by cutting out gluten, dairy, soy, corn, sugar, and more from her diet. "I healed my gut," she said. "I don't have pain when I wake up. I don't feel like I'm passing out. My stomach doesn't hurt. I don't have panic attacks today."

Mari Wilson
Singer

"In the early 90s, I used to have two outfits for my show – one figure-hugging, the other twice as big and very loose. I never knew from one day to the next what shape I would be.

I could be bloated to the point where my stomach felt like a balloon when I prodded it, yet at other times it would be flat.

There were days when I felt so tired, weak, depressed and in pain that I would lie on the floor unable to move, wondering how I was going to get out of the house, never mind up on stage.

To make things worse, my hair became lank and started to fall out in clumps. I was constipated and, without realising it, was suffering from anaemia.

In 1993, I finally told my doctor about my symptoms. He suspected Coeliac Disease.

After my diagnosis I thought 'OK, now I know what it is I can deal with it and get fit again!'

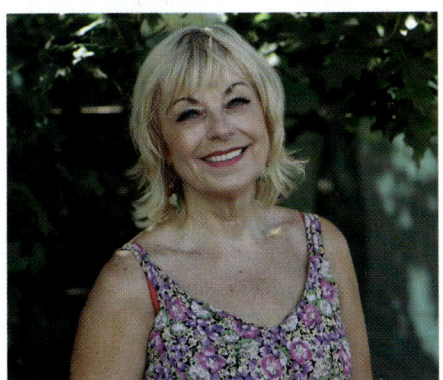

OTHER FAMOUS COELIACS

Lisa Snowden – TV and radio presenter and model

Peter Benenson – founder of Amnesty International and Coeliac UK

Cedric Benson – late Chicago Bears American footballer

Nick Hewer – presenter on *The Apprentice* and *Countdown*

Heidi Collins – CNN news reporter

Mandy Moore – singer/songwriter and actor

Josh Turner – country music star

Susie Essman – actor from *Curb Your Enthusiasm*

Megan McKenna – TV personality and *Celebrity Masterchef* finalist whose latest cookbook *Love Gluten Free* was published in March 2025

Finding out as much as possible about your condition allows you to be the boss – you control the disease; it doesn't run you."

Michael Obiora
UK actor from *Grange Hill*, *Hotel Babylon*, *Casualty*, *Robozuna* and, most recently, mini-series *Out There*

Michael finds if he eats anything with gluten in his energy levels drop. He says the diagnosis has made a big difference, despite the inconvenience of having to be disciplined about his diet.

"I love eating my food, so eating was always when I was at my happiest, but suddenly five minutes afterwards I would start feeling sluggish and bloated and tired, and I just thought something's wrong here."

Having been diagnosed he had to change a lot of things, and it has been a bit of an adjustment. "The most annoying thing is the cravings. The other day I had the biggest craving for pizza. And it kept me up at night. I said to myself the next day 'I am going to find pizza, whether I have to buy a gluten-free base and put on my own toppings, I need a pizza!'"

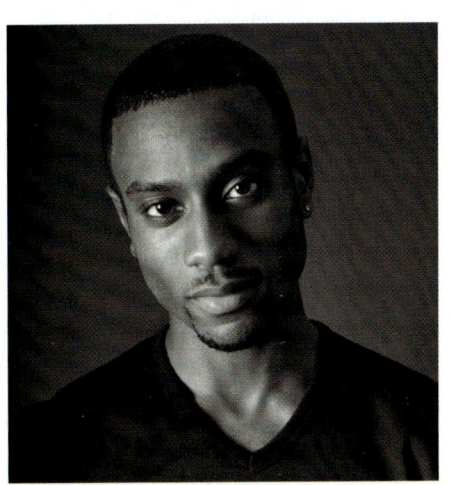

Jameela Jamil
UK actress and radio presenter

As a young child, I suffered all sorts of digestive problems and was constantly under the weather. The fatigue was so bad that I missed a lot of school days. If one of my friends had a birthday party, I would be first in line for a piece of cake. But within half an hour of eating it I would be bloated, suffering stomach cramps, and feeling sick.

Her worried parents took her to several doctors and Jameela underwent a battery of tests for everything from tonsillitis to anaemia. Finally, at the age of 12, the family was given a diagnosis of Coeliac Disease and told Jameela's diet would have to change forever. Avoiding gluten proved much more difficult than Jameela anticipated. "It's in so many foods," she has said. "Sometimes gluten is even added to chips, which is really annoying."

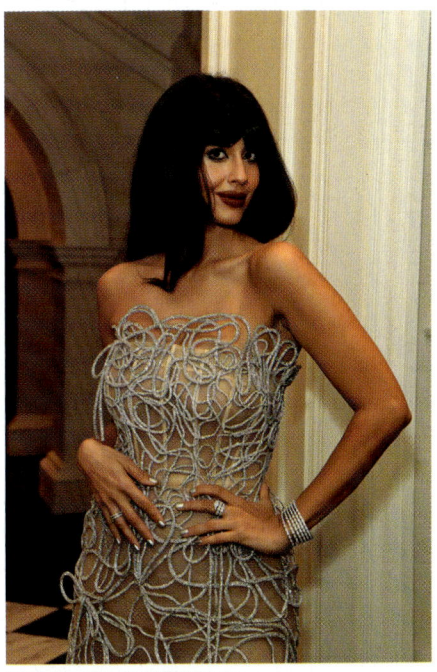

Coeliac Fact File

There are more than 200 symptoms that could indicate Coeliac Disease.

Any foodstuff that is labelled 'gluten-free' must not contain more gluten than 20 parts per million.

Coeliac Disease can develop at any age and to people of any race.

Children with Coeliac Disease are most likely to vomit, have loose bowel movements and refuse to eat.

Myth: Coeliac Disease is a food allergy.

Fact: Coeliac Disease is an autoimmune disorder, not a food allergy or intolerance.

Children can be slow to grow and develop a swollen pot belly.

Children can show signs of delayed development – sitting up, walking, talking, learning motor skills like holding a spoon or playing with toys, and interacting with others.

More children have Coeliac Disease than Crohn's, Ulcerative Colitis, and Cystic Fibrosis combined.

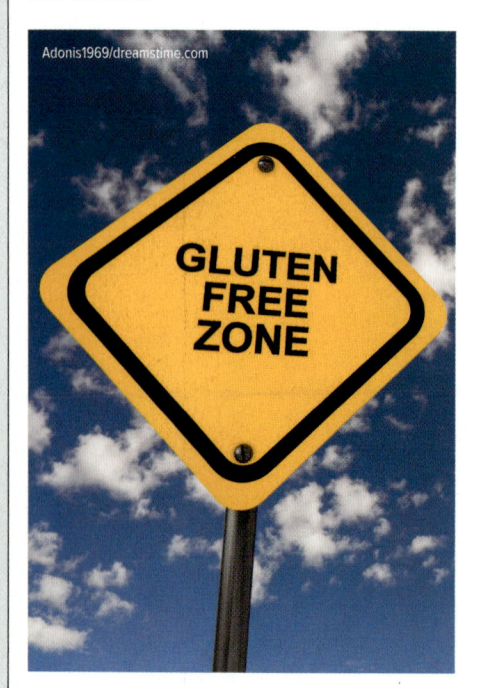

Infections, pregnancy and severe emotional or physical stress have been known to trigger the disease.

People with Coeliac Disease may also have a milk or fruit intolerance.

Coeliac Disease can cause miscarriage, infertility, thyroid problems, brittle bones, diabetes, and epilepsy.

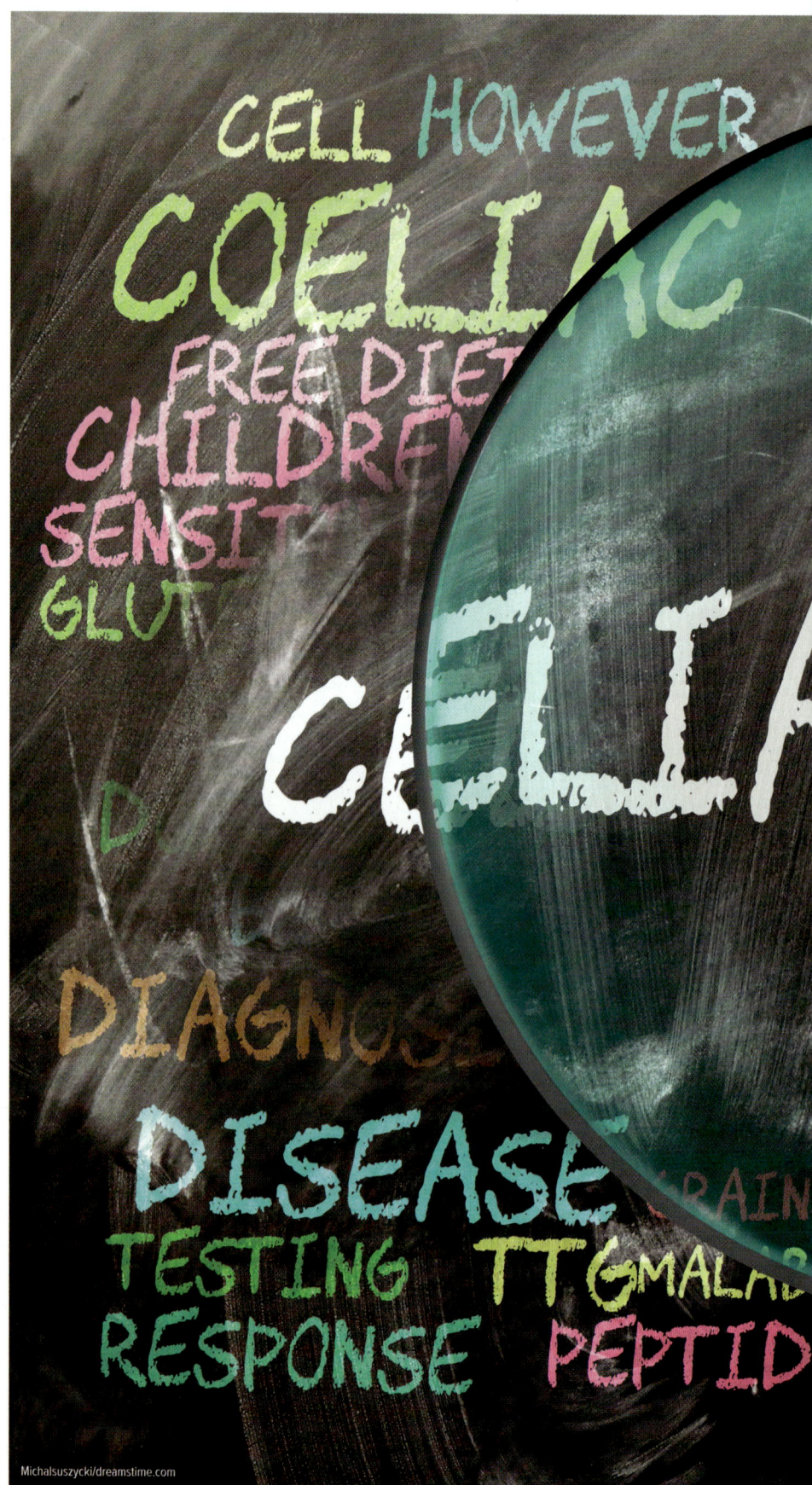

You cannot enlist for the Armed Forces if you have been diagnosed with Coeliac Disease.

Coeliac Disease, as well as all forms of gluten sensitivities and wheat allergies, should be listed under 'pre-existing conditions' when applying for travel insurance.

The global incidence of Coeliac Disease is rising, and this is thought to relate to environmental factors.

Undiagnosed Coeliac Disease costs a country's health service a lot of money. In a 2010 study in the United States, it was estimated that that amounted to an average $3,964 a year more than a normally healthy person.

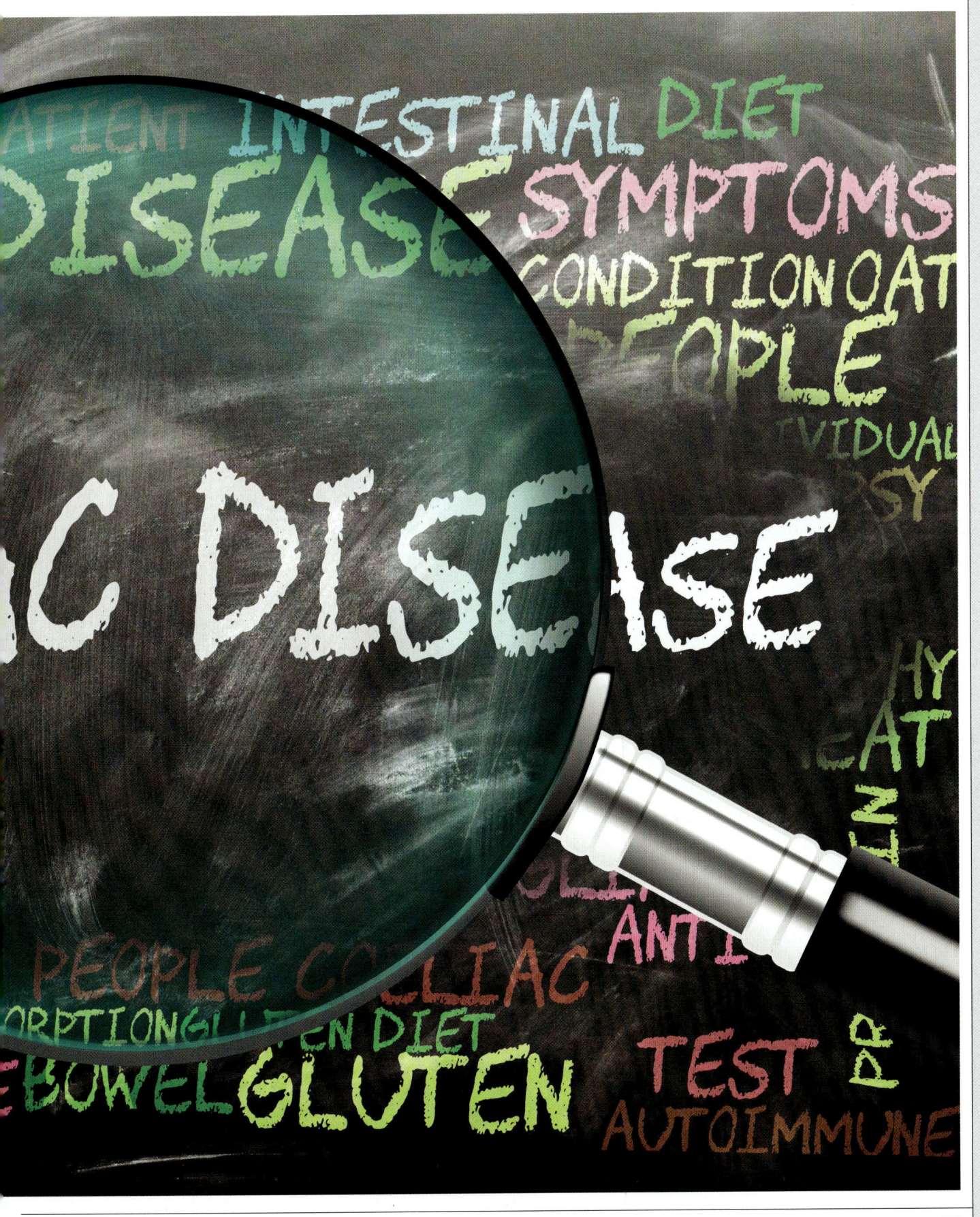

Non-coeliac Gluten Sensitivity

Although they do not test positive for Coeliac Disease, many people suffer similar symptoms that can be attributed to eating gluten.

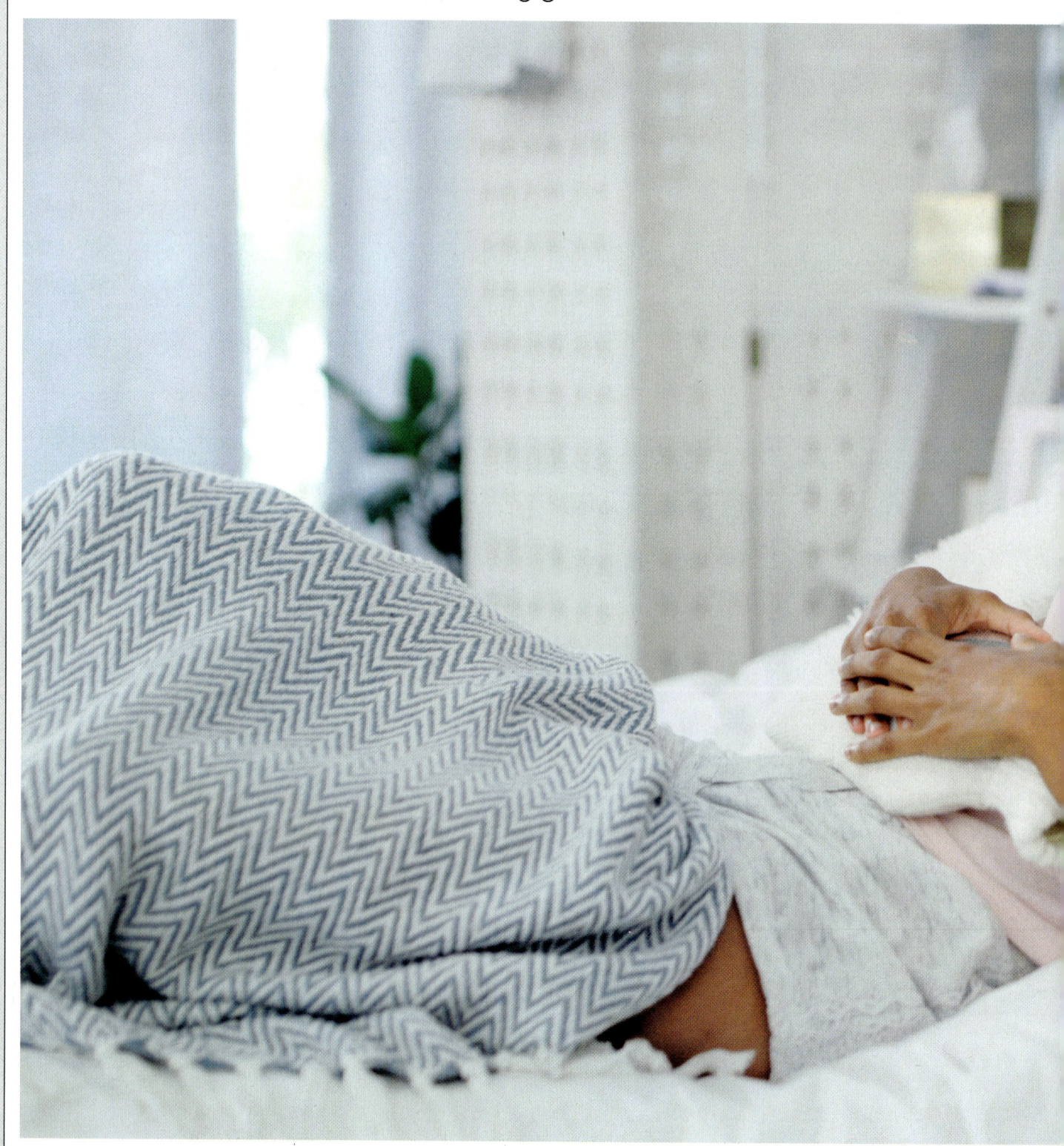

NON-COELIAC GLUTEN SENSITIVITY

Gluten is blamed by between 20% and 45% of people who find they are hypersensitive to something they eat. However, the term Non-coeliac Gluten Sensitivity (NCGS) has only as recently as 2012 been accepted as a condition in its own right.

It was also thought to be a condition only affecting adults but recent studies in New Zealand have directed suspicions at NCGS being a cause in school children who were found to be irritable, bad tempered and have development issues, as well as suffering with bouts of diarrhoea and having a low weight compared to their peers.

NCGS is different to irritable bowel syndrome (IBS), which also manifests itself as bloating, tummy pain, diarrhoea, and wind. NCGS patients exhibit all of the above, plus fatigue, headache, joint and muscle pain, numbness in the limbs, rashes, anaemia, and depression. In fact, these non-digestive tract symptoms are often more apparent in NCGS patients than problems with their abdomens.

Symptoms appear not long after food containing gluten is consumed and last for hours, or they can arrive a day or more later and take a few days to clear up after gluten has been excluded from the diet.

Also, NCGS is mainly only triggered by gluten, unlike IBS that can be activated by a range of foodstuffs. And it differs from Coeliac Disease in that the small intestine is not damaged and so the long-term good health of the individual is not threatened. The short-term effects, though, are highly unpleasant and debilitating and can affect mental health.

How can you tell if it's IBS or NCGS?

Irritable bowel syndrome and Non-Coeliac Gluten Sensitivity affect different parts of the digestive system. Whereas NCGS causes problems in the small intestine, or upper bowel, just below the stomach, an IBS reaction occurs in the colon, or large intestine, which is the final part of the digestive tract before waste is expelled.

Doctors are uncertain about exactly what causes IBS, but they consider various factors other than just food contribute, whereas NCGS is almost certainly food related. These other factors in IBS have been identified as a function of the digestive system passing food through too slowly or too quickly, oversensitive nerves in the gut, emotional stress, bacterial or parasitic infections, and some medications. IBS also includes inflammatory bowel diseases such as Crohn's and Ulcerative Colitis, which can be genetic and/or related to a faulty immune system.

Another point of differentiation is that NCGS always presents itself after eating suspect food, whereas IBS can come and go.

What is certain is that both conditions are difficult to diagnose and there are no tried and tested methods to ascertain either of the issues. So, an early consultation with your doctor is advised to begin the process to eliminate causes so that treatment can begin.

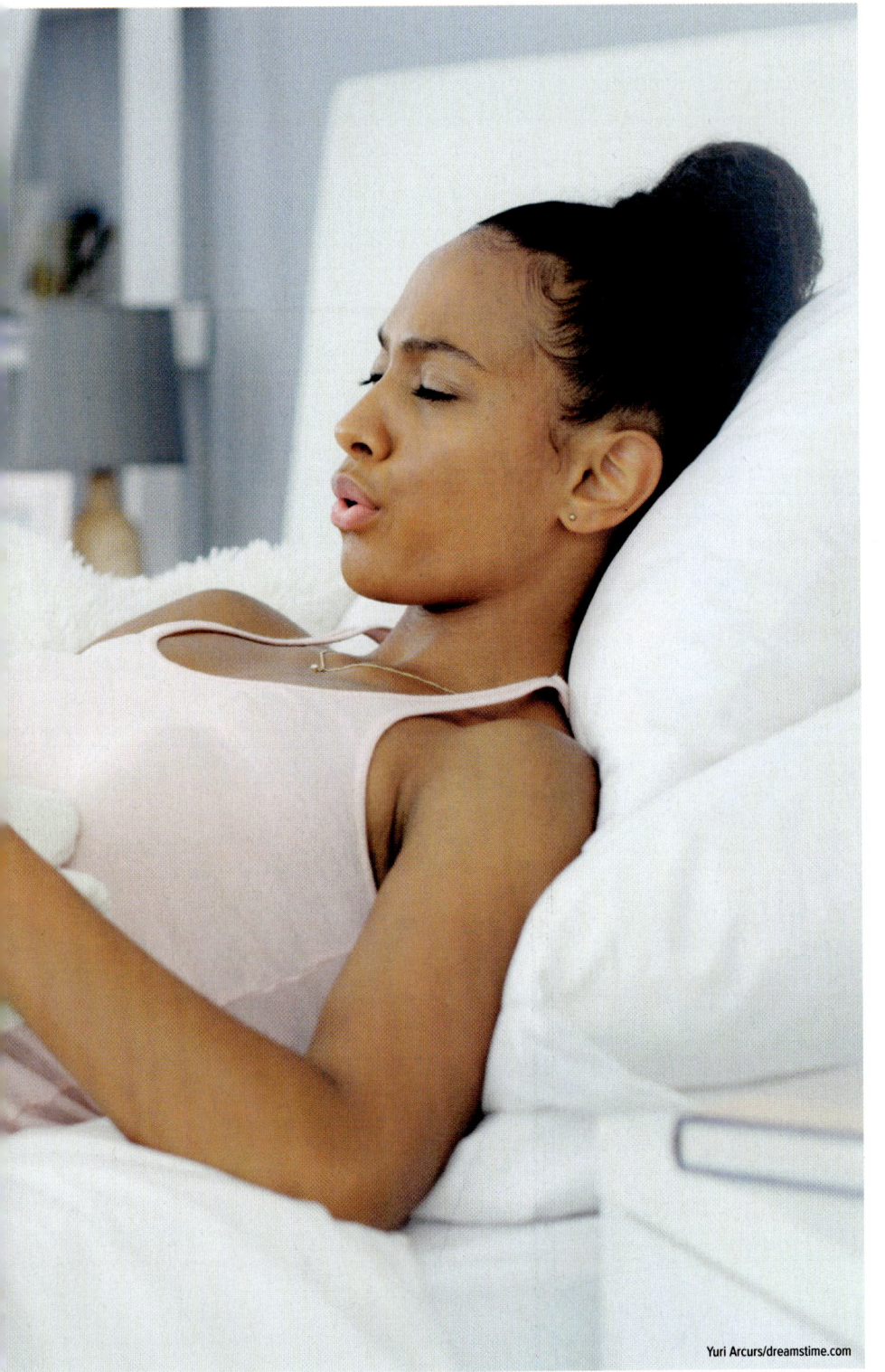

Yuri Arcurs/dreamstime.com

NON-COELIAC GLUTEN SENSITIVITY

Diagnosing Non-Coeliac Gluten Sensitivity

Since the symptoms of NCGS can closely resemble those of Coeliac Disease, it is important to exclude CD as a cause. The first step is blood tests to make sure the particular antibodies that characterise Coeliac Disease are not present. The patient needs to consume a gluten-containing diet for six weeks prior to the test. In a few cases, a small intestine biopsy will be needed to confirm that there is no damage and therefore it is unlikely to be Coeliac Disease.

The next step would be to try what's called a 'gluten challenge'. Researchers in the field of

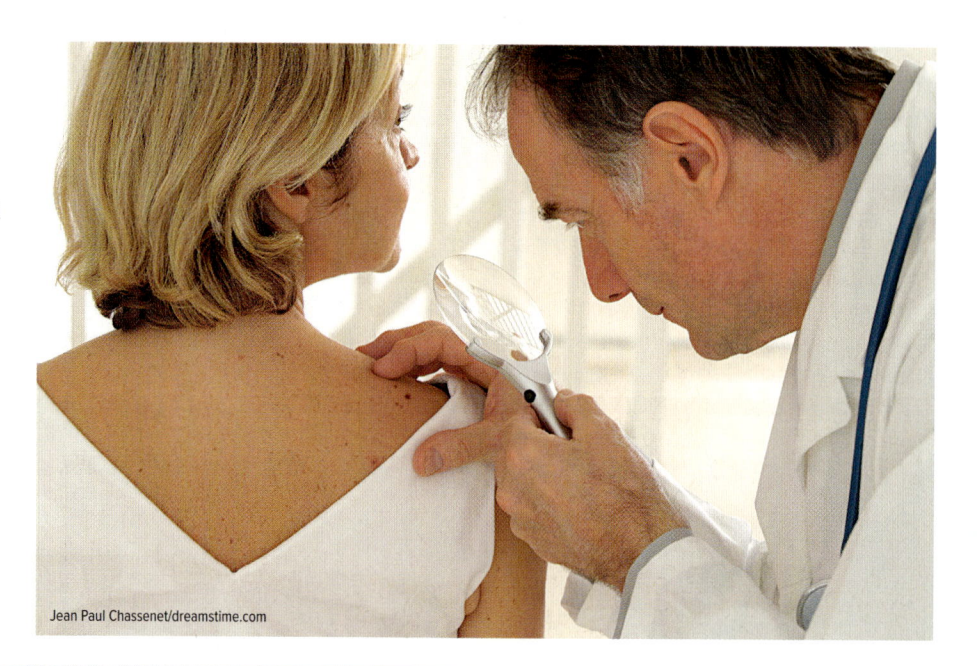

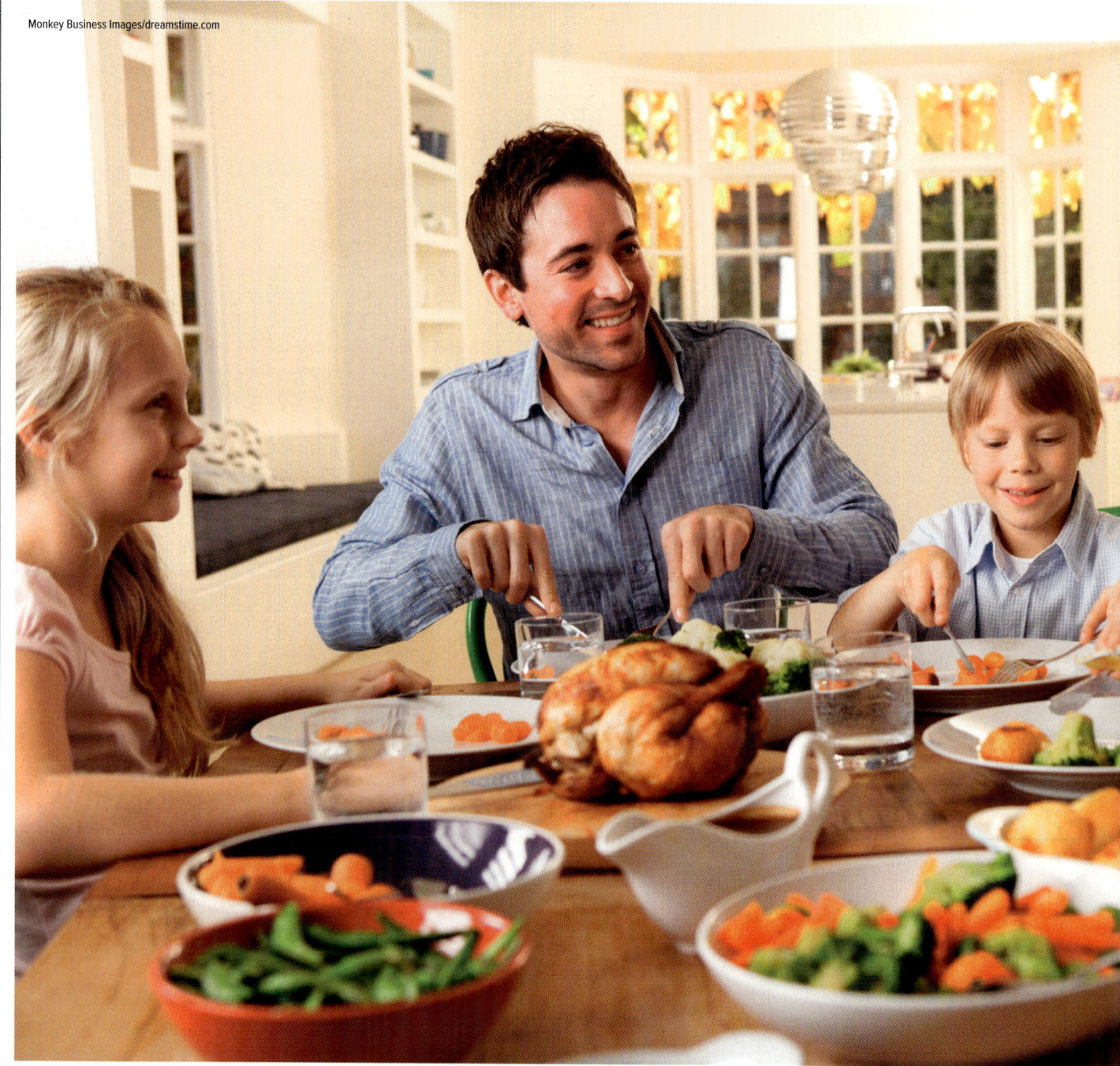

Jean Paul Chassenet/dreamstime.com

Monkey Business Images/dreamstime.com

gluten-related disorders at the 3rd International Expert Meeting on Non-Celiac Gluten Sensitivity in Italy in October 2014 set up guidelines that recommend a six-week challenge in which the patient eats 10 grams of gluten per day. The scientists agreed that in the absence of specific biomarkers, close monitoring of the patient while they eliminate and then reintroduce this small quantity of gluten foods in their diet is the best way of diagnosing NCGS.

Trial and error
The guidelines state that to do the challenge the patient has to identify between one and three common symptoms they experience and rate the severity of each on a scale of 1-10. This assessment should be carried out two weeks before starting the largely gluten-free diet, and then they should do the rating again every week thereafter.

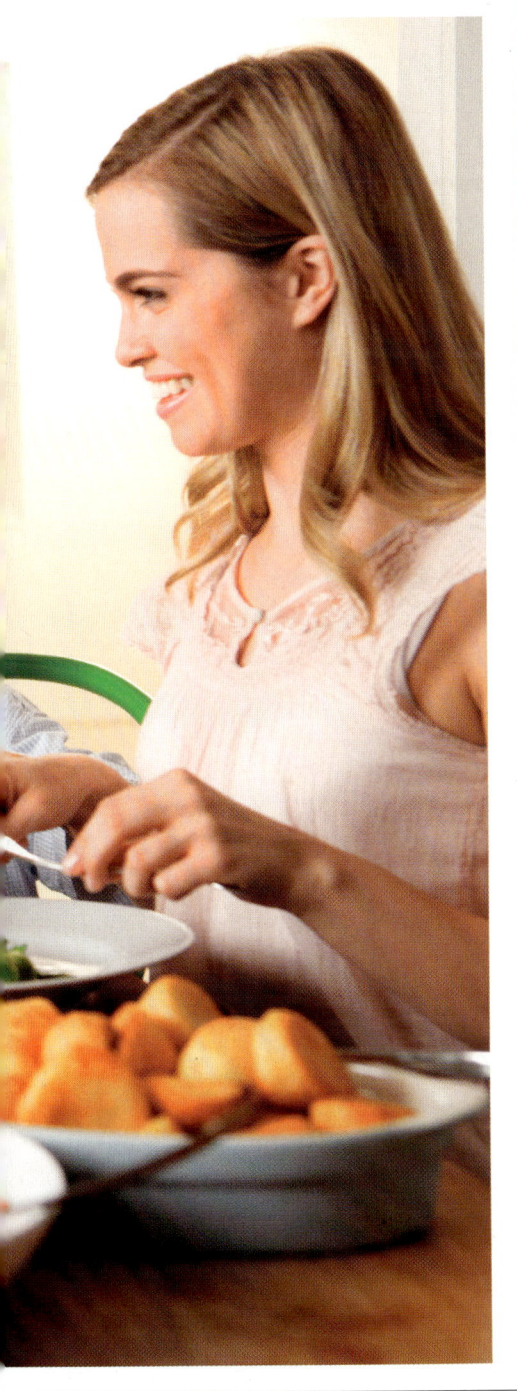

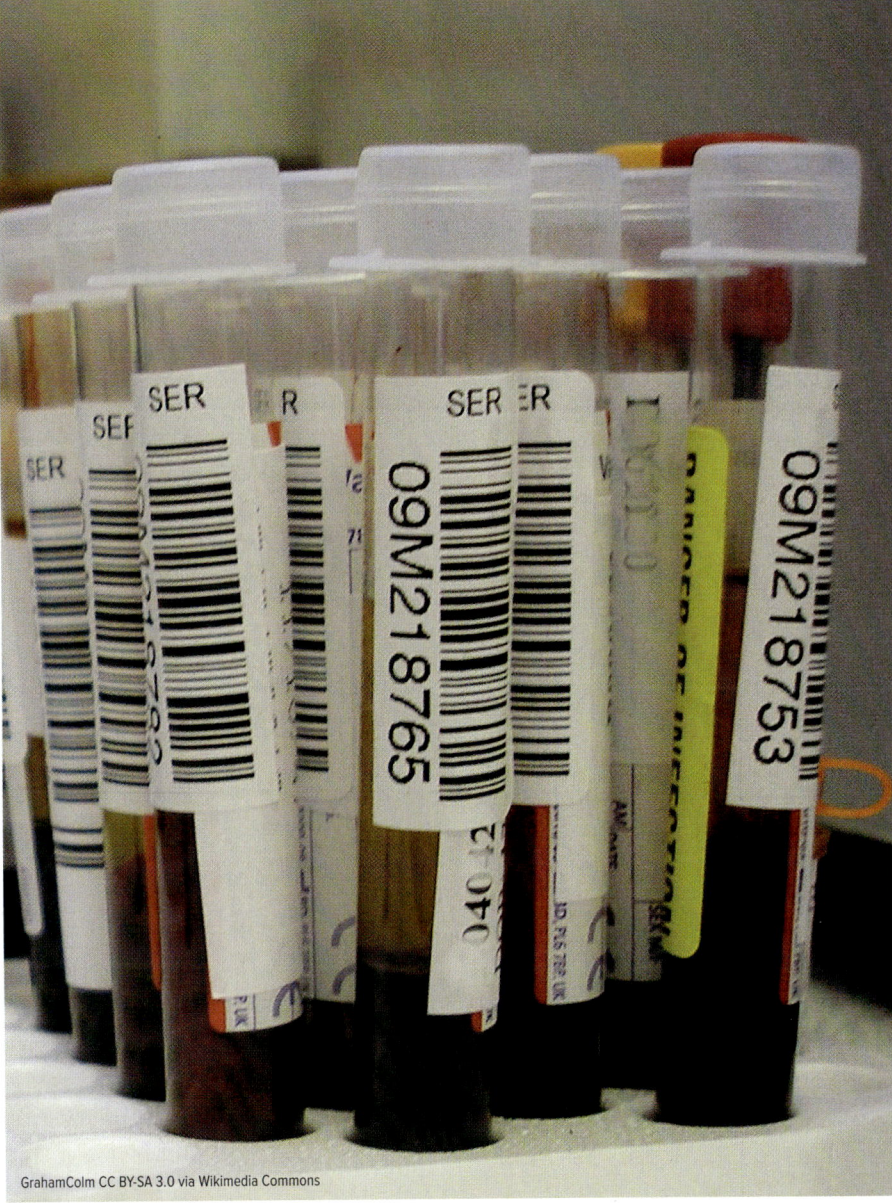

A good response is considered to be when the patient notices at least a 30% improvement in at least one of their three symptoms along with no deterioration in any of them. This improvement should be achieved for a minimum of at least three of the six weekly reviews.

As with testing for food allergies, a repeat of the challenge may be necessary for a definitive diagnosis of NCGS. After four weeks of being on a strictly gluten-free diet, patients should again take in 10 grams of gluten. If any of the symptoms recur within two days, they should go back on their gluten-free diet.

However, scientists later realised that some patients with NCGS might not be able to tolerate even that small amount of gluten, and recent evidence suggests that shorter challenges of two-weeks duration eating just three grams of gluten might work just as well to confirm diagnosis in a majority of cases.

On a completely gluten-free diet, the symptoms of patients with NCGS tend to improve or disappear within 14 days. Curiously, people suspected of having NCGS often do not test positive for a wheat allergy if they have a skin-prick test – see the chapter on Wheat Allergy on page 46 for more information on this. Another curious fact is that NCGS occurs more often in women than men.

NON-COELIAC GLUTEN SENSITIVITY

So NCGS is confirmed – what happens next?

If excluding gluten works to alleviate symptoms, then being gluten-free for life is the only way to stay symptom-free. A person with NCGS should, however, also have a conversation with a health expert/nutritionist about adopting a low FODMAP diet.

Those letters stand for a collection of short-chain carbohydrates – fermentable oligosaccharides, disaccharides, monosaccharides, and polyols. They are often the culprit in irritable bowel syndrome and are found in many of the same grains as the gluten protein but also in milk, kidney beans and baked beans, lentils, some nuts, cottage cheese, ice cream, yogurt, apples, pears, onions, garlic, cauliflower, mushrooms, sugar snaps, asparagus, honey, prunes, and some other sweet foodstuffs using fructose. This is not an exhaustive list as not all branded products have had their FODMAP content measured, so a nutritionist's advice is important as the subject is complicated.

But before anyone despairs of living a life on potatoes and nothing else, it has to be said that FODMAPs do not occur in pure protein food – i.e., fresh meat, fish, shellfish, and poultry – and are low in lots of other delicious fruits, vegetables and many nuts and cheeses, plus refined sugar, and sweeteners. And, of course, the full range of gluten-free products is safe.

In addition, a person may not necessarily be allergic to all of the short-chain carbohydrates so over time, and after trial and error, it is possible as well as highly desirable for good health, to refine your diet to include whichever FODMAP foods do not particularly affect you.

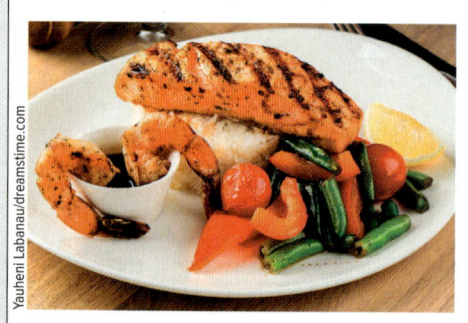

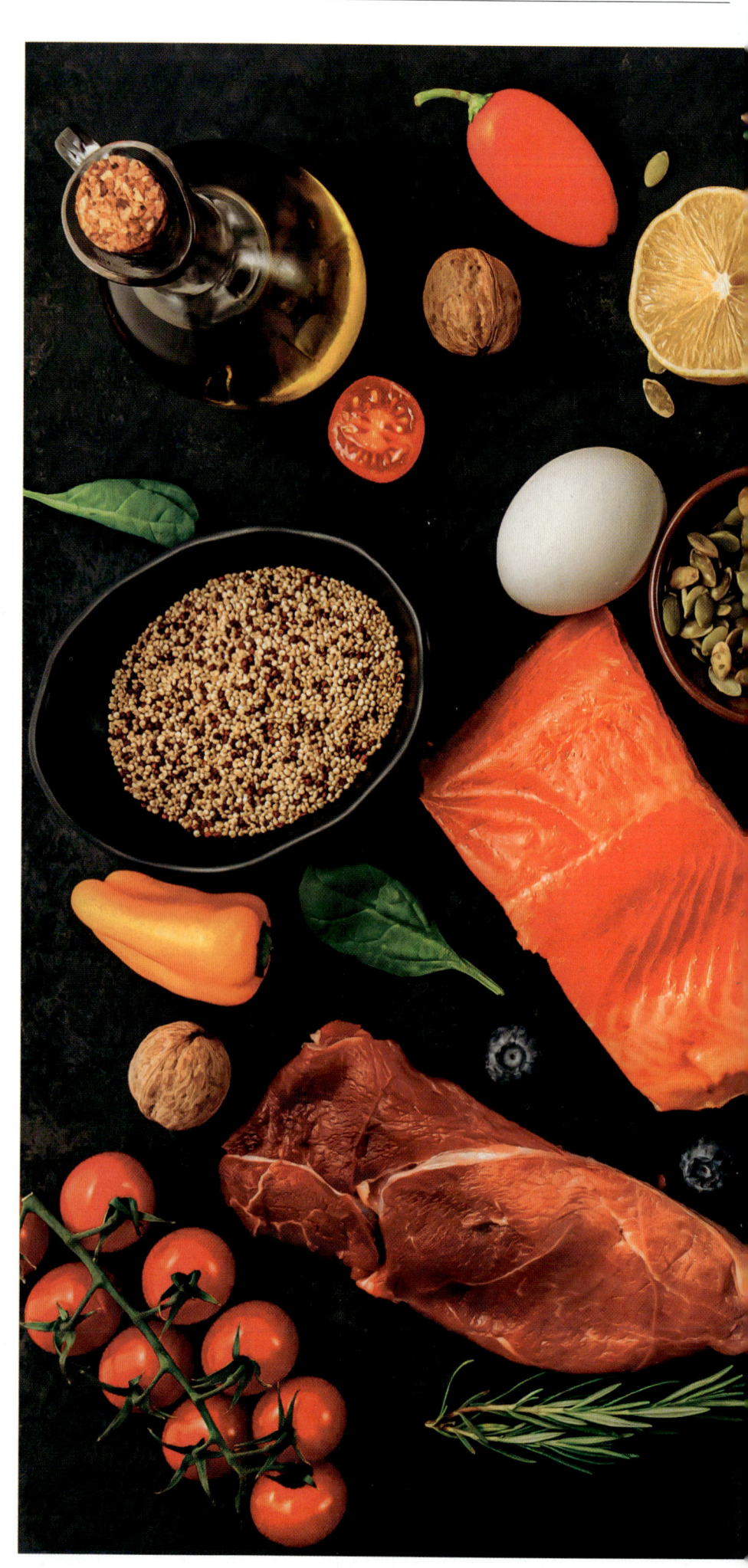

NON-COELIAC GLUTEN SENSITIVITY

LOW-FODMAP
GROCERY LIST

Colorful Vegetables
- Artichoke Hearts, Canned
- Baby Corn, Canned
- Bamboo Shoots, Canned/Fresh
- Bean Sprouts
- Beetroot, Canned/Pickled
- Cabbage, Red
- Carrots
- Celeriac
- Jicama
- Lettuce (Radicchio, Red Coral)
- Mushrooms, Canned or Oyster
- Olives, Green and Black
- Parsnip
- Radish
- Red bell Pepper
- Spinach
- Sweet Potato
- Tomatoes
- Turnip
- Water Chestnuts

Dairy
- Cheese (Manchego, Monterey Jack, Queso Fresco, Brie, Camembert, Cheddar, Colby, Feta, Goat, Havarti, Mozzarella, Pecorino, Swiss)
- Cream Cheese
- Sour Cream
- Grain/Noodles/Etc.
- Chickpea Noodle Pasta
- Gluten Free Pasta
- Polenta
- Quinoa (Black, Red, and White)
- Rice (Basmati, Brown, Glutinous, Red, White)
- Rice Noodles

Nuts
- Brazil
- Chestnuts
- Macadamias
- Peanuts
- Tiger nuts
- Pecans
- Pine nuts
- Walnuts

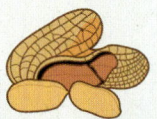

Protein via Meat, Fish, Eggs & Tofu
- Beef
- Bison
- Chicken
- Cod
- Lamb
- Pork
- Salmon
- Shrimp
- Tofu, plain and firm
- Tuna
- Turkey

Fruits
- Coconut, Shredded, Dried
- Dragon fruit
- Grapes (Red, Green, and Black)
- Lemon Juice
- Lime Juice
- Pineapple
- Rasberries
- Strawberries

Greens
- Alfalfa
- Arugula
- Bak choy
- Broccoli, Heads only/whole
- Broccolini, Stalks
- Cabbage, Comman
- Collard Greens
- Cucumber
- Edamame
- Green Beans
- Green Onion, Top
- Kale
- Lettuce (Romaine, Butter, Iceberg)
- Seaweed (Nori)
- Spinach, Baby and English
- Swiss chard
- watercress

Spices & Herbs
- Basil
- Cilantro
- Cinnamon
- Cumin
- Dill
- Ginger
- Lemon Grass
- Mint
- Oregano
- Paprika
- Parsley
- Rosemary
- Saffron
- Sage
- Tarragon
- Thyme
- Turmeric

Salad Dressing/Sauce/ Oils/Condiments
- Apple Cider Vinegar
- Avocado Oil
- Coconut Oil
- Miso Paste
- Mustard
- Olive Oil
- Red Wine Vinegar
- Rice Wine vinegar
- Sesame Oil
- Walnut Oil

Miscellaneous
- Capers
- Fish Sauce
- Kelp Noodles
- Nutritional Yeast Flakes

Seeds
- Hemp Seeds
- Pumpkin Seeds
- Sesame Seeds
- Sunflower Seeds

©ThriveClique

This and a range of useful dietary charts can be found at www.etsy.com/shop/thriveclique.

Yuliya Mikhaylova/dreamstime.com

THE GLUTEN-FREE HANDBOOK

Celebrities who cannot eat gluten

Although not diagnosed as Coeliac, these famous faces nonetheless suffer from the effects of gluten in their diets.

Billy Bob Thornton
US actor from *Fargo*

Thornton once claimed bananas are his only sweet indulgence. "I'm vegan and eat extremely healthy," he told *People* magazine. "For me, something indulgent would be to cut two bananas into my gluten-free oatmeal instead of one. I don't eat junk at all."

However, the 69-year-old actor admitted he sometimes wished he could enjoy a wider variety of food rather than having no option but to follow a strict diet. "I wish I could have that stuff, but I'm allergic to wheat and dairy." So, because of these allergies he said he leads an "extremely healthy" lifestyle and has been forced to cut out numerous different foods from his diet.

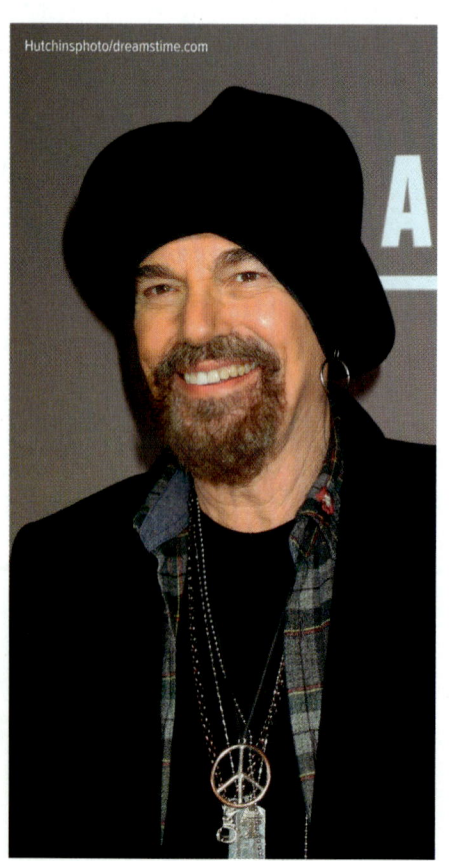

Bill and Chelsea Clinton
Former US President and his daughter

It has been rumoured that Bill Clinton is a late-diagnosed NCGS, but he has only confirmed that he follows a strict plant-based diet. His daughter, though, is on record as not being able to eat wheat products. Chelsea's upstate wedding to Marc Mezvinsky in 2010 featured a vegan menu and a gluten-free wedding cake. She chose her menu based on both personal preferences and health needs. She has been vegan since her teen years and has a gluten allergy. The head of the New York City catering firm that arranged her wedding breakfast said at the time: "This will empower people to make these requests [for gluten-free]. Prior to this, they might have thought it was not mainstream enough to even talk about, but now that they see it being done by such a public persona it becomes acceptable."

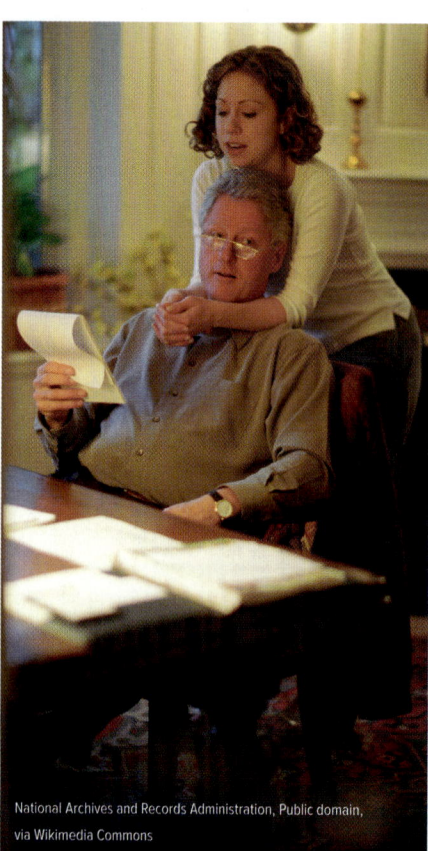

Miley Cyrus
US singer, songwriter, and actress

Faced with claims that she was too thin, Miley Cyrus took to Twitter in 2012 to say she wasn't anorexic but had a gluten allergy. The then 19-year-old star said she switched to a gluten-free diet for health reasons. "For everyone calling me anorexic, I have a gluten and lactose allergy. It's not about weight, it's about health." She followed up with another tweet saying everyone should try to go gluten-free for a week, saying: "The change in your skin, physical and mental health is amazing! U won' go back!"

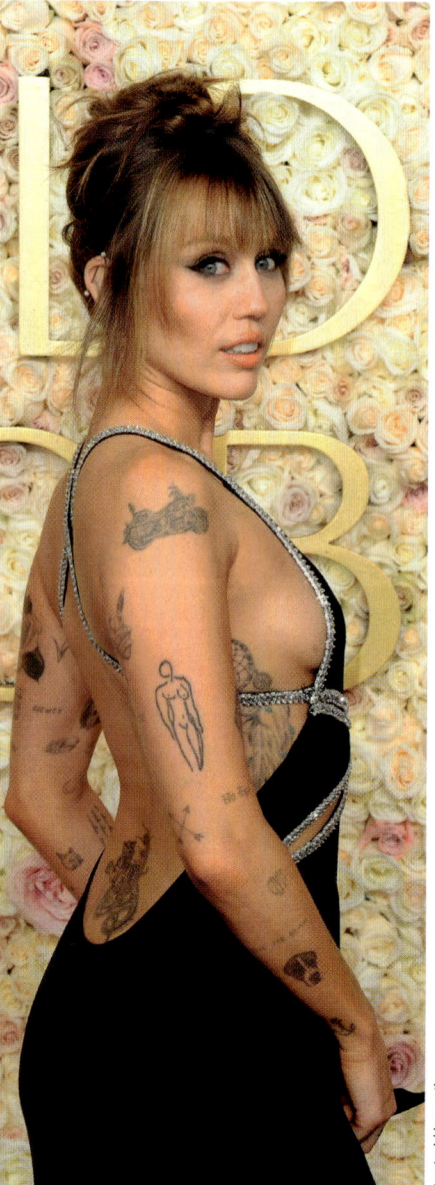

Novak Djokovic
Tennis champion

Prior to the Australian Open Men's Quarter Final in 2010 against Jo-Wilfried Tsonga, Djokovic found that he was struggling with breathing difficulties. "I had an inability to cope with the heat, endurance issues, even though I was training hard."

Then during the match things got much worse as he described in a film interview for the *Food Matters* website (www.foodmatters.com). "I was feeling weaker and then all of a sudden, the vision became different. I couldn't catch breath after each point was finished. I remember between the fourth and fifth set I went out to throw up, and felt my stomach was aching. I came from a culture where food is based a lot on gluten and so I would have different breads each day. Even eating pizza, I would have a little bread on the side, that's how integrated that kind of culture of eating was in our region. I didn't know that all of these things would cause that kind of feeling of being helpless on the court and feeling of being powerless."

Then he met fellow Serbian Dr Igor Cetojevic, who contacted him having watched the Australian Open match. He conducted a curious test: he applied pressure to Djokovic's racquet arm both before and after he asked him to hold a bread loaf in his left hand. When he was holding the bread his playing arm became noticeably weaker. This led to blood tests.

"He received the data that I have a great sensitivity to gluten, to dairy products and refined sugar," said Djokovic. "I had to sit down and rethink what is going on." After refining his diet, Djokovic was back on his winning streak.

Ryan Phillippe
US actor, most recently seen in *Saint Clare* and *Prey*

When doctors told him he has trouble digesting wheat, Phillippe had a choice: modify his diet and ditch things he loves (like beer on football Sundays) or eat the same foods as before and deal with the consequences. As he told *Men's Health* magazine, he has broken down and had the occasional Sunday brew, but it doesn't go down well. So now he knows; you eat badly, you suffer. He's recognised that he can make a situation better by taking a different route, by controlling what he can. "Can't eat wheat? Learn to cook and thrive within your restrictions, just like a guy on a belly-flattening diet." And he sees the example he's setting for his children. Instead of buying easy takeout dinners, he makes homecooked meals.

"There's something about the kids knowing the parent is making the food for them with love," he said. "It's worth it to me to do that extra work whenever possible because I see the benefit it has. My kids think I'm an amazing cook, and that's all that matters."

Other Gluten-free Followers

Terence Stamp – UK actor and author of *The Stamp Collection Cookbook*

Victoria Beckham – model and former Spice Girl

Jessica Simpson – US singer, actor, and fashion designer

Drew Brees – American former football quarterback for the New Orleans Saints

Rachel Weisz – UK TV and film actor

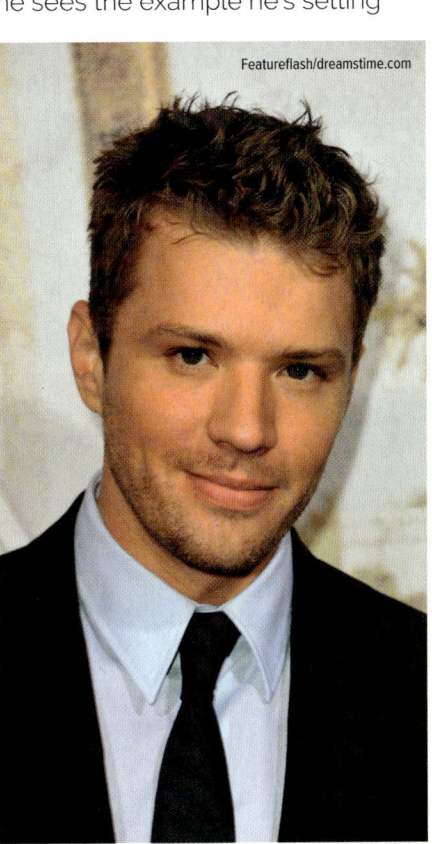

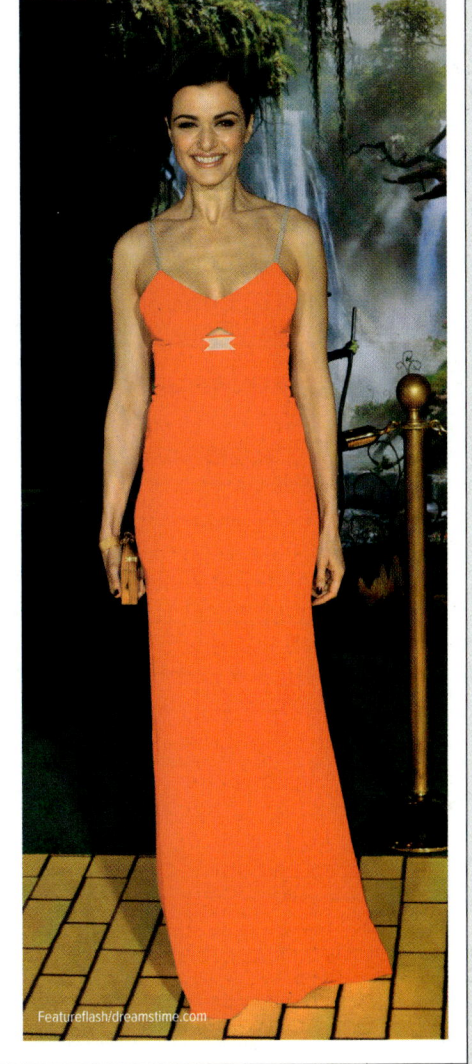

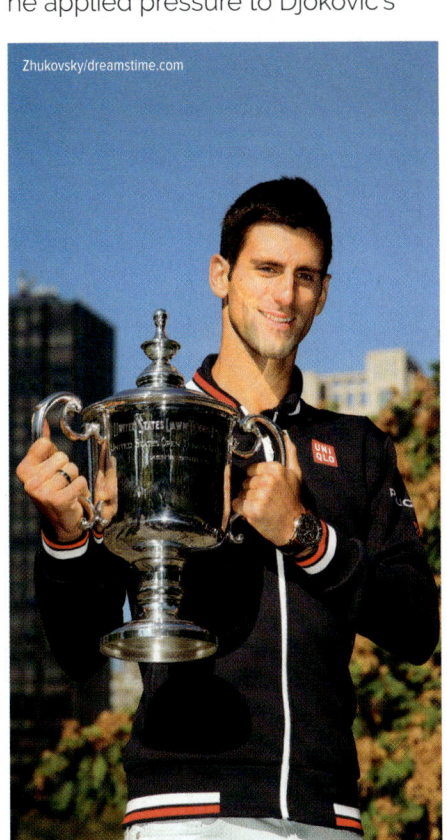

WHEAT ALLERGY

Wheat allergy

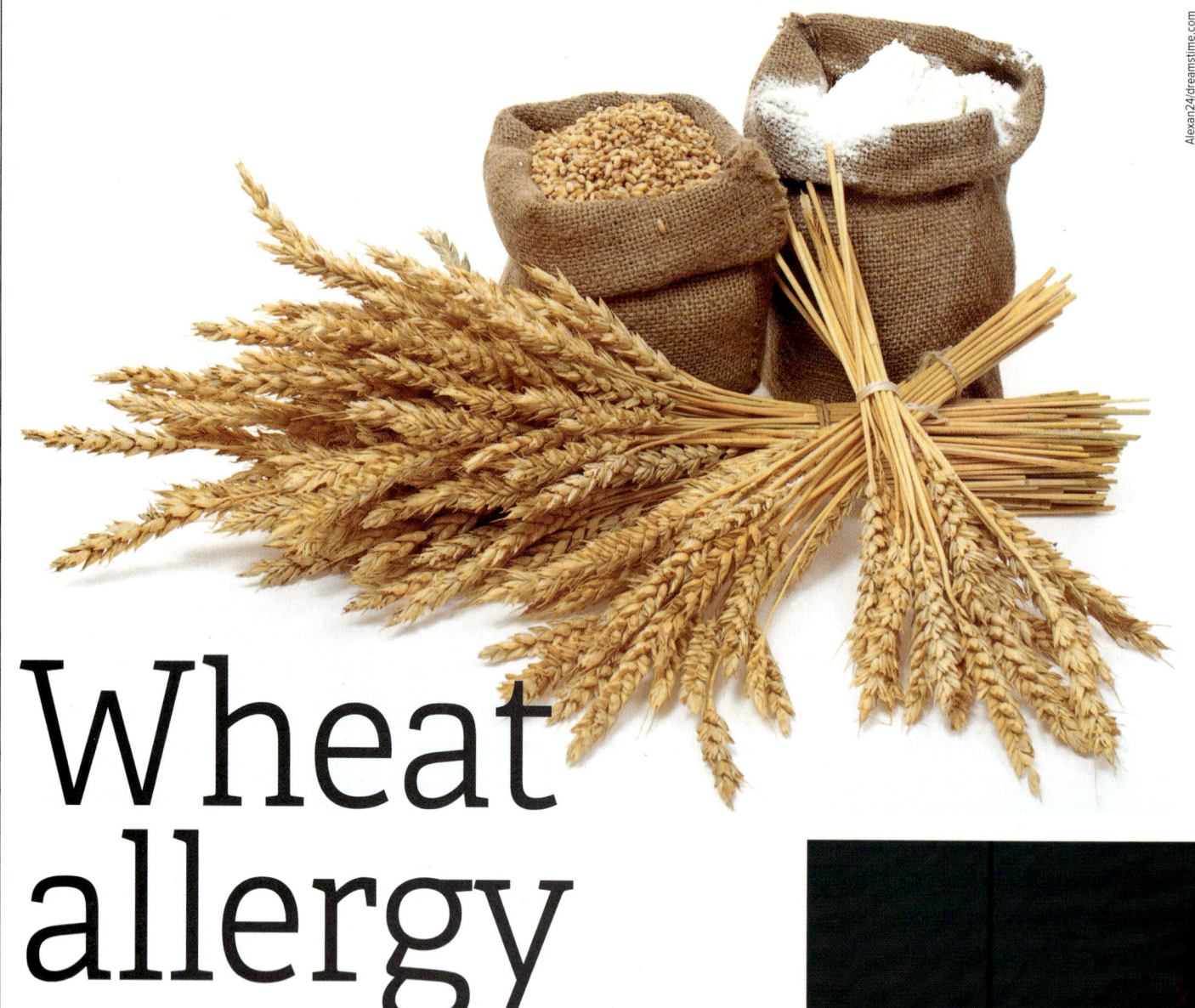

Like Coeliac Disease, this condition has a single trigger – wheat protein – but unlike Coeliac Disease it is not only experienced when eating wheat.

A food allergy is when your body's immune system reacts negatively to a specific protein in a food. In the case of a wheat allergy, that is not necessarily just to the gluten content of wheat, as you get with Coeliac Disease and Non-Coeliac Gluten Sensitivity, but to one or more of the other proteins present in the grain as well.

There are four types of protein to which you can react. And, like a nut allergy, minute particles from wheat can be present in the air and can enter the body via the lungs or skin.

The body's immune system regards these wheat proteins as it would an invading bacteria or virus and swings into action to safeguard internal systems and force out the irritant. These reactions can be mild and slightly uncomfortable, or they can be as severe as to restrict breathing and lead to death.

Wheat allergies are experienced by all ages and in all parts of the world. Up to 1.3% of the world's population has some form of intolerance to wheat products. That's approximately 104 million people. In the US just under one-and-a-half million children are affected by the condition.

What are the symptoms?
Some of these are similar to Coeliac Disease and NCGS, but there are

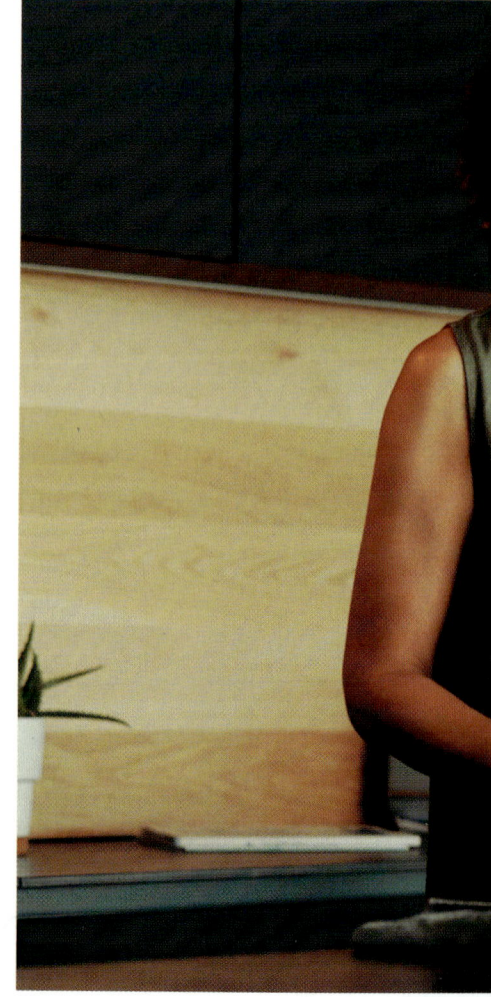

additional signs that point to wheat in particular being the problem.

- Nausea
- Vomiting
- Indigestion
- Stomach cramps
- Diarrhoea
- Bloating
- Flatulence
- Mouth ulcers
- Sore throat
- Hives
- Rashes
- Blocked nose
- Irritated eyes
- Breathing difficulties
- Feeling of dread

Not everyone will experience all of these unpleasant symptoms, and they will vary in severity from person to person. On the plus side, there is no damage to the small intestine so even if the allergy has not been properly diagnosed and has been affecting a person over a long period of time, there should be no lasting effects once wheat has been excluded from the diet.

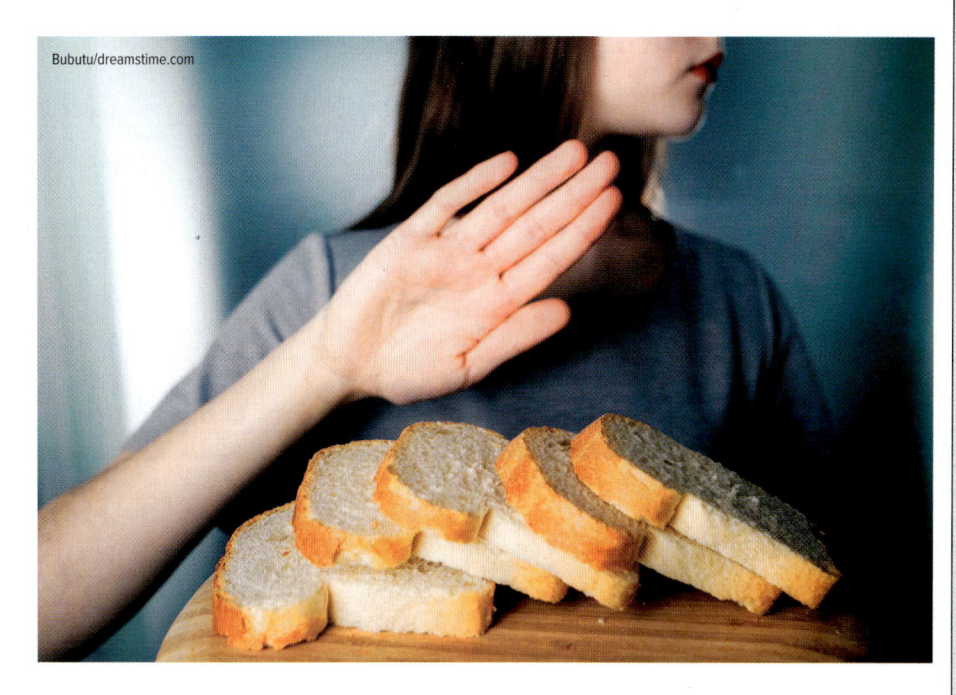

The one symptom to be most wary of is if a person has swelling in the throat and is experiencing breathing difficulties, increased heart rate, tight chest and trouble swallowing.

In that case a call to emergency services and a swift trip to hospital is essential. This reaction is known as anaphylaxis, and it occurs when the immune system releases a flood of chemicals in response to an allergen and that puts the body into shock. This effect seriously lowers the blood pressure and causes the tissues of the lungs and throat to narrow, affecting the ability to breathe.

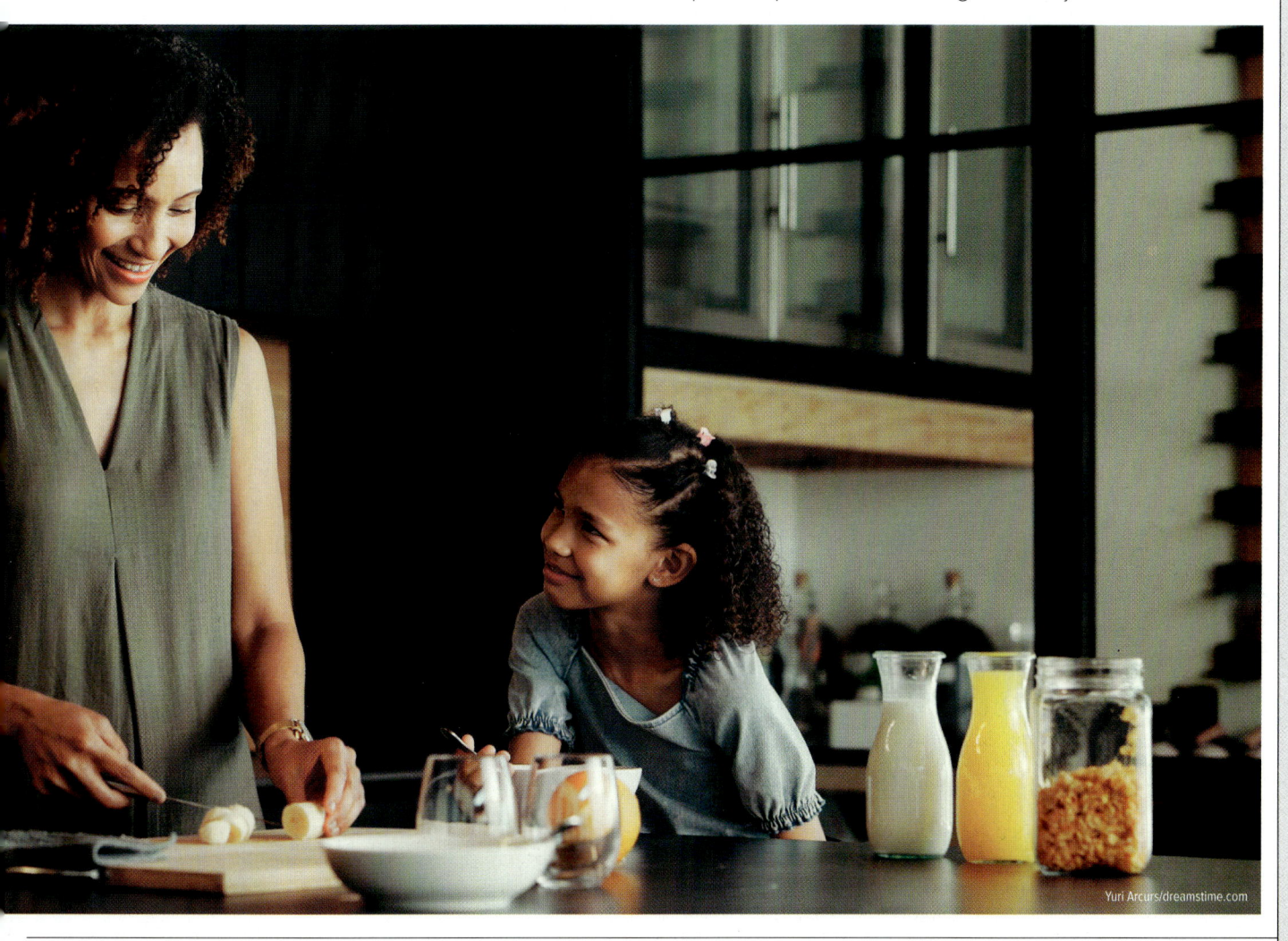

WHEAT ALLERGY

How do you find out if it's a wheat allergy?

With a wheat allergy your body can react in two different ways. Either it creates a substance called Immunoglobin E, which kicks in very quickly – a few minutes to four hours after wheat protein has been eaten or inhaled – or it causes white blood cells to collect and set up an inflammation in your oesophagus between your mouth and your stomach, or in the stomach itself. In the latter case it can take a day or two to be felt after wheat has been encountered.

An allergy specialist can conduct a variety of tests to discover if you have a wheat allergy. They will also likely ask you to keep a food diary to rule out other types of food being the cause of your symptoms.

Skin prick (scratch) test

A fine needle is used to place a small amount of liquid containing wheat proteins under a thin layer of your skin on your lower arm or your upper back. Alternatively, a small drop is placed on the surface of the skin and then that area is gently scratched so the liquid penetrates. If you are allergic to any of the wheat proteins, the skin where the liquid was applied will rise up in wheals, like the reaction to an insect bite.

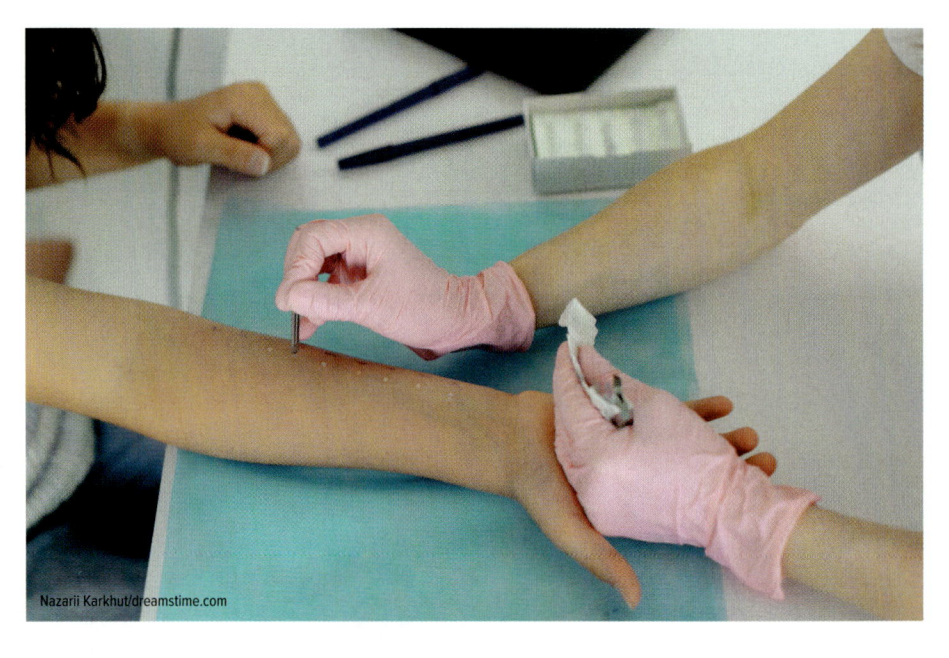

Blood test

A medical laboratory adds wheat proteins to a sample of your blood and then it is inspected under a microscope to see if it contains Immunoglobin E antibodies.

A graded oral test

This involves eating a small amount of a wheat product in the allergy specialist's office while they record any reactions. The patient may be asked to increase the amount they eat over a period of an hour or more.

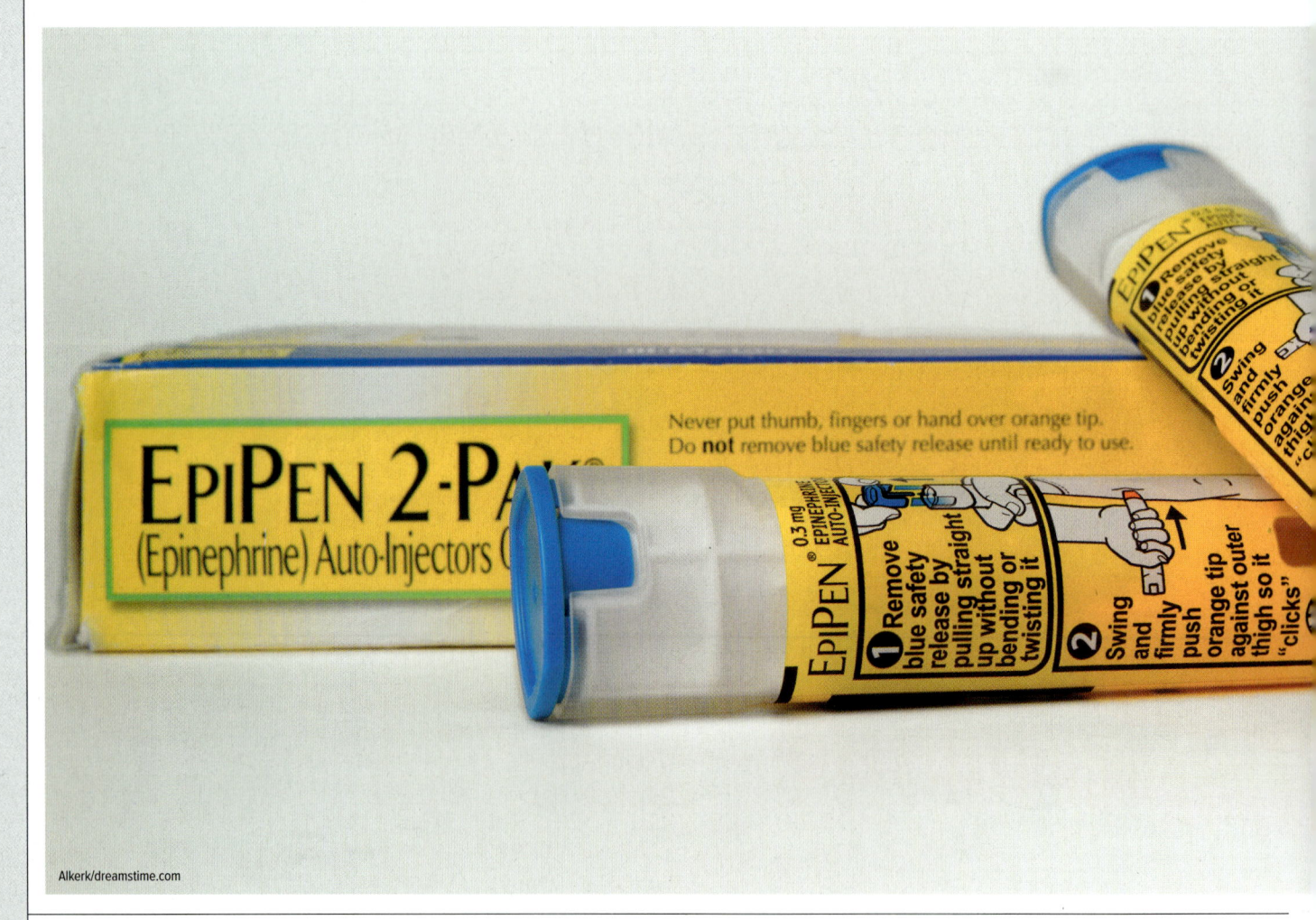

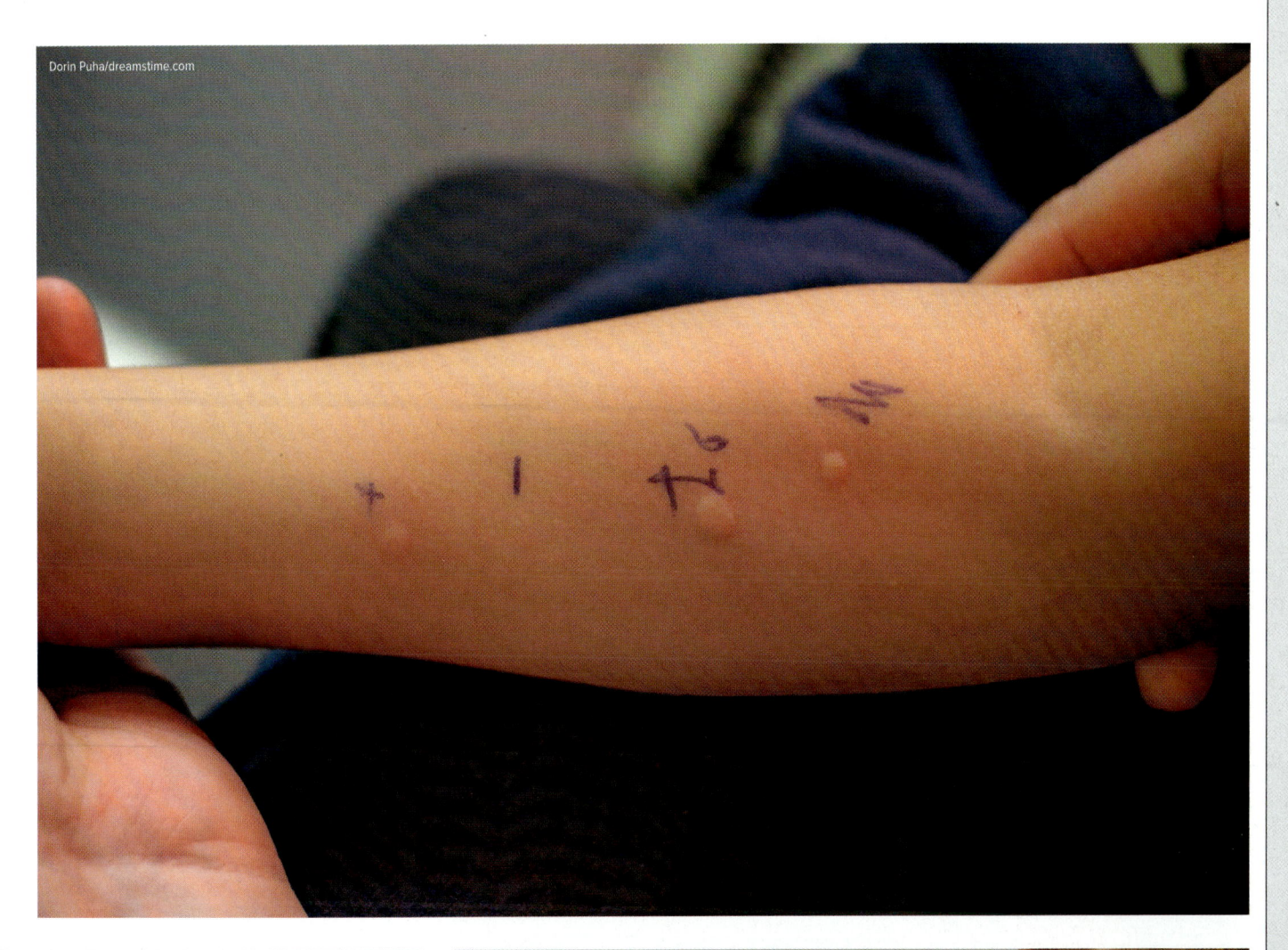

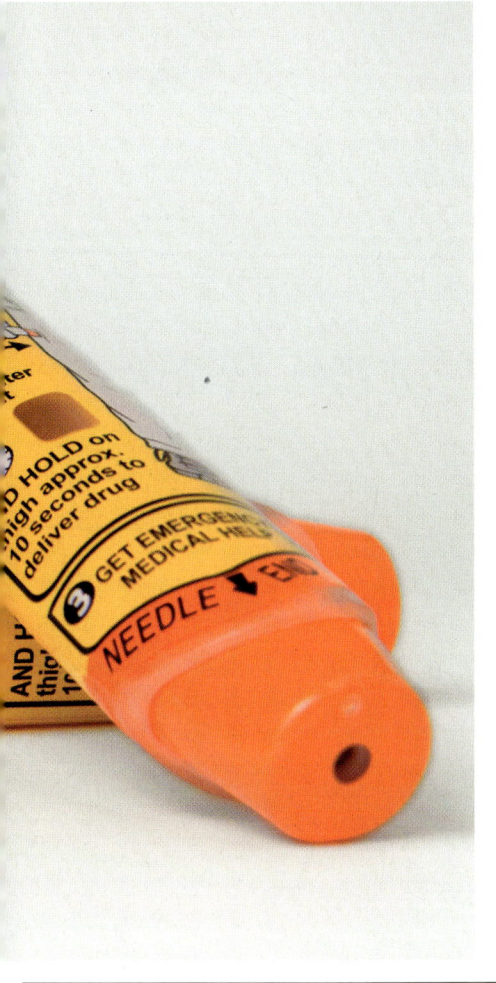

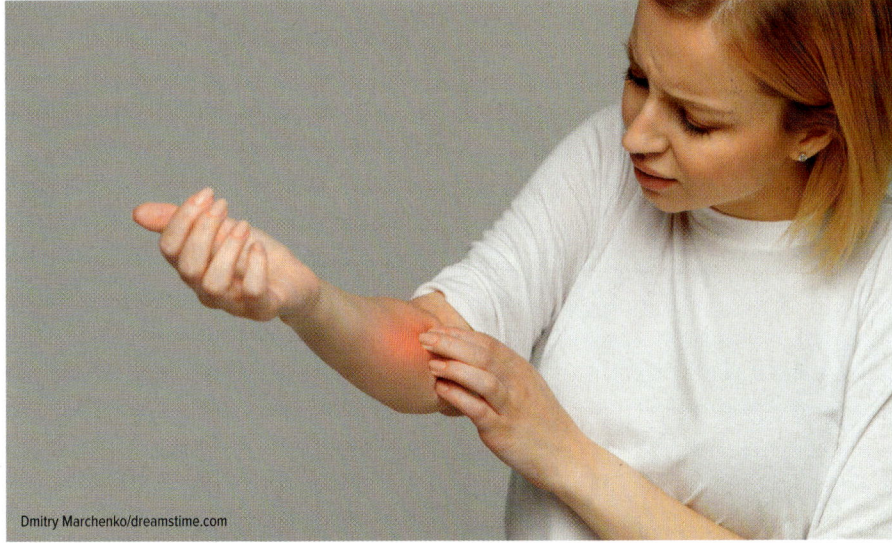

What happens next?

Apart from excluding wheat from the diet, there is no sure-fire way of treating a wheat allergy. However, it is possible to outgrow it, and it is thought that up to 66% of children do just that over a period of time.

If the reaction is generally mild then an antihistamine medication can sometimes help, as it does with hay fever, for instance. These medicines start working after about 20 minutes. Or short-term corticosteroids can be used, which take about an hour to start doing their work.

If the allergy is so severe the person is at risk of anaphylaxis, then it is important that they carry two epinephrine injectors (such as an EpiPen) with them at all times. A swift injection into the thigh will begin to take effect immediately and then the patient should take themselves to hospital to be checked over.

WHEAT ALLERGY: BAKER'S ASTHMA

What is Baker's Asthma?

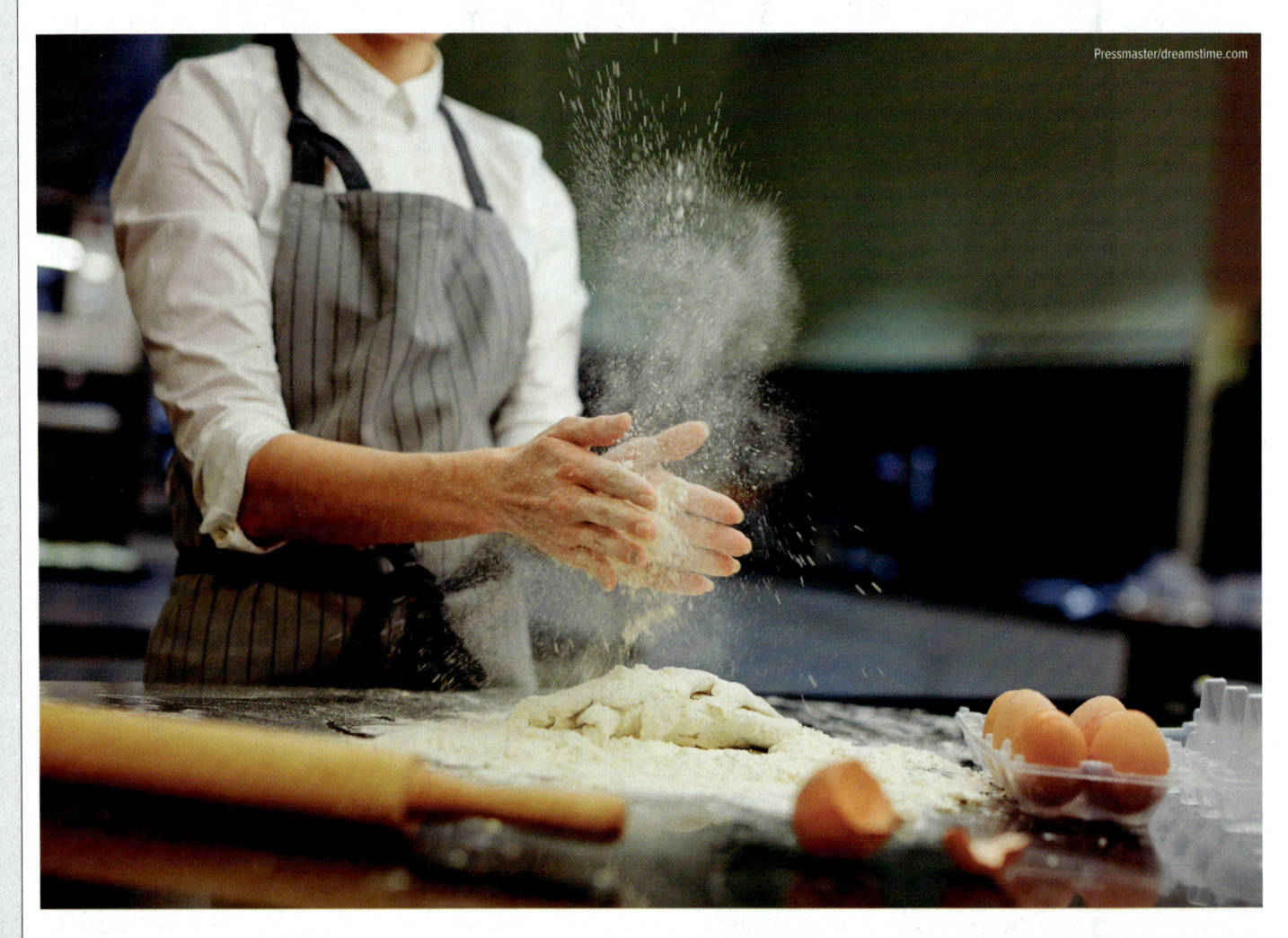

The asthmatic symptoms that occur in people who spend large amounts of time in an environment filled with flour and grain dust represent one of the most common forms of occupational asthma. These include grain millers, elevator workers and farmers who are exposed to wheat dust at harvesting, pastry chefs in industrial kitchens and, of course, anyone working at a bakery.

It has been recorded that the incidences of Baker's Asthma have been rising in recent years, particularly among supermarket bakery staff. The prevalence of this type of asthma has been attributed, essentially, to an allergic reaction to wheat proteins when they are inhaled into the body with the flour dust. Surprisingly, wheat can beat smoke, fumes, gasses, and various types of organic and metallic dusts as a cause of long-term asthma.

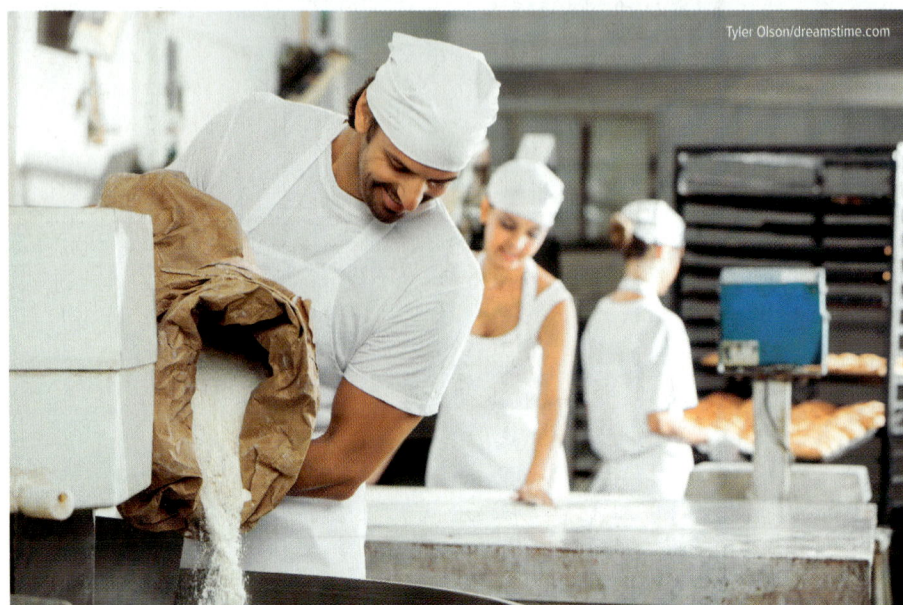

With Baker's Asthma, though, it is not just wheat proteins that are the culprits. The proteins in the flour of other cereal grains can also trigger the lung condition as can the egg powder, sesame seeds, nuts and yeast that are also usually found in bakeries. The allergens can also cause sore, red hands in people who are frequently handling flour and dough.

Curiously, scientists studying the condition have found that many of

WHEAT ALLERGY: BAKER'S ASTHMA

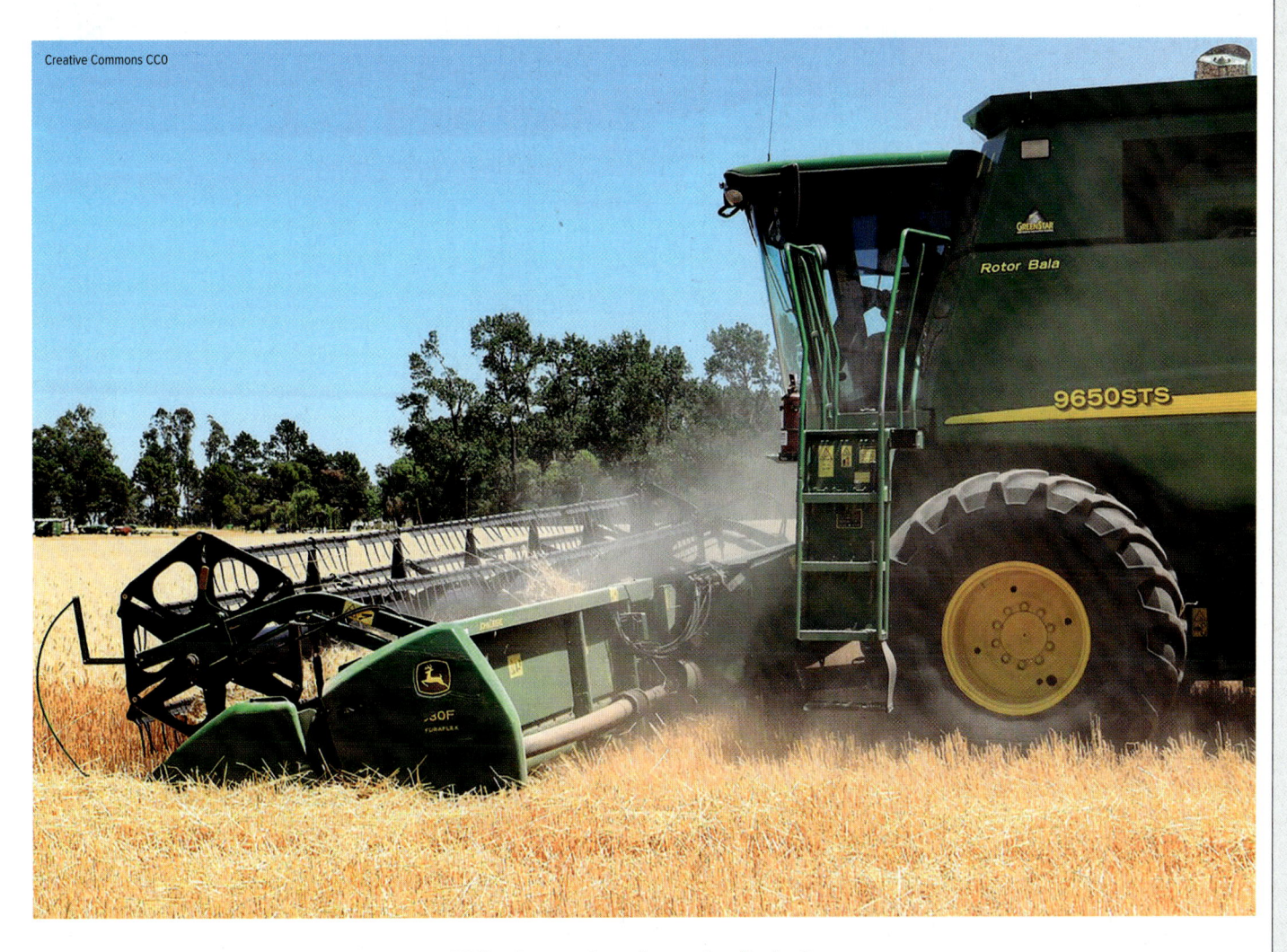

the people with asthma do not have an adverse reaction when they eat wheat or other grains. It has been speculated that something in the cooking process alters the proteins in such a way that they become intolerable for those with the various types of gluten sensitivities.

What are the symptoms?
These don't necessarily appear while the person is at work, instead they can begin some hours after. At first, they may only be apparent during the working week, subsiding or disappearing at the weekends and during holidays. But gradually they can become chronic and the asthma debilitating for life unless steps are taken to reduce exposure. The symptoms are:

- Coughing
- Tight chest
- Shortness of breath
- Wheeziness
- Sneezing and stuffed up or runny nose
- Conjunctivitis
- Dermatitis of the hands and arms

What can be done to help?
As with gluten intolerance, avoiding the triggers is the only way to effectively treat the condition in sensitive individuals. Asthma medication can alleviate symptoms but not end the issue.

A lot can be done to protect the airways, though. Good ventilation and protective equipment, from a Covid-style mask that is always worn in the workplace to a purpose-built respirator and goggles in more serious cases. It goes without saying that avoiding any other lung irritants, such as cigarette smoke and bonfires, is a good idea.

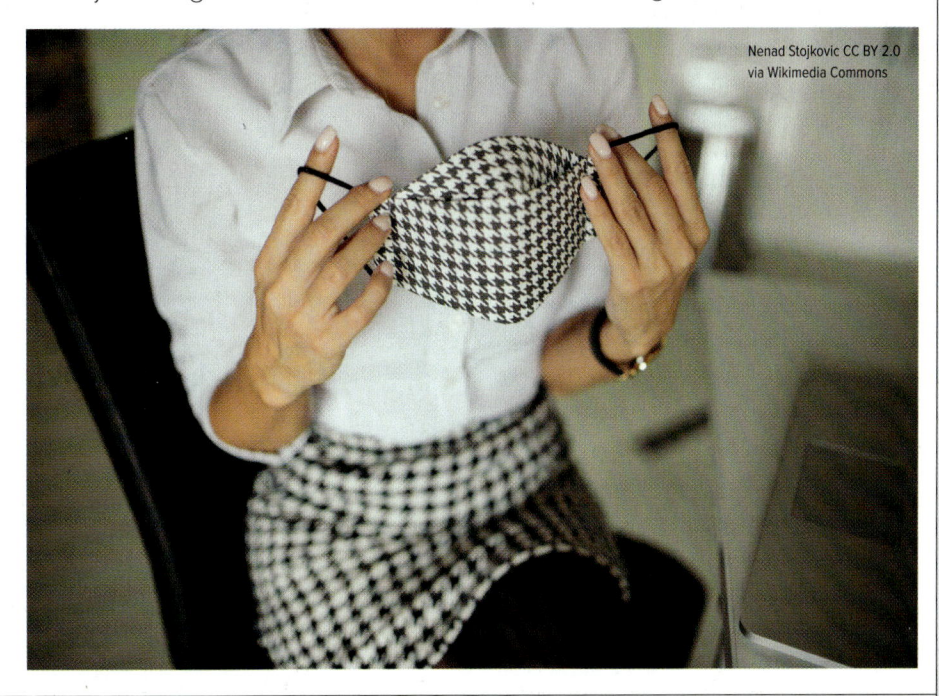

THE GLUTEN-FREE HANDBOOK

WHEAT ALLERGY: ANAPHYLACTIC REACTION

Exercise, gluten and severe reactions

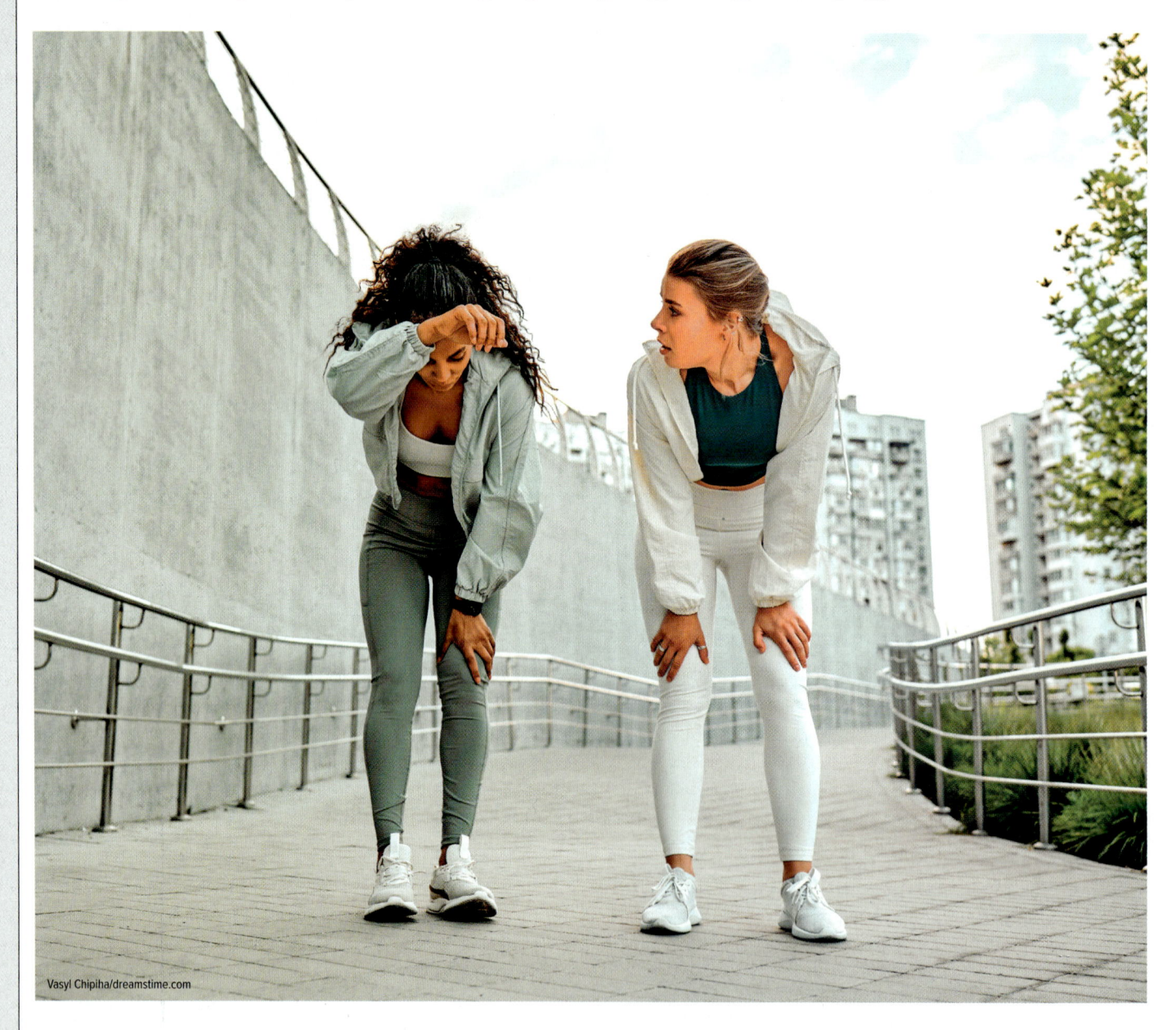

Vasyl Chipiha/dreamstime.com

There is a rare but dangerous form of gluten sensitivity that can induce an extreme reaction in a person who eats a trigger substance and then does a physical activity. Its full name is Wheat-dependent Exercise-induced Anaphylactic Reaction (WDEIA).

A particular wheat protein has been identified as the guilty party. Called Omega 5 Gliadin, it is not strictly gluten but a much smaller protein compound that, together with substances called glutenins, help bread dough to rise. The condition is not yet fully understood but what seems to be certain is that gliadin provokes the body into releasing chemicals such as histamine, and these flood the tissues and bring on the allergic reaction.

What happens if you have WDEIA?

In people who are susceptible to the condition, taking exercise within six hours of eating a wheat product can result in symptoms that range from mildly uncomfortable to life-threatening. These symptoms may not manifest themselves immediately and may develop overnight:

- Swelling of the throat and tongue
- Tingling in the mouth and swollen lips
- Difficulty swallowing and speaking
- Breathing difficulties
- Dizziness

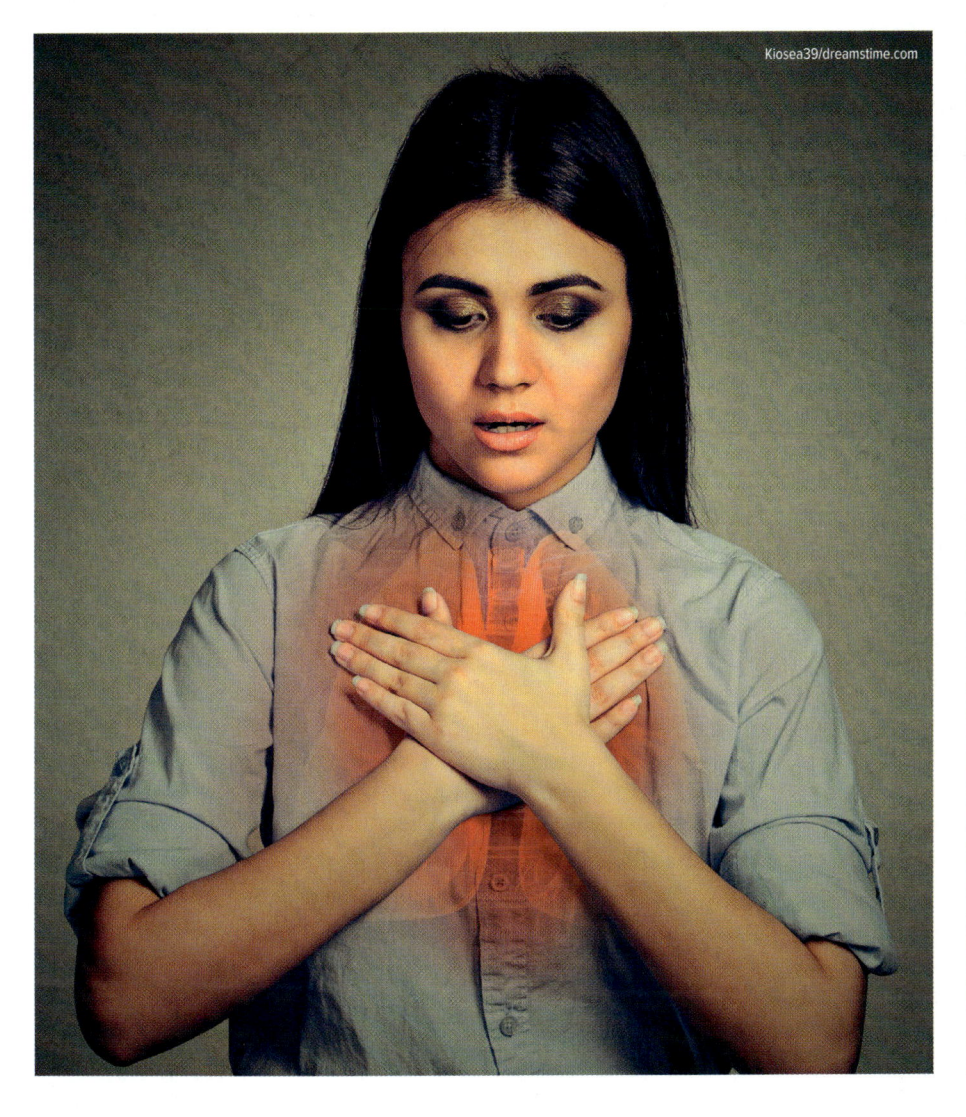

WHEAT ALLERGY: ANAPHYLACTIC REACTION

COLLAPSE AFTER BREAKFAST

A 30-year-old patient, who was the subject of a study published in *Sage Open Medical Case Reports* in 2023, had been suffering from chronic urticaria (hives) for five years. On the way to work one day, having had toast and some other wheat-containing foods for breakfast, she suddenly felt restless, irritated, itchy and then she fainted. She was treated for anaphylaxis and kept in hospital for 12 hours under observation, by which time she had recovered satisfactorily. Her blood test revealed Omega 5 Gliadin.

The patient went on to a gluten-free diet and had no further episodes of anaphylaxis symptoms, although her urticaria remained, but under control. It was thought by the scientists conducting the study at the Tbilisi State Medical University in Georgia that this rash condition may have been an indication that the patient was allergic to wheat.

- Sudden sleepiness
- Confusion
- Clammy skin
- Sense of dread
- Fainting
- Raised rash
- Stomach ache and sickness

If you join wheat-eating together with other factors, such as drinking alcohol, menstruation, being under stress, having an infection or having asthma, the results can be amplified. In all cases, it is a combination of events that causes the condition, unlike Coeliac Disease or wheat allergies.

The exercise involved in causing the reaction is generally aerobic – running, dancing, cycling, climbing, etc – but it does not necessarily have to be vigorous. Even going for a walk after a wheat-based meal can be a problem for some. But to make things even more confusing, the effects may not be seen every time exercise is taken.

It really is a mysterious state of affairs that scientists are still studying, but the remedy for all the various permutations of the condition is the same – eliminate wheat from the diet and you greatly reduce the chances of falling prey to WDEIA.

As a footnote: wheat is not necessarily the only foodstuff to result in this extreme reaction. Other common triggers are nuts, eggs, dairy products, and shellfish. In the case of these items the condition is known as Food-dependent Exercise-induced Anaphylaxis (FDEIA).

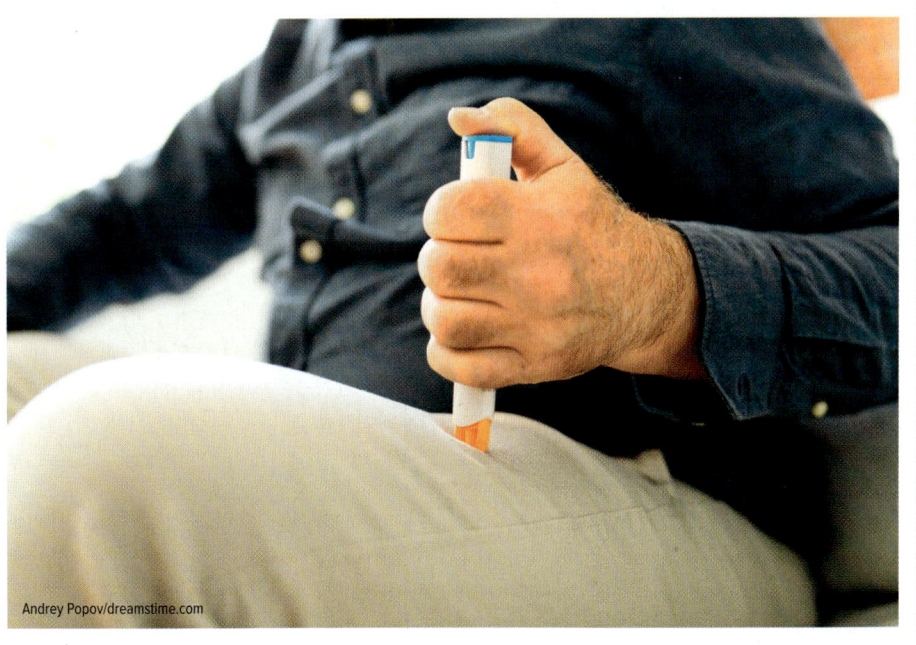

THE GLUTEN-FREE HANDBOOK

Gluten Ataxia

A relatively new condition that has been linked to an autoimmune response to gluten.

This is a rare situation where the antibodies your body produces when it is affected by gluten mistakenly attack your nervous system as well as the digestive system. In particular, the antibodies target the part of the brain called the cerebellum, which is the area that controls motor skills and balance.

Compared to the number of people with Coeliac Disease or Non-Coeliac Gluten Sensitivity, the proportion with Gluten Ataxia is quite small but anyone with CD and NCGS should be aware of the link and therefore alive to the possibility of symptoms.

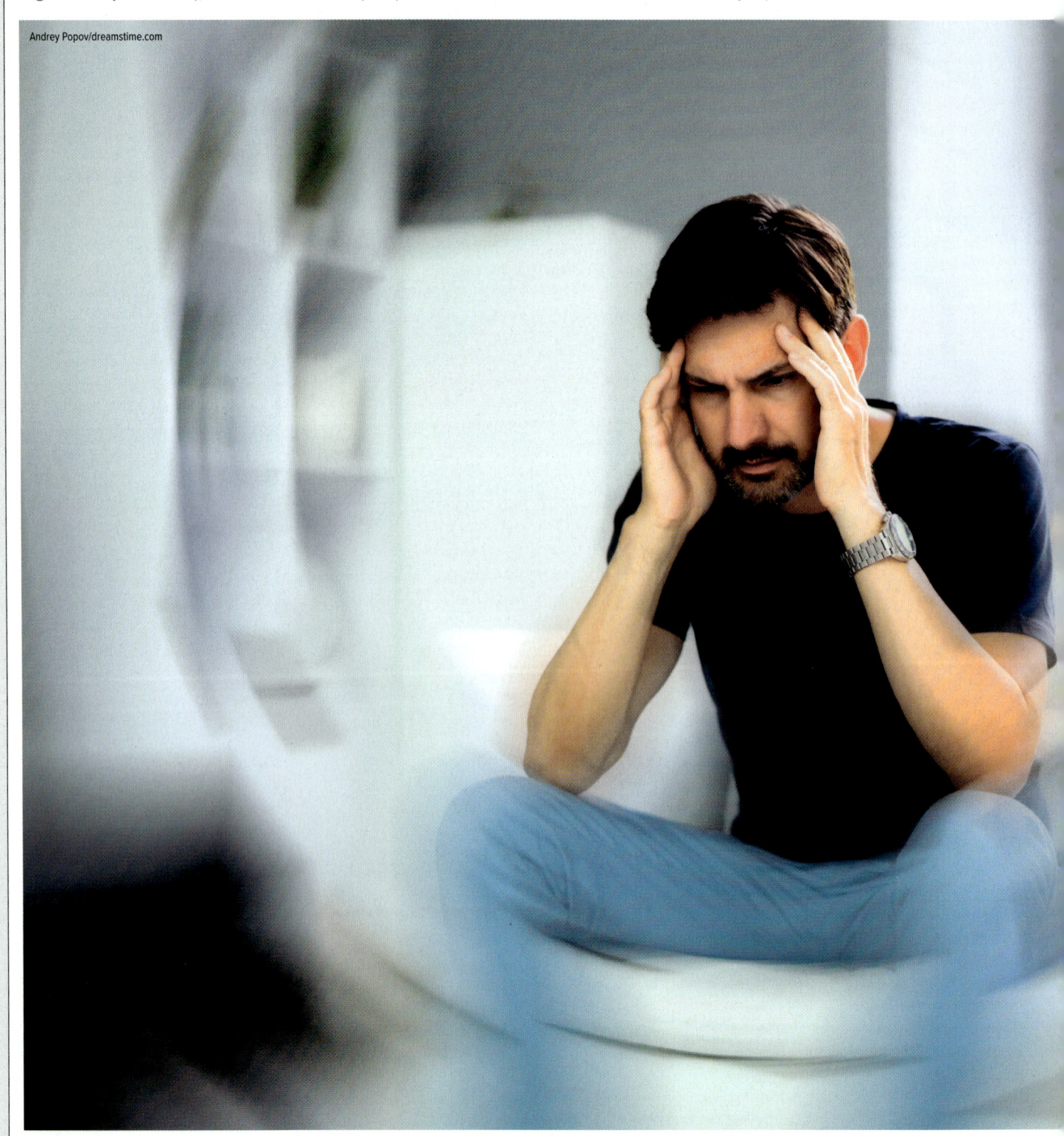

GLUTEN ATAXIA

Giving it a name
The term ataxia itself has long been used to describe poor muscle control and problems with walking, co-ordination, and speech but until recently the various possible causes have not included a reaction to gluten or wheat. This relationship was first defined in the late 1990s by Professor Marios Hadjivassiliou and his colleagues, who have been working at the Department of Neuroscience at The University of Sheffield in northern England on a variety of gluten-related nerve issues.

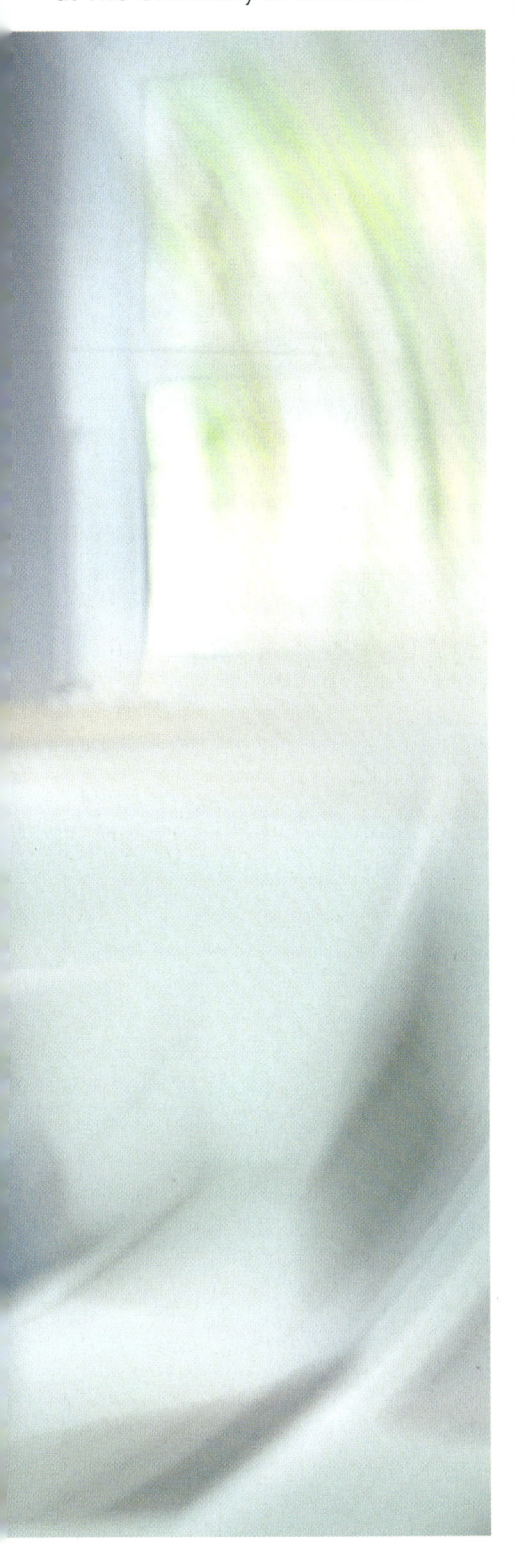

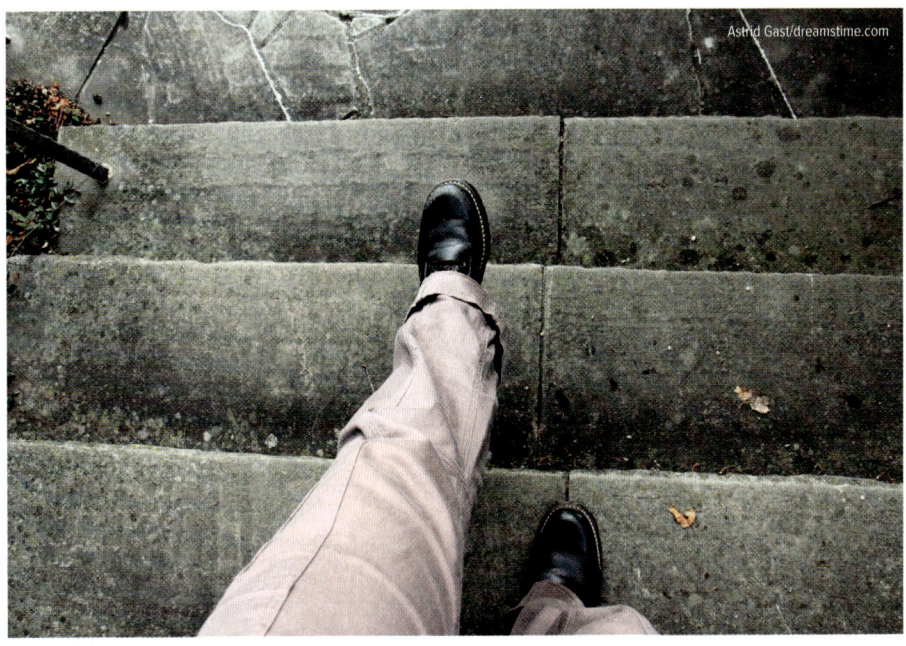

In a paper published in *The Lancet* in 1998 they stated that "Ataxia is the commonest neurological manifestation of Coeliac Disease." They went on to say that some individuals who were found to be genetically predisposed to develop Coeliac Disease showed no signs of inflammation in the small intestine. They did, however, exhibit evidence of ataxia.

Of the 28 patients they studied, all had some degree of trouble with walking and tremors in their limbs, and the ones who had had the disease longest had the most severe symptoms. They concluded that their ataxia had resulted from their immune systems damaging the cerebellum, the nerve fibres at the back of the spinal cord and the nerves that connect the brain to the spinal cord. They said: "Gluten sensitivity is an important cause of apparently idiopathic ataxia and may be progressive… We propose the term Gluten Ataxia to describe this disorder."

Is it widespread?
Because Gluten Ataxia is such a newly described condition it's hard to estimate what proportion of people who have been diagnosed with ataxia have Coeliac Disease as the cause of their issues. If their Coeliac Disease is undiagnosed, and they do not have any digestive symptoms, the autoimmune damage of Gluten Ataxia could eventually become irreversible because the cerebellum has shrunk. Dr Hadjivassiliou has been quoted as saying that he believes as many as 41% of people who have developed ataxia but do not know why, may actually have Gluten Ataxia.

What are the symptoms?
In the early stages, possibly only your balance may be affected. You could become a little unsteady and have trouble picking up your feet. Later, speech may be affected, and people may accuse you of being tipsy. You may also develop muscle spasms and uncontrolled eye movements. The full list of symptoms can be as extensive as:

- Difficulty walking
- Uncoordinated movements
- Clumsiness in simple tasks such as using a pen, doing up buttons, tying shoelaces or using a knife and fork.
- Slurred speech
- Blurred vision and rapid eye movements
- Limb tremors and muscle jerks
- Fatigue
- Dizziness
- Headaches
- Ringing in the ears
- Tingling, burning, or shooting pains
- Hearing loss
- Numbness in the hands and feet
- Feeling of unease and loss of confidence

Can anything be done?

Diagnosing the condition is the most important first step to improving matters. However, being a new discovery, there isn't medical agreement on the best way to test for it.

On the plus side, blood tests have been established as the initial method for establishing if Coeliac Disease and Non-Coeliac Gluten Sensitivity are present. Given that Gluten Ataxia is only known to affect people who have one of those two, a blood test for those is a reasonable starting point.

If the distinguishing antibodies are found, the next step is to adopt a strict gluten-free diet. If improvements are seen, then the likely cause can possibly be guessed at.

At the same time, though, it is not unknown for someone to have Coeliac Disease and another condition, other than a gluten sensitivity, which is causing their ataxia. So, a doctor may decide to refer their patient to a neurologist to rule out those other possible causes.

What are the treatments?

Apart from the exclusion diet, there are many ways forward to help improve Gluten Ataxia symptoms. Physiotherapy can assist to correct movements and build up strength and control of the muscles. Speech therapy can be employed to help communication to be clearer. And there are specialists who can train people on how to prevent falls and what to do if they accidentally inhale food.

If Gluten Ataxia is discovered early enough, full, or at least partial recovery is possible but may take a few years. In a dietary study of individuals with Gluten Ataxia reported in the *British Medical Journal* in 2003, Dr Hadjivassiliou's team followed the progress of 26 patients who stuck to a strict gluten-free diet. They found that after a year the patients' bodies were no longer showing signs of the gluten antibodies and their ataxia symptoms had improved significantly, compared to a control group that had voluntarily refused to be put on the diet.

FROM WHEELCHAIR TO WALKING

The experience of a 19-year-old British man was described in a paper co-authored by Laurence Newrick, Nigel Hoggard and Marios Hadjivassiliou and published in 2021. The man had been referred to the Sheffield Ataxia Centre because he had a 12-month history of slurred speech, unsteadiness, vomiting, weight loss and mobility issues. He had been getting steadily worse to the point that he had to use a walking frame and wheelchair and was having trouble speaking and keeping his balance. After a battery of blood tests, scans, and biopsies he was diagnosed with Gluten Ataxia. He was given drugs to reduce inflammation and suppress the overactivity of the immune system and was put on a gluten-free diet. Two years into his treatment he was able to walk without assistance and scans revealed an improvement in his brain tissue. To the date of the paper, he had remained stable.

Javiindy/dreamstime.com

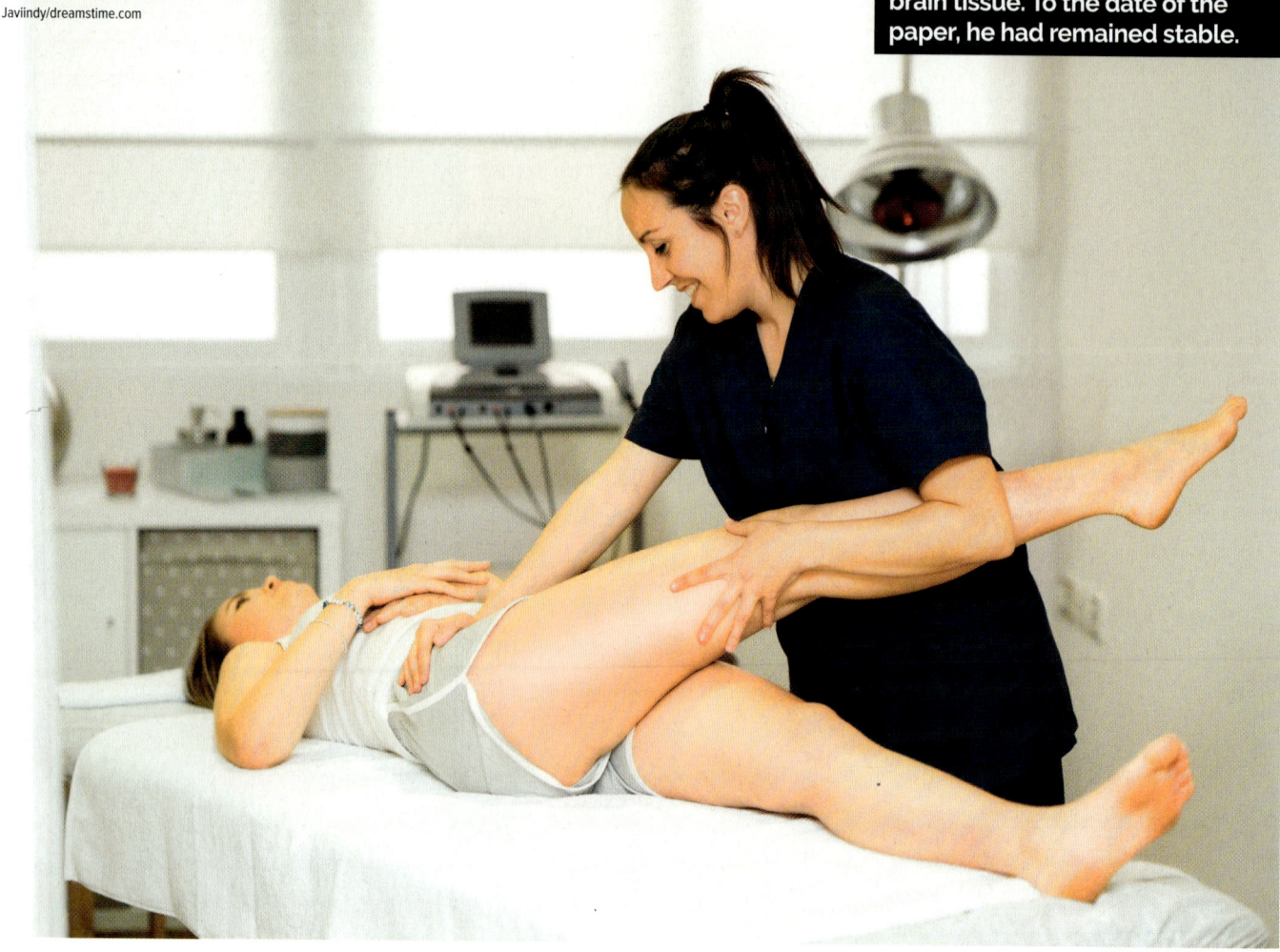

Lightfieldstudiosprod/dreamstime.com

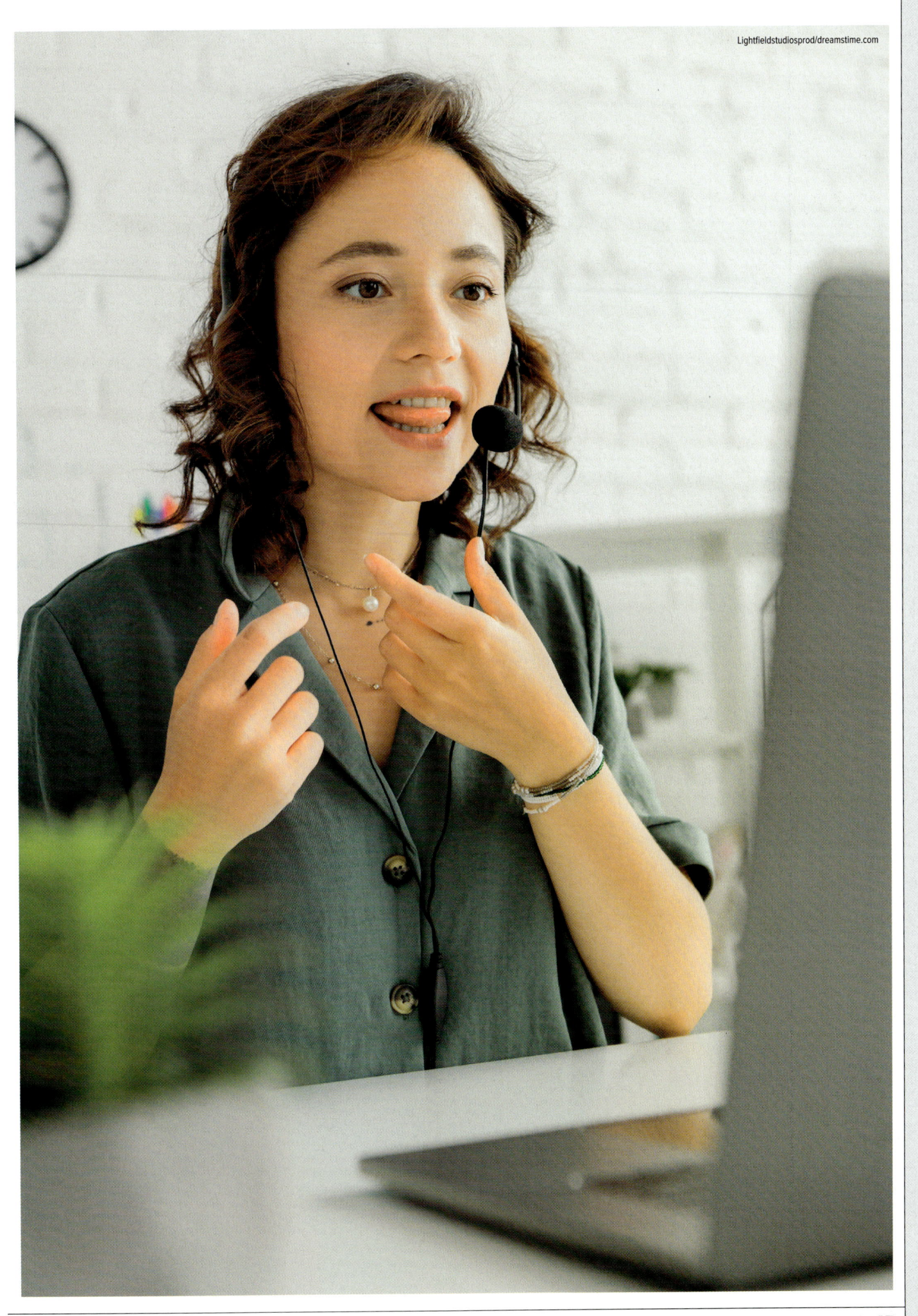

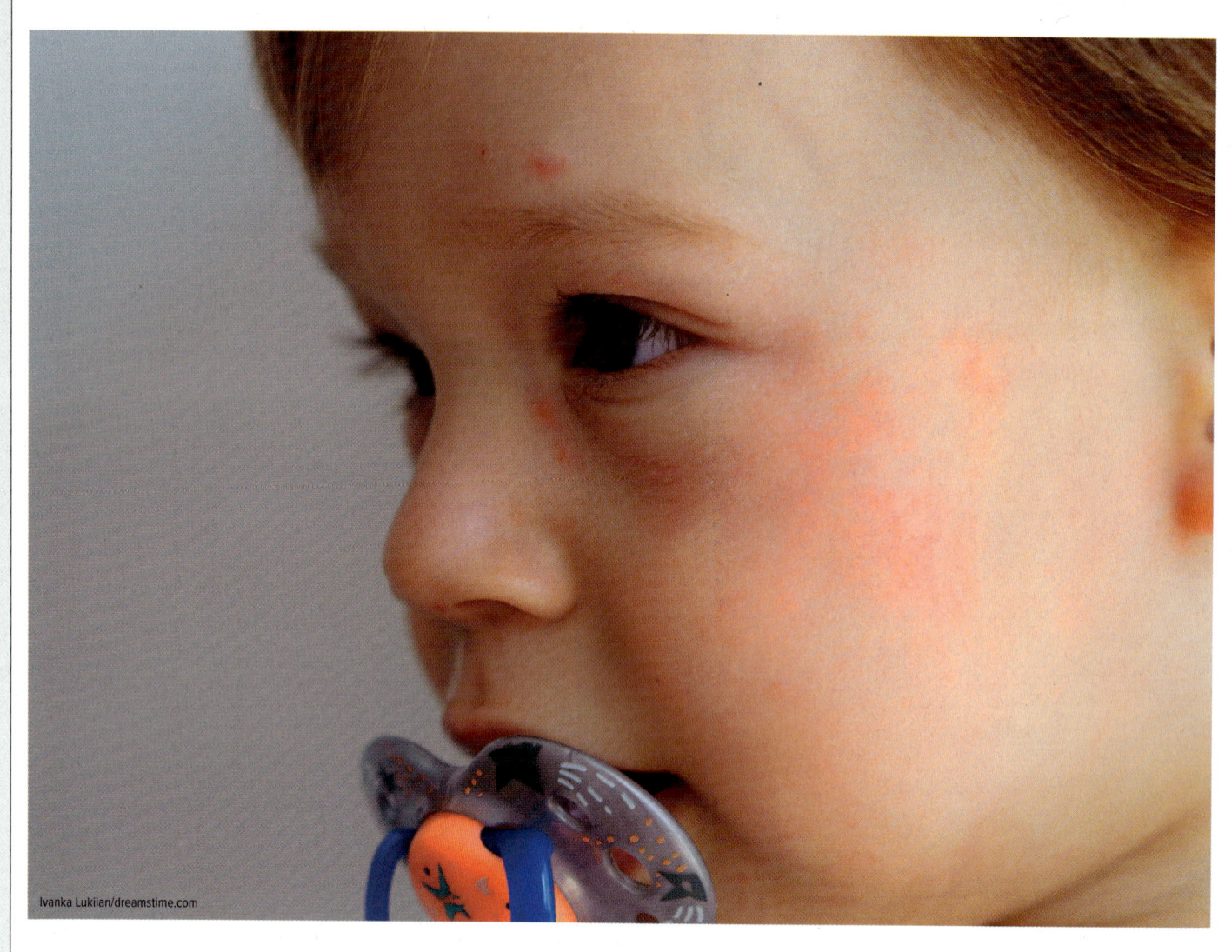

Dermatitis Herpetiformis

Not everyone with Coeliac Disease and Non-Coeliac Gluten Sensitivity will develop these irritating and painful blisters but it is a possible complication.

What happens with this condition?

The appearance of Dermatitis Herpetiformis (DH) can happen at any age, even in children as young as a few months if they have been started on a solids diet that includes gluten products. A majority of instances occur in people much older, though, typically between 50 and 70 years of age.

Antibodies that flood the body from the immune system after gluten has been ingested gather in the layers under the top skin and cause raised, red and extremely itchy patches of skin. Often there are blisters that rupture when the person scratches and these can then get infected and pus-filled. Sometimes, the first signs that all is not well appear in the fingers.

Most people get the rash on their elbows and knees, on both sides simultaneously, and also on their shoulders, around their buttocks and sometimes on their scalp. If they have had the condition for a long time the patches may have thickened and become very rough.

Around 15-25% of patients who have DH also have quite marked intestinal damage compared to those who don't have any symptoms on their skins. However, it is possible for a coeliac patient to only have dermatological signs and no symptoms from their digestive systems. Some 60% of

DH sufferers don't experience any bloating, stomach pain, loose bowels, or constipation. However, they can nonetheless be subject to intestinal damage.

How is DH confirmed?

In order to verify that a skin condition is being caused by a gluten sensitivity, a small sample of skin must be taken from an area that hasn't been affected by a rash. It is then checked under a microscope to detect if there are any signs of an antibody called Immunoglobulin A (IgA). If this is found, the next step is for blood tests and the small intestine being biopsied for evidence of Coeliac Disease. Patients are encouraged throughout the testing period to continue eating gluten products otherwise they run the risk of their immune system's reactions not being picked up.

ITCHY SKIN BUT NO SICKNESS

A team of dermatologists from Florida and Pennsylvania, Drs Julie Templet, John Patrick Welsh and Carrie Ann Cusack, reported in the clinical journal *Cutis* in 2007 the case of a six-year-old boy who had been suffering from itchy skin lesions since the age of nine months. He had previously been diagnosed with a form of eczema and repeated outbreaks of hives but none of the creams and tablets his paediatrician prescribed seemed to have worked.

The team found that although he had some signs of dry, cracked, and itchy skin, he lacked the thickened, leathery skin patches normally associated with long-term eczema. His mother said that he had been small for his age at first but had more recently caught up. He had not been suffering from sickness or diarrhoea.

Nevertheless, a sample of his skin that was biopsied revealed that he had antibodies that respond to eating gluten. They had accumulated in the inner layers of his skin, where the blood vessels run that nourish the outer layers. Tests of his gut showed that there was some damage to the villi in his small intestine, even though he hadn't had digestive symptoms.

The boy was put on a gluten-free diet and his skin condition was much improved. The scientists noted that restricting a child's diet was challenging and could take months to yield results and so referral to a dietician could be helpful.

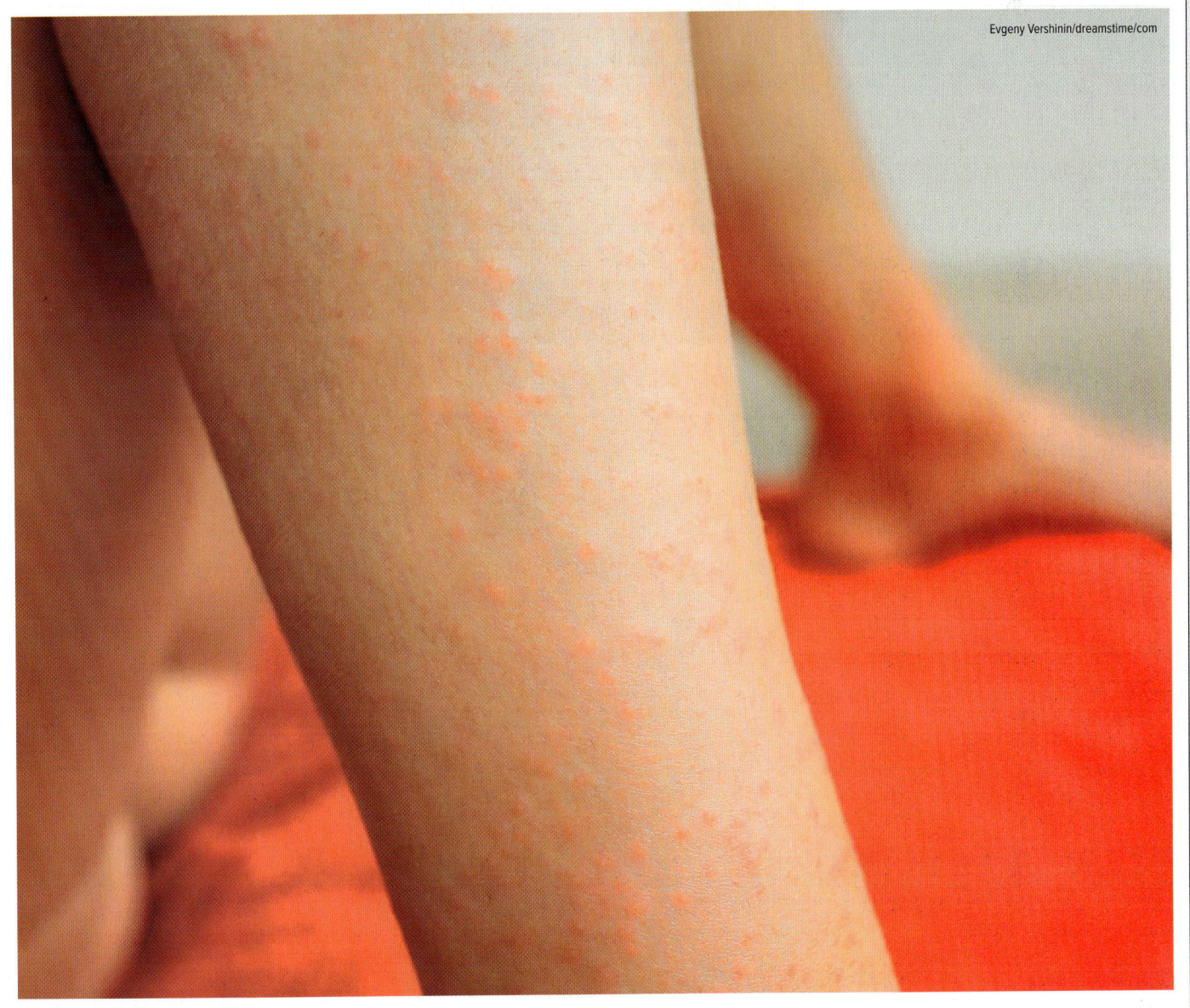

Evgeny Vershinin/dreamstime/com

How is DH treated?

As with all conditions caused by gluten, the ultimate cure is a gluten-free diet for life. But while intestinal symptoms can disappear quite quickly, even if the areas already damaged take a few years to properly heal, the skin symptoms of DH take longer to clear up. On average, it will be two years before most people find they have a significant improvement in the appearance and feel of their skin.

Because the DH skin condition is so irritating, the knock-on effects caused by scratching and the risk of infection can not only be disfiguring and embarrassing but also hazardous to skin health in the long term. So, while the patient is waiting for the gluten-free diet to work its magic there are drugs, primarily one called Dapsone that is also used to treat leprosy, that can be taken to lessen the DH symptoms. These control the development of the blisters and help to lessen the itching. They do not, however, have any effect on the digestive system symptoms – only the strict gluten-free regime can do that.

What happens if it is not treated?

The consequences of not following an exclusively gluten-free diet if you have DH are the same as if you have Coeliac Disease. You are at risk of brittle bone disease, small bowel cancer, Non-Hodgkin Lymphoma and developing other autoimmune conditions such as Type 1 diabetes and thyroid problems. You can lessen the chances of progressing to all these by changing your eating habits.

In addition, repeated eruptions of DH can leave permanent marks, as the skin further reacts by making extra melanin that darkens the affected patches.

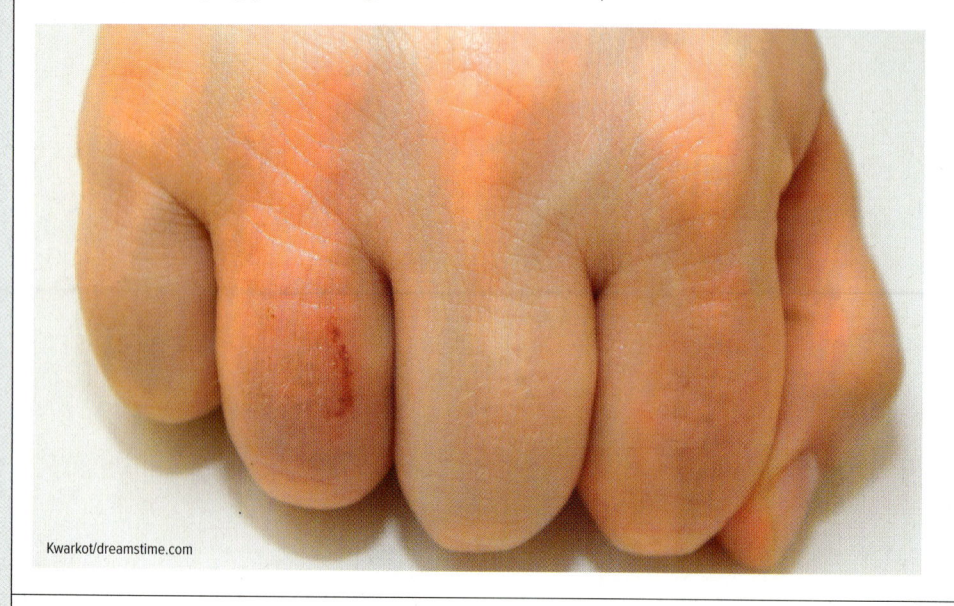

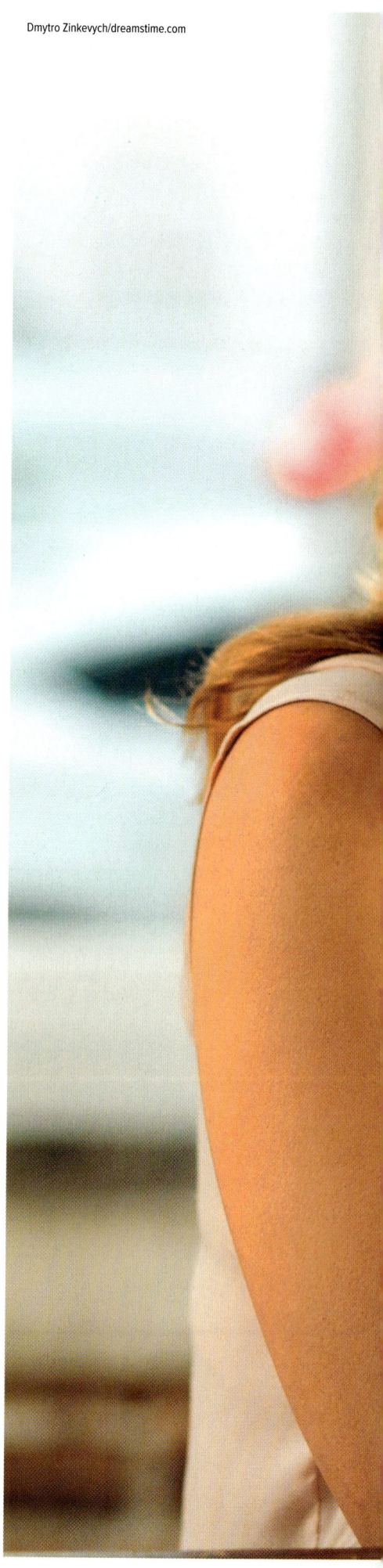

RASH ON FINGERS

A team comprising members of the Dermatology and Gastroenterology departments of the Hospital de Salut Mar in Barcelona, Spain, examined a 38-year-old man in 2013. The findings of Drs Daniel López Aventin, Lucas Ilzarbe and Josep Herrero-González were reported in a journal of the AGA Institute.

The man had been suffering with rashes on his fingers, blood blisters on the fingertips and occasional stinging pains over the course of seven months. He said he had not suffered any traumatic damage to his fingers in the past, nor had they been subject to repetitive pressure.

At the same time, over the previous three months he had been losing weight for no apparent reason. In all other respects he was quite healthy.

Studies of samples taken from the patient revealed the presence gluten-related antibodies and a biopsy of the top end of his small intestine showed signs of Coeliac Disease damage. A gluten-free diet resulted in the rapid disappearance of the rashes on his fingers and the patient progressively regained the weight he had lost.

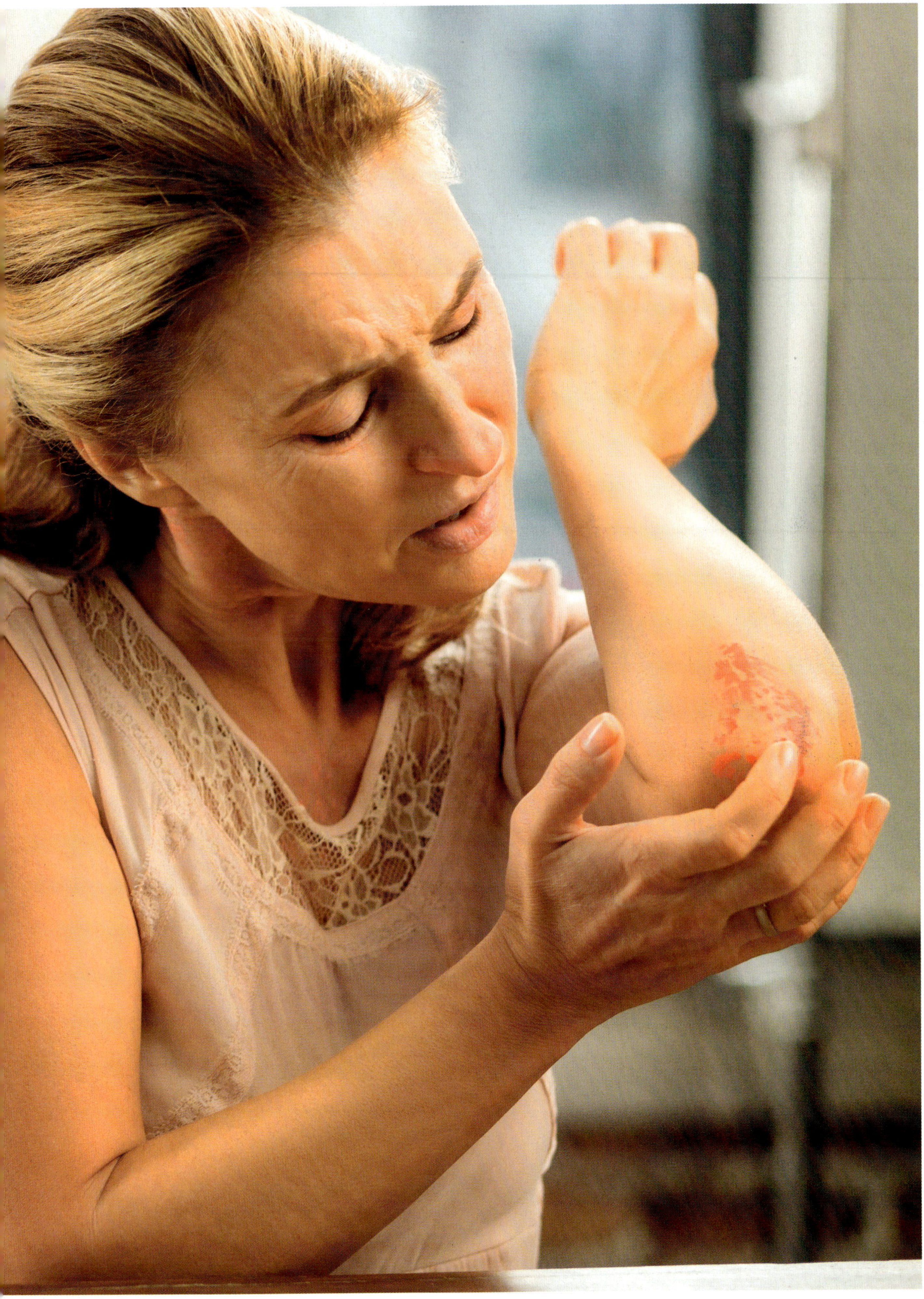

COELIAC AWARENESS MONTH

Coeliac Awareness Month – May 2025

The month of May has been designated around the world as a time to draw attention to the existence of Coeliac Disease and just how many people are living with it.

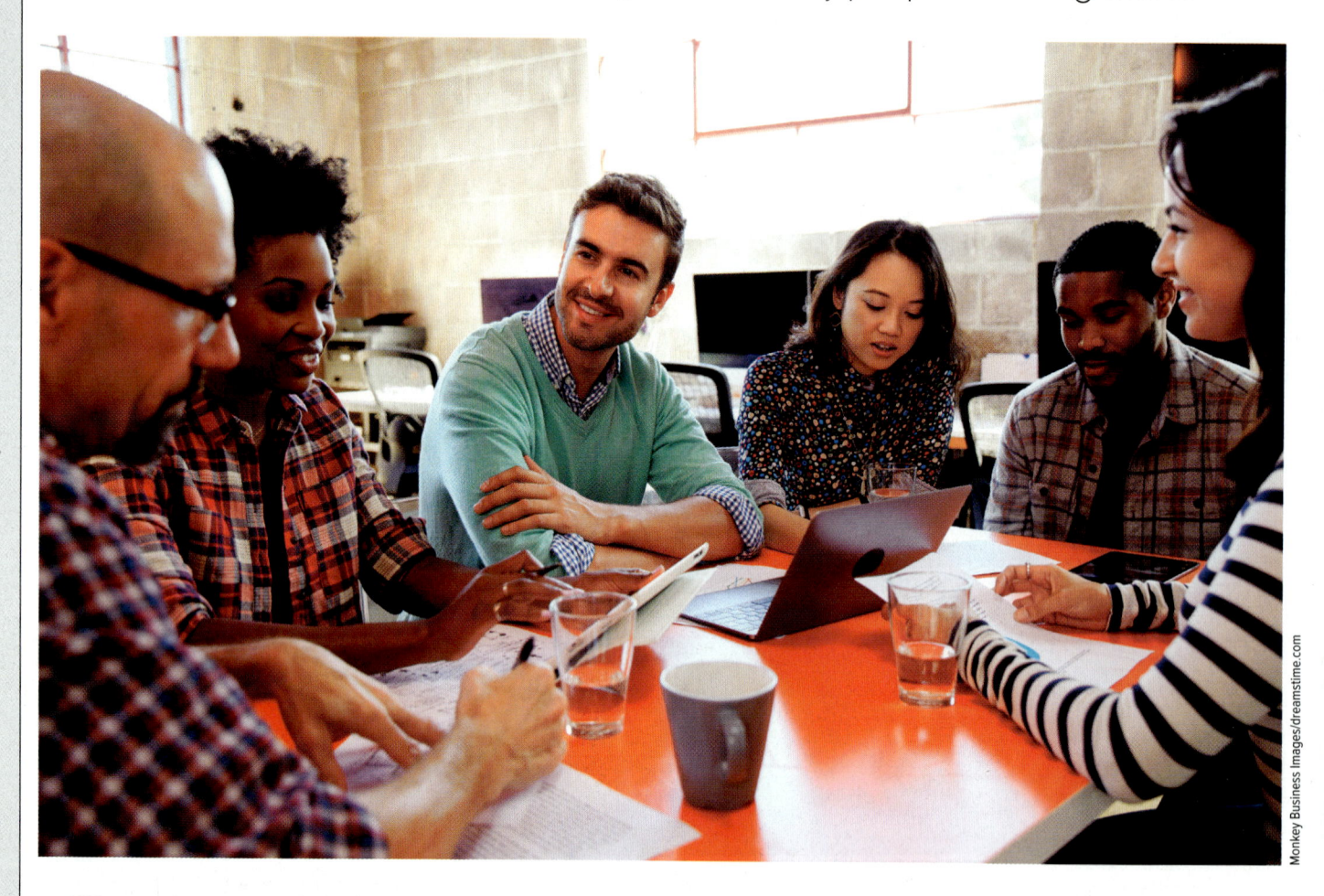

Monkey Business Images/dreamstime.com

One in 100 people in the UK have Coeliac Disease but only 36% of them have been properly diagnosed. That leaves 64% living with the disease but with no support and possibly facing a future of permanent damage to their digestive systems. In the United States the figure is one in 141 and 60-70% undiagnosed, and in Australia one in 70 and 80%.

That's a huge number of people who could be helped if they, their families, and their friends knew what might be causing their symptoms, how to call on medical help and what's involved in getting a proper diagnosis.

Internationally, there will be events going on in many different countries to bring Coeliac Disease to everyone's attention and raise funds for research and support for those who need it.

Around the UK
In the UK, the theme of the 2025 campaign will be the number 64, to represent the 64% of undiagnosed cases in the country. Coeliac UK is issuing a Virtual Challenge to raise much needed funds and suggests some fun activities to get involved in during May and raise money for Coeliac UK, all based on 64:

- Bake 64 of your favourite cupcakes, cookies or treats to sell
- Get sponsored to read 64 pages of your favourite book, or 64 chapters of lots of different books, or even 64 whole books!

64

www.keypublishing.com

COELIAC AWARENESS MONTH

Supporting Coeliac Awareness Month
May 1-31 2025
coeliac uk

- Hold a quiz with eight rounds of eight questions each
- Walk, run, or cycle 64km or 64 miles throughout the month
- Get active with 64 star jumps every day in May

To take part, order your free fundraising pack from www.coeliac.org.uk/get-involved/fundraise-for-us/join-the-coeliac-uk-64-challenge The pack has balloons and bunting, posters and lots more. You can also sign up for the Coeliac UK 64 Challenge via Enthuse, an online fundraising platform for charities where you can create a fundraising page and be automatically added to a team page. https://enthuse.com

Anyone raising over £64 using the fundraising platform will get a Coeliac UK T-shirt.

You can contact the fundraising team by emailing fundraising@coeliac.org.uk or call 0333 332 2033 and press option 0.

North America
Fundraising events will be held throughout May across the US and Canada. And within the month, May 16 has been picked out especially as International Celiac Awareness Day. For the past five years groups of supporters have come together to Shine a Light and get local signs, prominent buildings, bridges, and other edifices illuminated in coloured lights on that day to bring Celiac Disease to the public's attention.

Information on how you can lobby your governor or state official to issue a proclamation recognising May 16 as Celiac Awareness Day is at https://celiac.org/proclamations

Other events suggested by Beyond Celiac are:

- Holding a gluten-free party so your family and friends can learn more about your diet and find out that gluten-free food can be delicious
- Forming a 5k team and taking part in a run sometime in the month
- Sending in your story to its Voice of Celiac section to encourage others to know that every experience is unique. www.beyondceliac.org/voices-of-celiac-disease/tell-your-story
- Take part in a social media campaign. The Beyond Celiac website offers sample posts that can help spread the word during May. www.beyondceliac.org/celiac-awareness-month

Australia's Special Week
Australia opted for a full-on Awareness Week in March and also celebrates Coeliac Awareness Day on May 16. Coeliac Australia encourages people during that week and on the special day to:

- Talk to family and friends, particularly children, about Coeliac Disease and teach them how to make a gluten-free meal
- Hold a coeliac-friendly bake sale to raise awareness as well as funds to help support people with the disease and research into it
- Encourage anyone experiencing mystery symptoms to visit the doctor and ask the question, "Could it be Coeliac Disease?"

WORRIED IT COULD BE COELIAC DISEASE?

There are online assessment tools available on coeliac support websites that are aimed at helping people identify whether their symptoms could indicate Coeliac Disease. At the end of the quick and easy questionnaire there will be a recommendation on whether to seek out a medical diagnosis. The results of the test are also emailed to the respondent so they can be printed out and taken to the doctor.

In the UK visit https://isitcoeliacdisease.org.uk

In the US visit www.beyondceliac.org/celiac-disease/symptoms-checklist or https://celiac.org/about-celiac-disease/symptoms-assessment-tool

In Australia visit https://coeliac.org.au/self-assessment-tool

In Canada visit www.celiac.ca/celiac-disease-symptom-checklist

---

THE GLUTEN-FREE HANDBOOK

How to live gluten free

The steady growth in the availability of gluten-free food and beauty products has gone hand-in-hand with growing awareness of the condition, but the real explosion in branded gluten-free products began in the early 2000s.

Coeliac Disease (CD) had been identified in the 1940s as an allergy to wheat and then in the 1950s to the gluten component of many grains, not just wheat.

A number of bespoke gluten-free manufacturers came into being to cater for people who could not eat wheat and grain products and improve the lives of everyone for whom gluten was a problem. In the 1970s the condition of Non-Coeliac Gluten Sensitivity was first described and in the 1980s it was accepted by the medical community that CD was an autoimmune condition. But it was not until 2012 that the full range of gluten-related issues was formalised.

Finding their own cure
In the meantime, people suffering from mysterious gastrointestinal

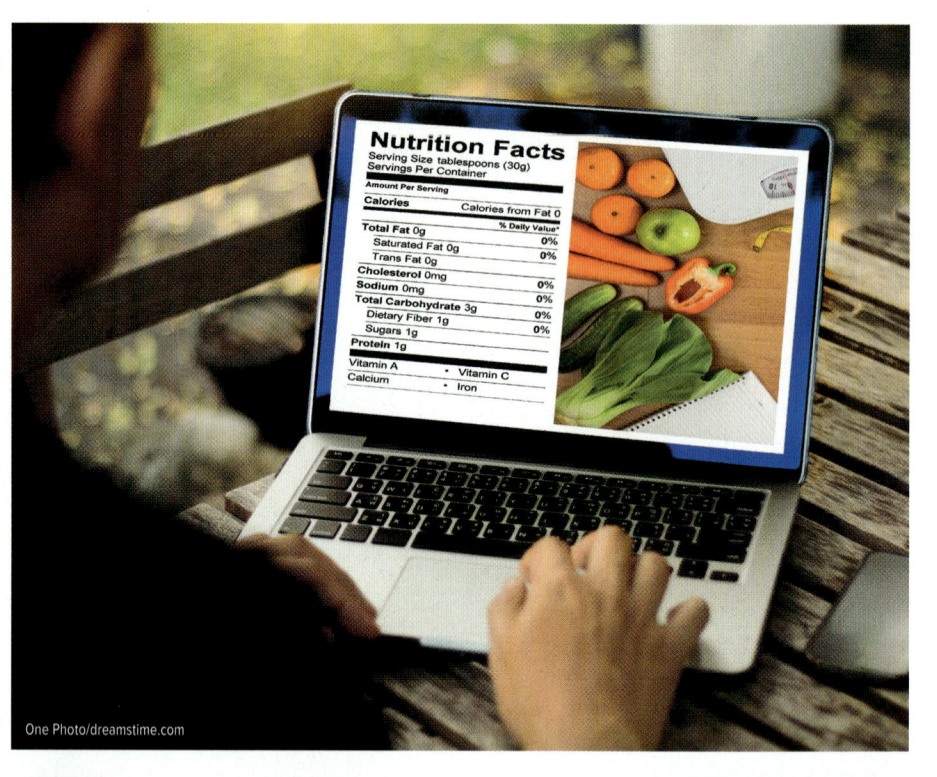

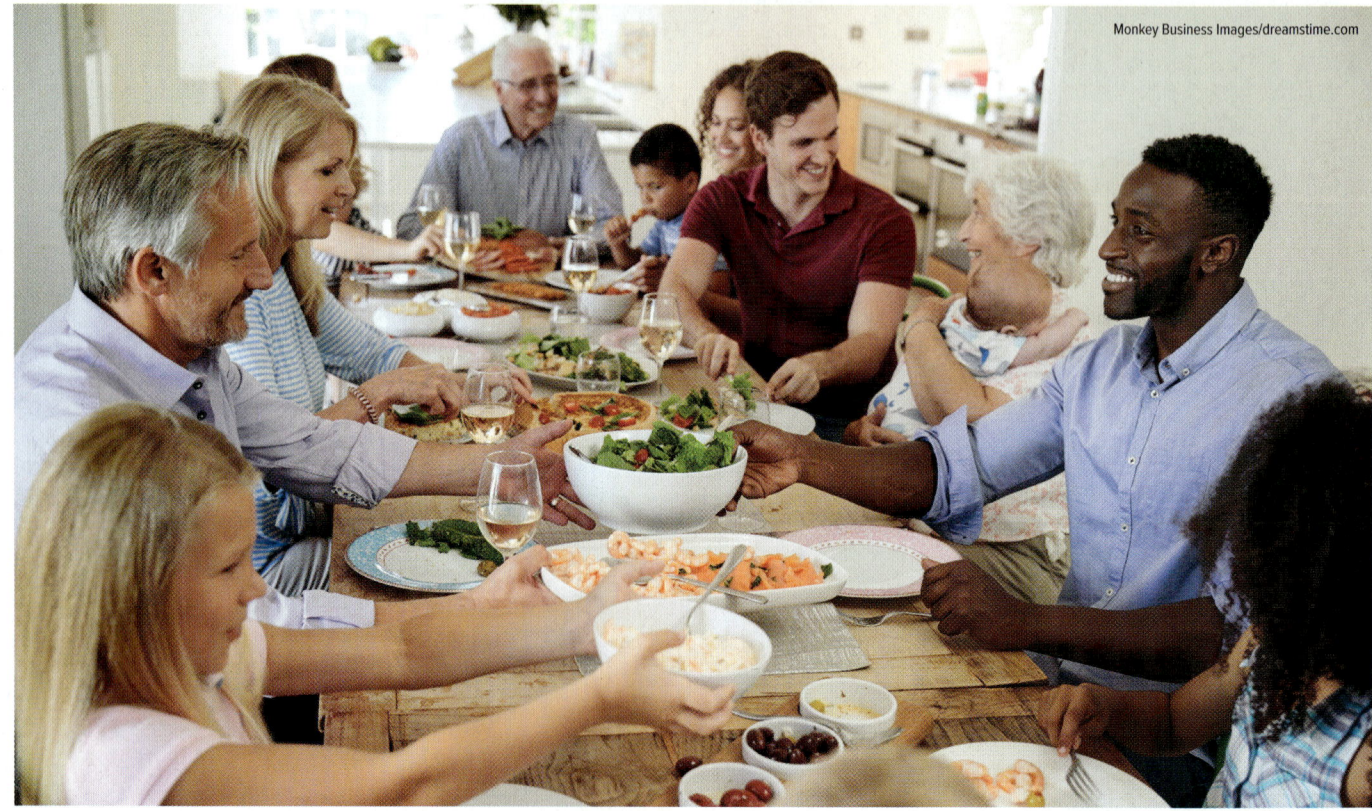

HOW TO LIVE GLUTEN FREE

symptoms for which the medical profession had no diagnosis were experimenting with their diets and lifestyle in an effort to find a cure for themselves. As a result, articles began to appear in magazines and word of mouth spread that eating bread and bakery products could be the cause of many unpleasant side-effects. This was picked up by some celebrities who advocated gluten-free living as a health benefit even for people who did not have a particular sensitivity, although gluten-free food can be just as fattening as any other.

The trend on the internet and social media was closely followed by mainstream manufacturers recognising an opportunity and producing gluten-free alternatives to their popular food, drink, and beauty products. Much more resource has also been ploughed into research and development.

Today, supermarkets and grocery stores have dedicated gluten-free sections displaying a wide range of suitable foodstuffs, bakers create interesting alternatives to conventional bread and pastries, restaurants and takeaways include tasty gluten-free items on their menus, and there are a growing number of specialist establishments that cater specifically for the gluten-free customer.

EATING OUT IS A CHALLENGE
Najett from Denmark

"Having been diagnosed with chickenpox three times in a year, I went to a dermatologist. He decided I had 'herpes dermatica', which he thought was a skin reaction due to gluten. He sent me to hospital and tests revealed I had the two variants of Coeliac Disease – gut and skin – and malnutrition as a result.

There are many challenges with my condition because I am quite gluten intolerant. Some people I visit get a little uncomfortable when I cannot eat what they serve, which in turn makes me feel uncomfortable. When I know people well enough, I call to ask what they will be cooking, and I then bring the same meal in a gluten-free version.

When we're travelling it also affects my husband and family as we cannot just drop into the first restaurant we see but have to search for gluten-free places.

Once, in a sports health resort, I got my own 'Chef de Cuisine'. I told him I could eat potatoes, rice, and cornstarch-based sauces. In his view any kind of 'starch' was obviously not good for me, so he prepared beautiful dishes with fish and steamed vegetables. And he came to the table dressed in his chef's hat and loudly presented me with the dishes. The resort had a large buffet for all other guests, so they were amazed. They seemed to think I was a VIP!"

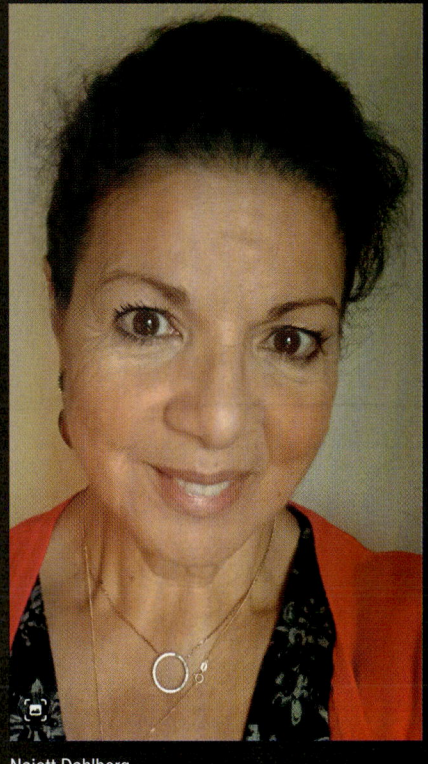

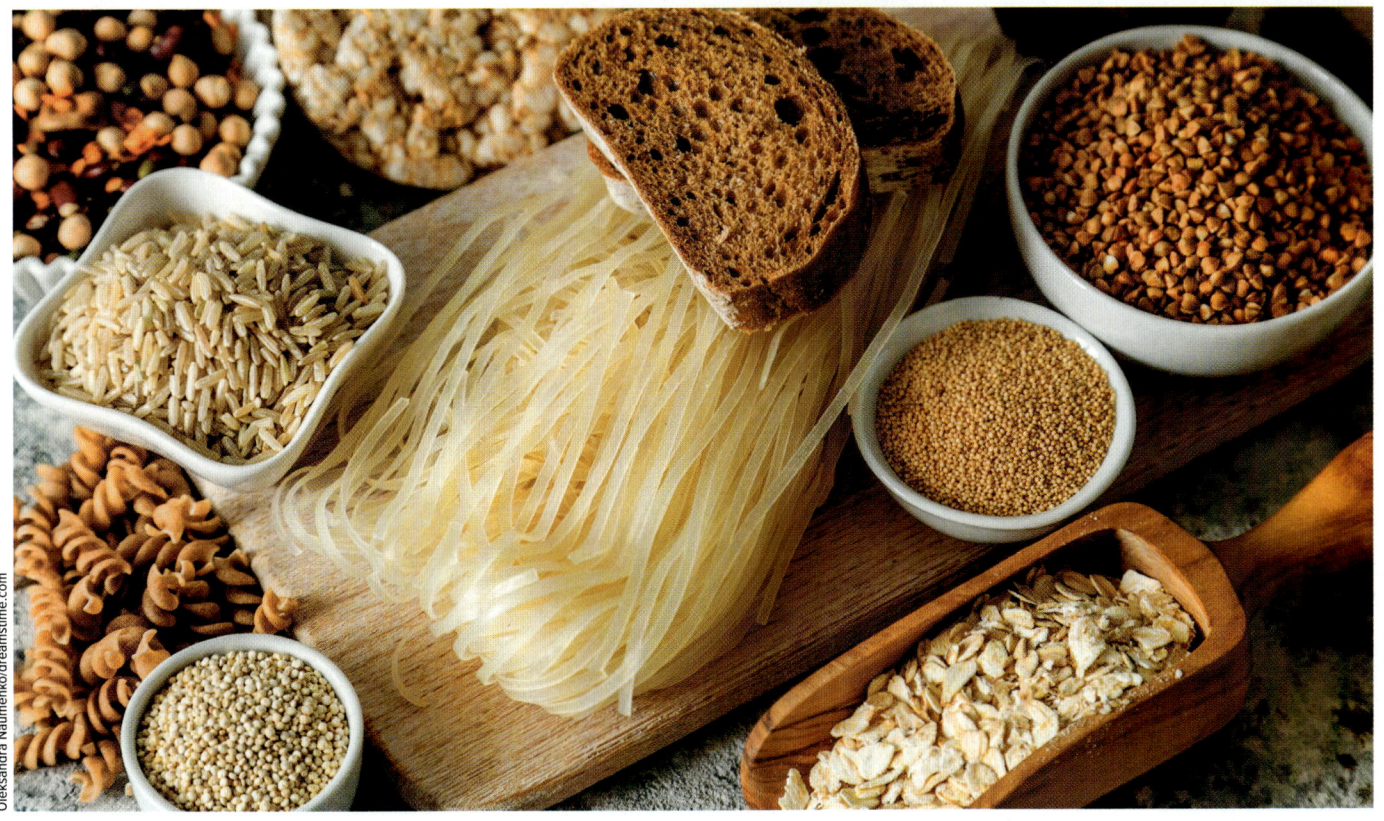

Najett Dahlberg

THE GLUTEN-FREE HANDBOOK

Shopping and food swaps

A gluten-free diet doesn't have to be a boring one, or a worrying challenge for anyone catering for friends and family who can't eat gluten. There are lots of gluten-free equivalents for recipe ingredients and gluten-free ranges that can be bought instead of those using wheat and other grains.

Some gluten-free foods are more expensive than their gluten equivalents because they are not produced in such great quantities, but there are lots of safe ingredients for home cooking. A gluten-free diet can also be a healthy one as it naturally consists of low carbohydrate and an abundance of vegetables and fruit; you just have to beware of too much fat and sugar, particularly in processed meals.

So, what is safe to eat?

Grains
Quinoa
Brown rice
Wild rice
Buckwheat
Sorghum
Tapioca
Millet
Amaranth
Teff
Polenta
Arrowroot
Oats – although these are often produced in a factory where gluten is present, so it is best to choose those oats labelled gluten-free

Flours
Almond
Gram (chickpea)
Amaranth
Buckwheat
Teff
Rice
Sorghum
Corn and cornmeal

Meat and fish
All types of fresh meat, poultry, fish, and shellfish
However, check ground meats, for instance pre-prepared hamburgers, which may have additives such as breadcrumbs

Meat alternatives
Tofu
Quorn – but check if buying pre-prepared dishes using Quorn as these may contain gluten

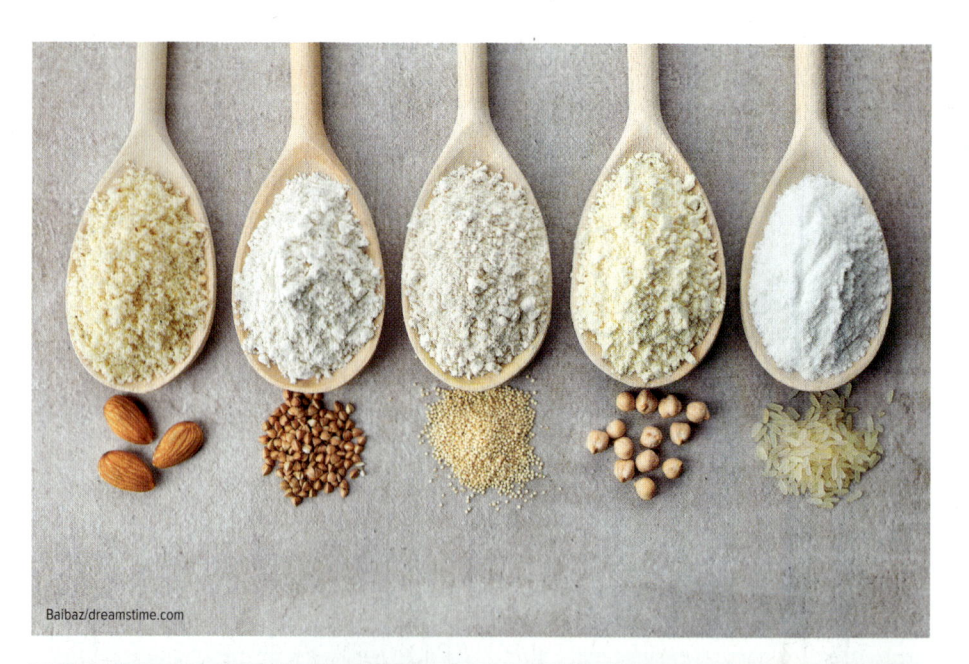

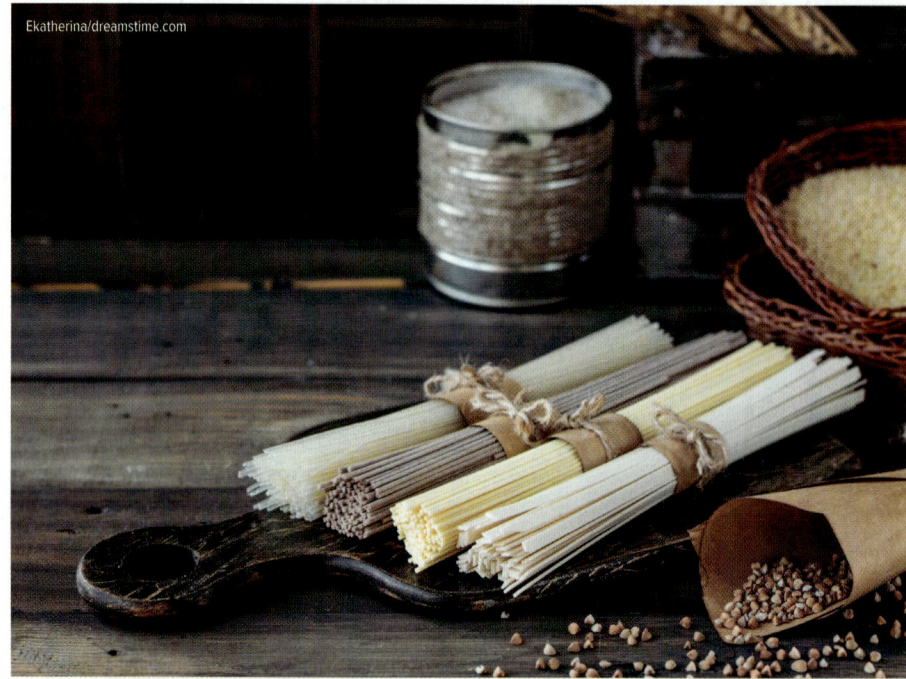

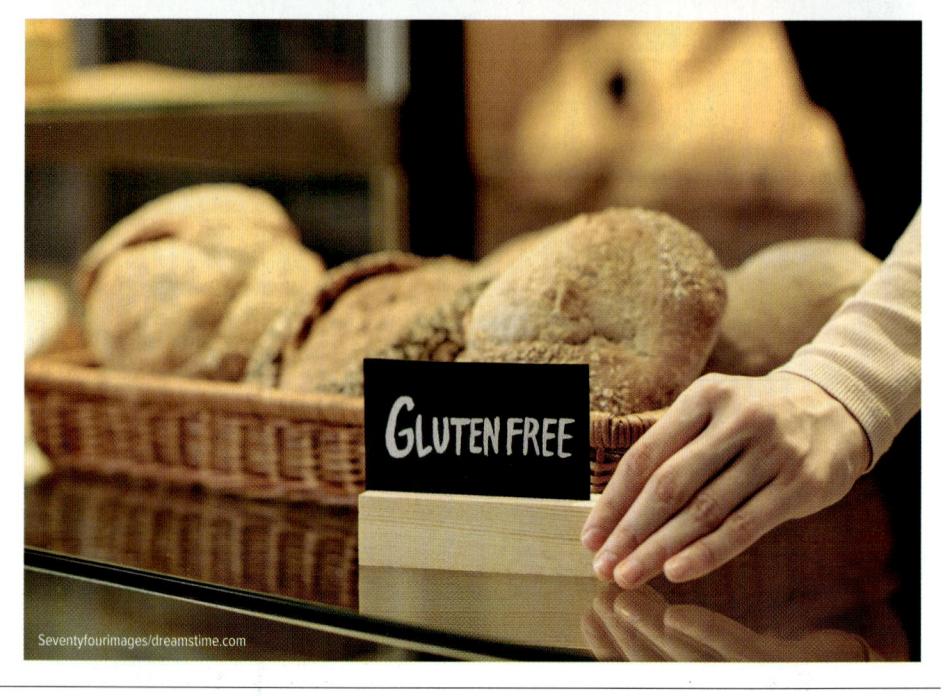

HOW TO LIVE GLUTEN FREE

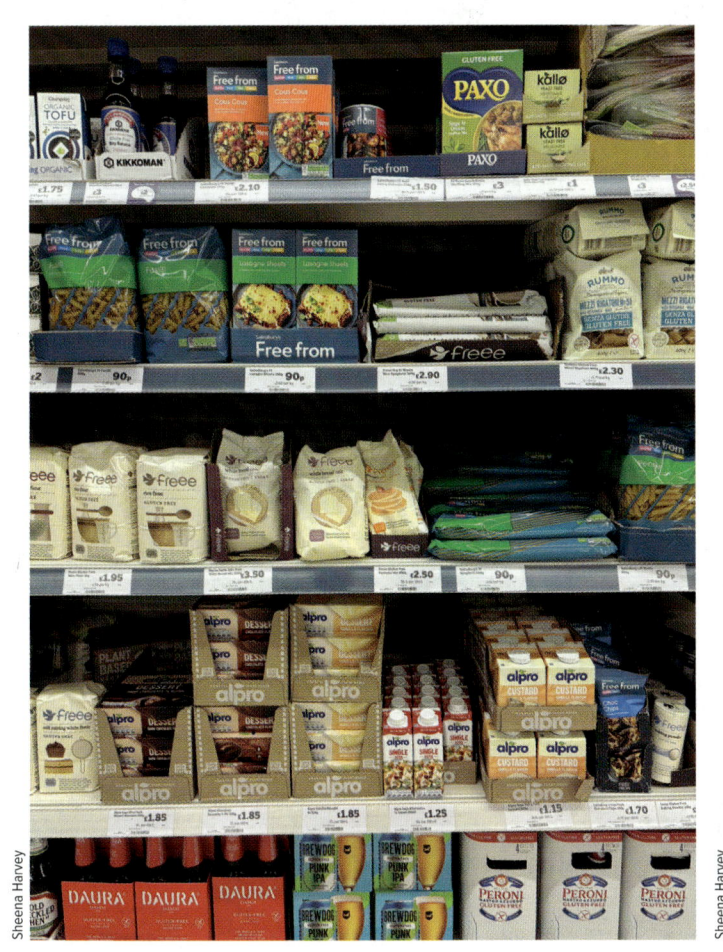

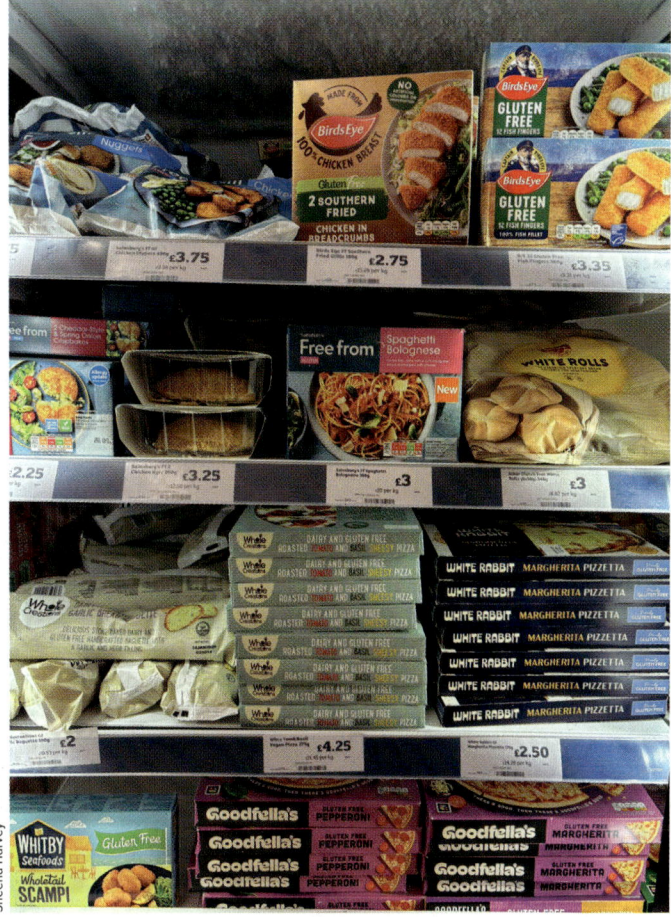

Soya protein – but check processed soy products
Tempeh

Vegetables and Fruit
Brassicas – cauliflower, broccoli, cabbage, Brussels sprouts, kale, cavolo nero, pak choy, collard greens, kohlrabi
Root vegetables – potatoes, parsnips, turnips, swede (rutabaga), carrots, radishes
Sweetcorn
Squashes
Mushrooms of all types
The onion family – red and Spanish onions, spring onions, chives
The pepper family – green, red, orange, and yellow bell peppers, chillis
Legumes – green beans, runner beans, fine beans, mange tout, sugar snaps, lentils, split peas, chickpeas, haricot beans, borlotti beans, black beans, soybeans, and edamame

All types of nuts and seeds, apart from coated peanuts and flavoured nuts. Check dry roasted nuts as they may contain wheat flour or other ingredients containing gluten.

Fresh fruit of all varieties
However, anyone who has, or suspects they have, a Non-Coeliac Gluten Sensitivity should also be aware that they may be sensitive to FODMAP fruits (see page 42).

Where you need to check
There are some fruit and vegetable products that have hidden gluten. These are:

Tinned products – these can have juice and sauce that has been thickened with gluten. Choose those tinned in water or natural juice.
Frozen products – they can have added flavouring or coatings that contain gluten.
Dried fruit – can contain gluten derivatives. Look for natural, unsweetened varieties.
Pre-prepared fruit and vegetables – can be cross-contaminated with gluten depending on the factory where they were processed.

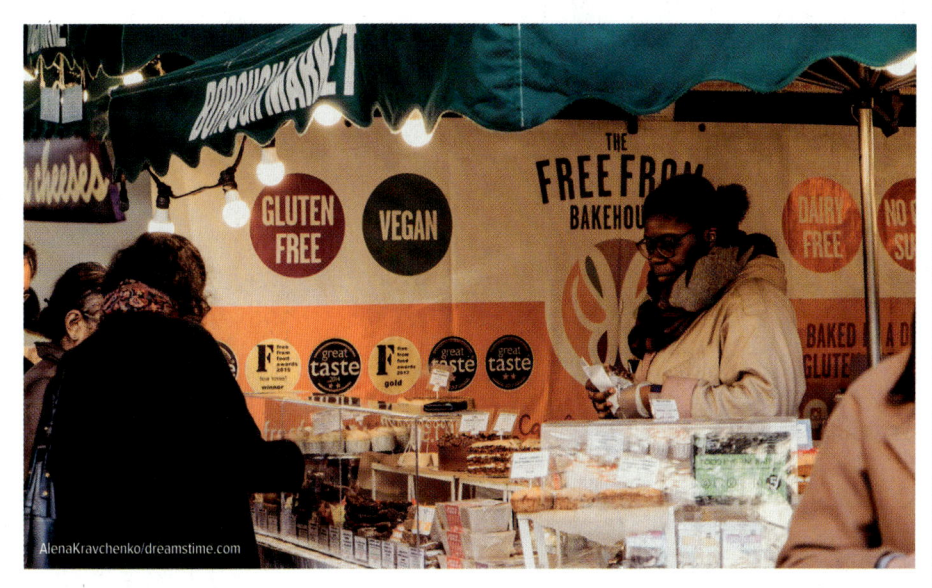

THE GLUTEN-FREE HANDBOOK

67

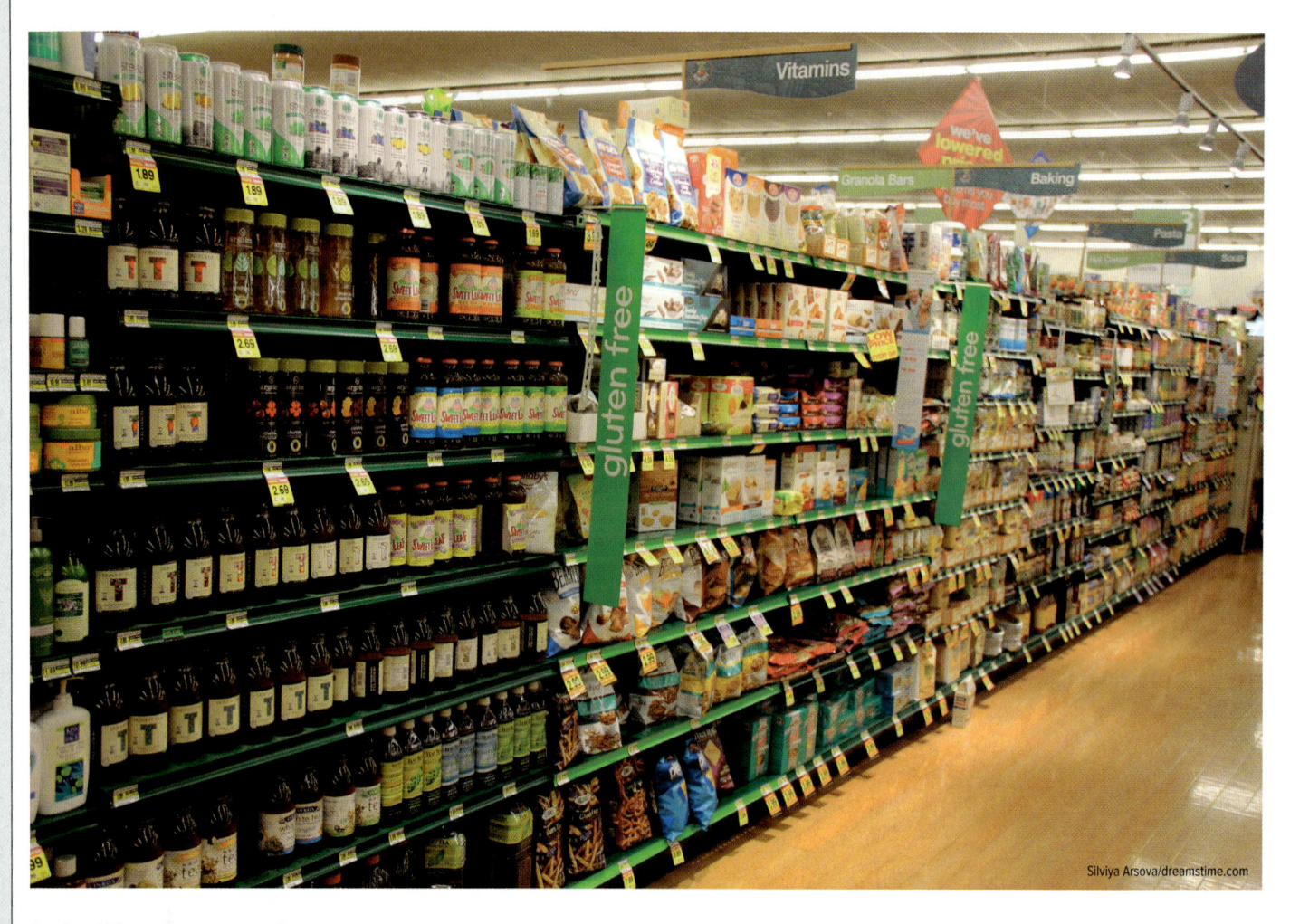

Labelling laws and guidelines

There are regulations in place in many countries to ensure only foods that are truly gluten-free can use that label on their packaging. Products must contain fewer than 20 parts per million of gluten or they cannot be labelled 'gluten-free'.

There are no requirements for manufacturers to put their labelling in a particular place on the product or in a particular size, so you must be prepared to do some searching in many cases.

United Kingdom and European Union

All packaged foods in the UK and the EU are covered by labelling laws, which include rules around the allergen information that must be provided on the label. There are two types – 'prepacked' and 'prepacked for direct sale'.

Prepacked

Refers to food that has been encased in packaging before it is put on sale, i.e. a bag of sugar or a packet of bacon.

Prepacked for direct sale

Refers to food that is presented unwrapped at the point of sale but is wrapped when it is handed to the customer, i.e. a sandwich or a salad box in a delicatessen.

In all cases of prepacked food, the 'deliberately used' (not accidentally introduced by cross-contamination) must be listed in order of the highest to lowest quantities. If something containing gluten, or another known allergen, is in the ingredients it must be highlighted in bold or in some other way emphasised.

If there is a risk of cross-contamination, manufacturers have been given the option by the UK Food Standards Authority to print a warning on the label such as 'made on a line/in a factory handling wheat' or 'may contain traces of gluten'.

Coeliac UK has a scheme whereby their scientists thoroughly check a food item and its manufacture and issue the food producer with a Crossed Grain Trademark symbol they can print on their labels for that product.

North America

The United States Food & Drug Administration (USFDA) rules

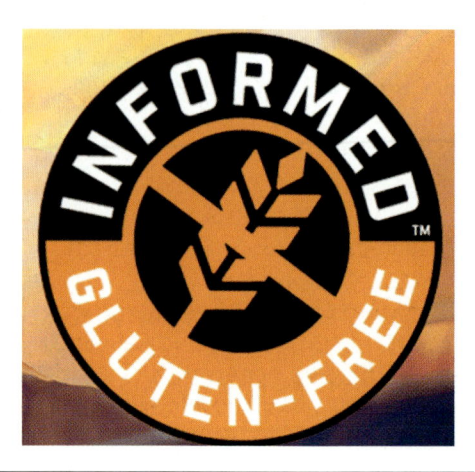

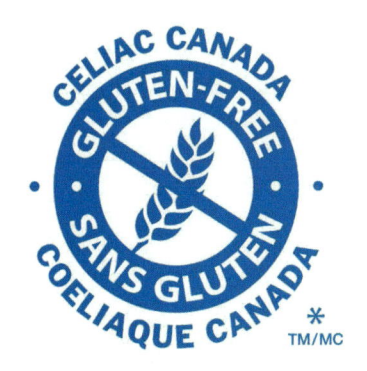

establish the requirements for the voluntary use of 'gluten-free' on a manufacturer's products. It defines the term 'gluten-free' to mean that the food bearing the claim does not contain an ingredient that is a gluten-containing grain (i.e. spelt wheat).

It should also not contain an ingredient that is derived from a gluten-containing grain that has not been processed to remove gluten (i.e. wheat flour). And it should not contain an ingredient that is derived from a gluten-containing grain that has been processed to remove gluten (i.e. wheat starch), if the use of that ingredient results in the presence of 20 parts per million or more gluten in the food which equates to 20 milligrams or more gluten per kilogram of food.

The USFDA also applies the same parts-per-million rule to fermented and hydrolysed foods, such as pickles, soups, and sauces, if they are labelled as gluten-free.

The US National Celiac Association and the Celiac Sprue Association have certification labels for food manufacturers and catering establishments. They certify products and processes as being safe for anyone with a gluten sensitivity.

In Canada, Celiac Canada provides a similar certification programme with a logo that manufacturers can put on their labels once approved.

Australia

Food Standards Australia New Zealand (FSANZ) requires food businesses to meet Plain English allergen labelling for the way certain foods known to be common allergens are declared. A bolded, separate allergen summary statement starting with the word 'contains' also has to be provided near the ingredient list to help identify any allergens present quickly. For example, 'Contains milk'.

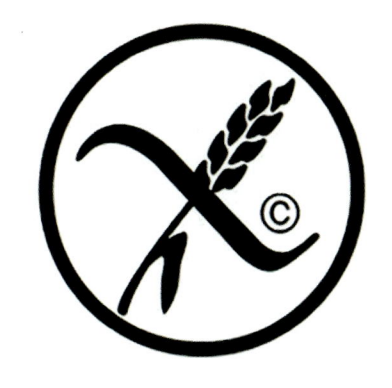

If a cereal containing gluten – wheat, barley, oats, rye, and hybrids of these cereals such as triticale – is present, the label will have to identify this in the summary statement using the word 'gluten'.

If the food is not in packaging or does not need to have a label, the information must be displayed with the food or be available on request from the supplier. A note on the label about the unintended presence of gluten from cross-contamination is voluntary and not a requirement.

The Celiac Australia Gluten Free Accreditation Program licenses businesses to use its Trademark endorsement symbol.

Mystery ingredients

There are a number of lesser-known ingredients on a label that sound like they might be a problem but are actually safe. Although in the case of anything labelled 'starch' it would be prudent to also check for 'gluten-free' wording or a certification logo as well.

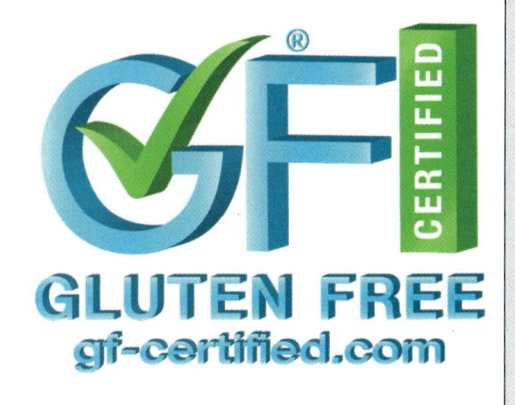

Codex wheat starch (this has been washed to remove most of the gluten to trace levels)
Cornstarch
Diglycerides
Distilled alcohol
Guar gum powder – used as a thickener
Linseed
Maltodextrin – despite having malt in the name, it is refined to remove gluten
Modified starch (this is different to modified wheat starch as it comes from a different grain)
Monoglycerides
Whey concentrate
Whey hydrolysate
Whey isolate
Xanthan gum

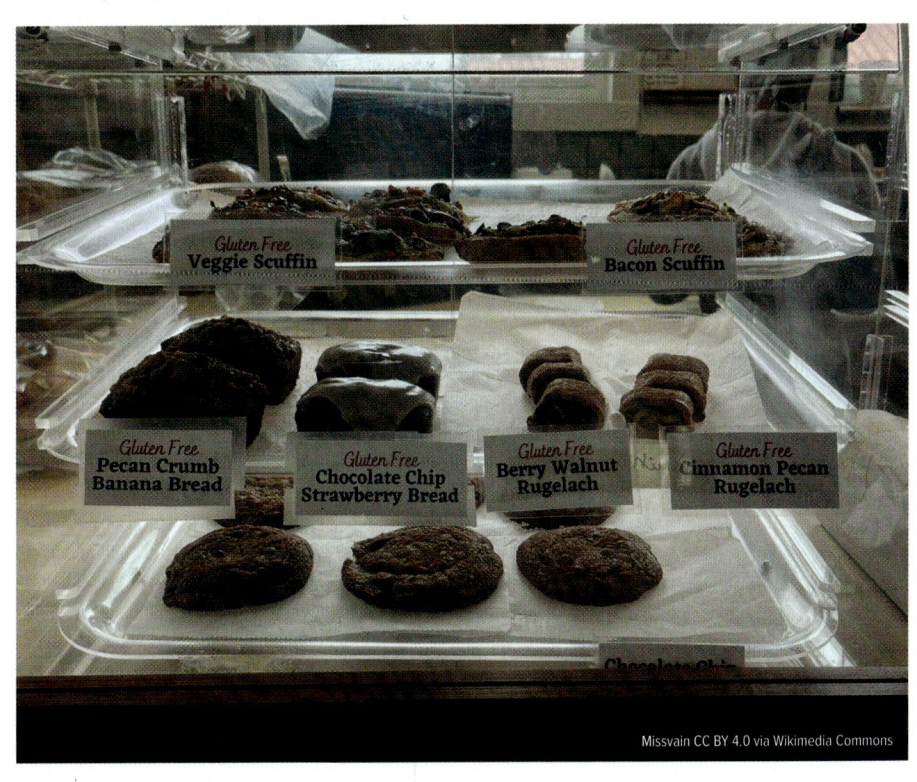

Missvain CC BY 4.0 via Wikimedia Commons

HOW TO LIVE GLUTEN FREE

Gluten-free food manufacturers

Nowadays there are quite a number of bespoke gluten-free food manufacturers – some that have been in existence for many years – as well as mainstream manufacturers that have branched out into producing gluten-free versions of their products.

All of the following companies supply their products worldwide either in stores or by mail order, apart from where stated. There are also lots of local manufacturers producing gluten-free for their home markets.

Schär
The gluten-free food brand of the Dr Schär company has been producing specialist food products for a variety of conditions for many years.

BFree
A global gluten-free food manufacturer based in Ireland that produces loaves, rolls, flat breads, wraps, pizza bases and pitta breads. Different ranges are sold in supermarkets and grocery stores depending on whether you are in the UK, Europe, the US, or Australia.

Hain Celestial
A company producing gluten-free food among other products and sold through brands such as Arrowhead Mills, Imagine, Rice Dream and Soy Dream, DeBoles and Hain Pure Foods.

Kraft Heinz
This famous manufacturer now produces some gluten-free products and versions of its popular lines.

Kellanova
The well-known Kellogg's cereal and Pringles crisp company produces many of its breakfast brands in gluten-free versions.

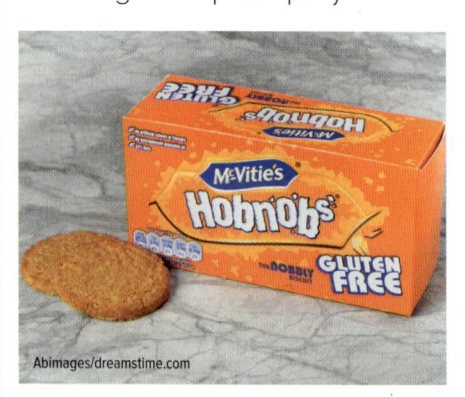

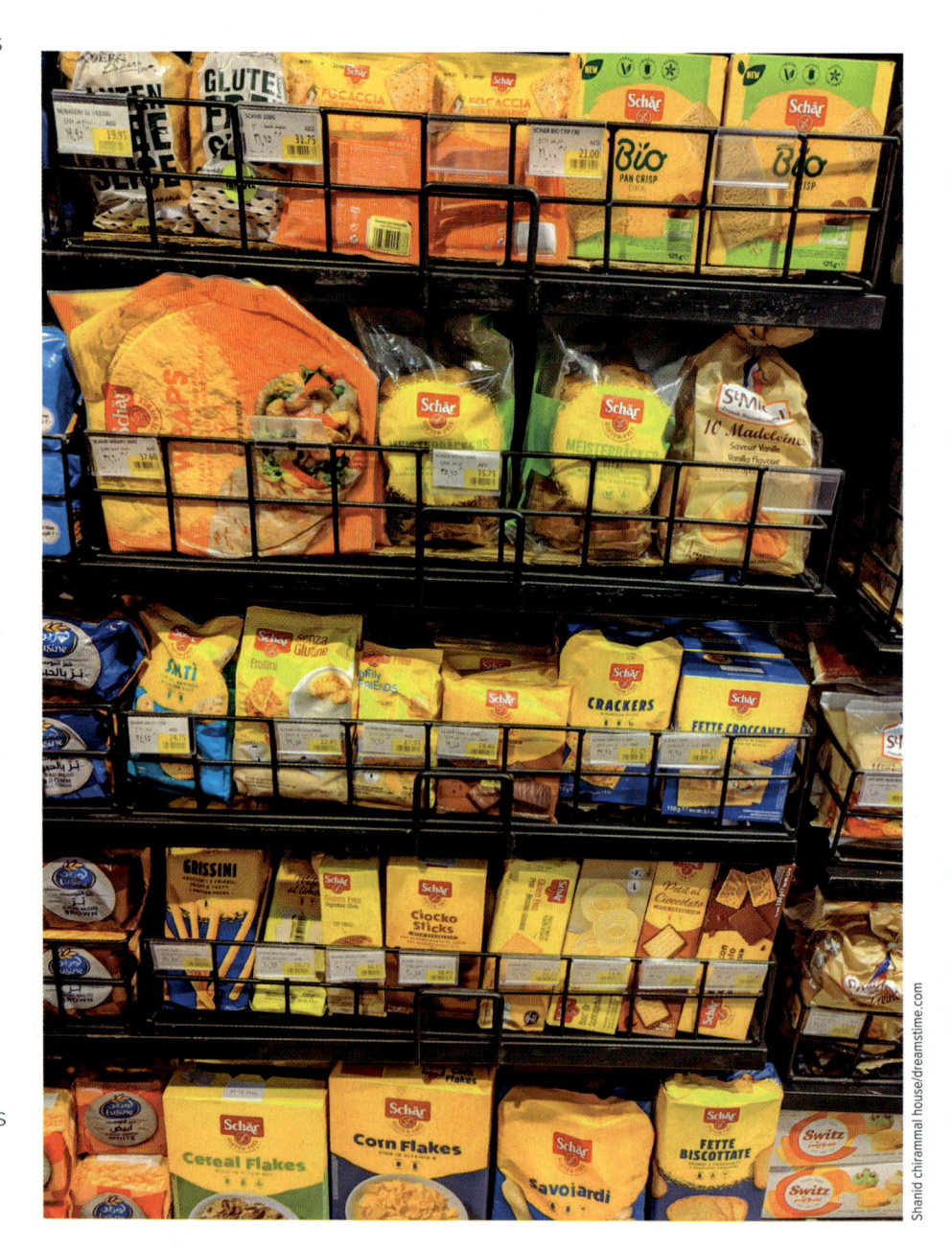

Barilla
A pasta company that produces an extensive gluten-free range.

Mondelez
The international company producing Cadbury, Belvita, Daim, Oreo, Philadelphia, and Ritz, among many others snack and sweet brands, it also manufactures gluten-free products under the brand names Enjoy Life Foods and Tate's Bake Shop.

Amy's Kitchen
US food manufacturer that sells gluten-free products in the UK, US, Canada, and Australia.

Freee by Doves Farm
A dedicated gluten-free manufacturer specialising in flours, pancake mixes, pizza bases and grain bars. UK only online orders.

www.keypublishing.com

HOW TO LIVE GLUTEN FREE

Claudiodivizia/dreamstime.com

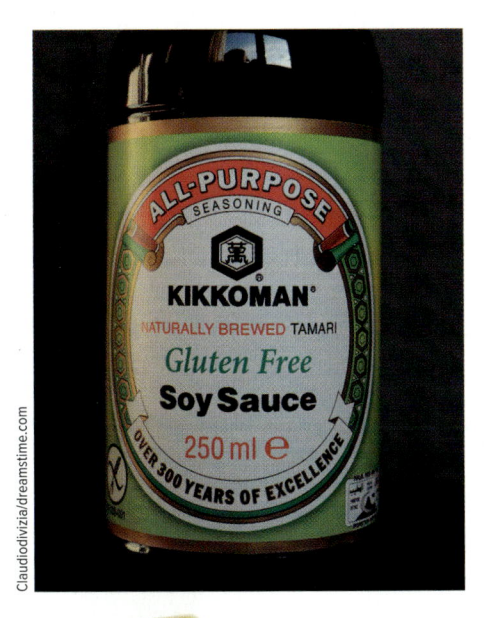

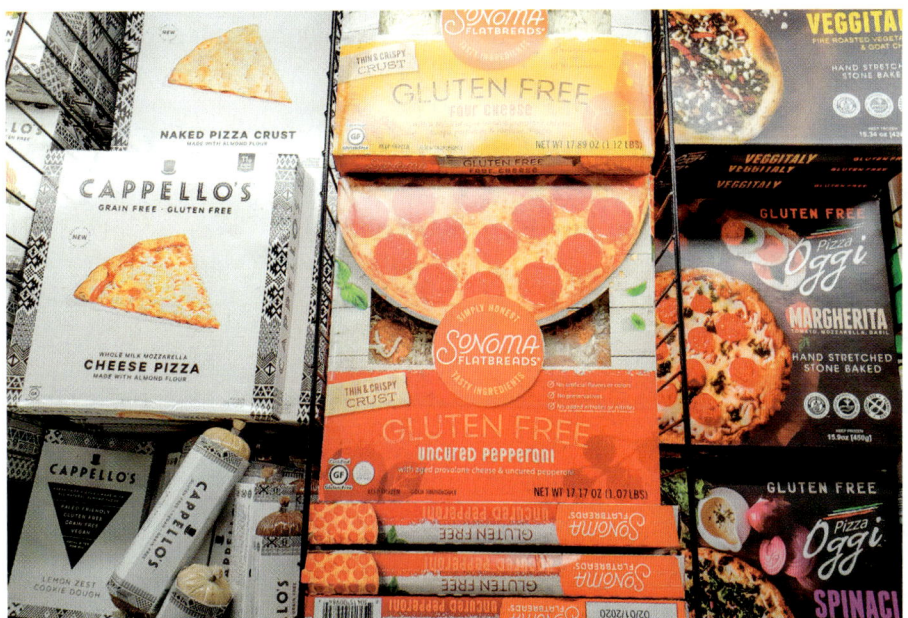

David Tonelson/dreamstime.com

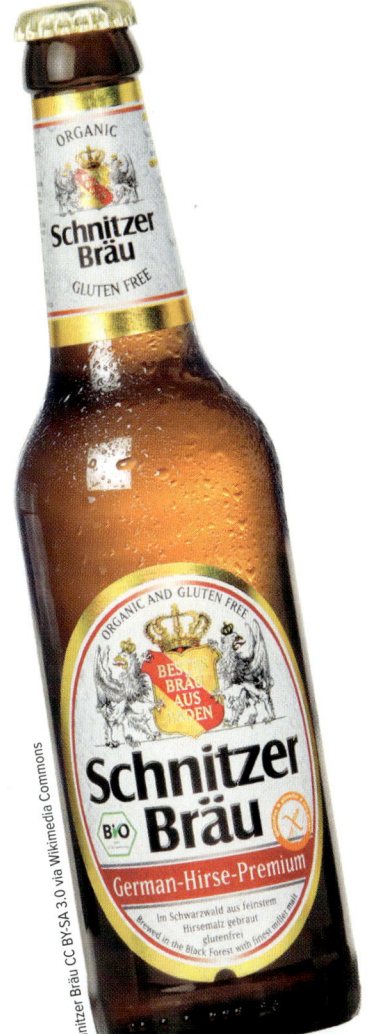

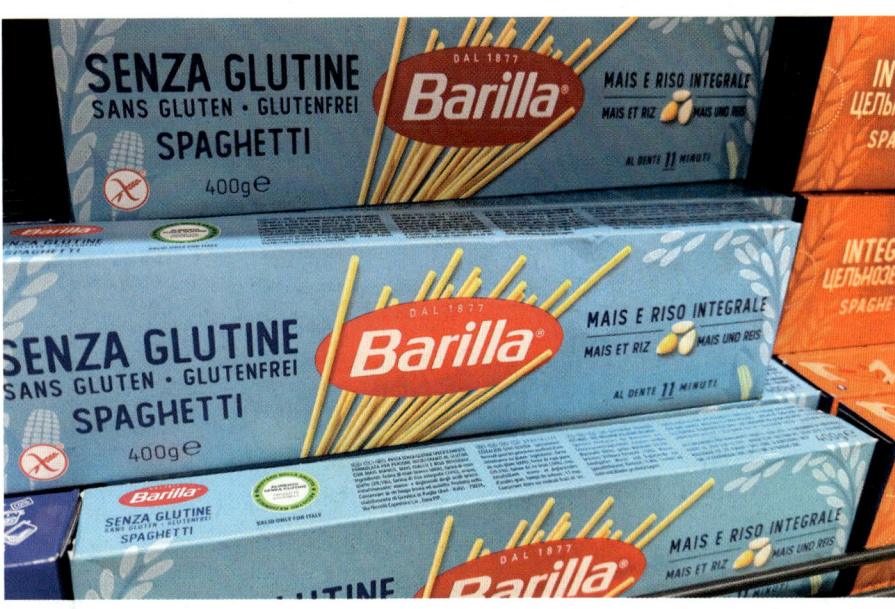

Dzmitry Skazau/dreamstime.com

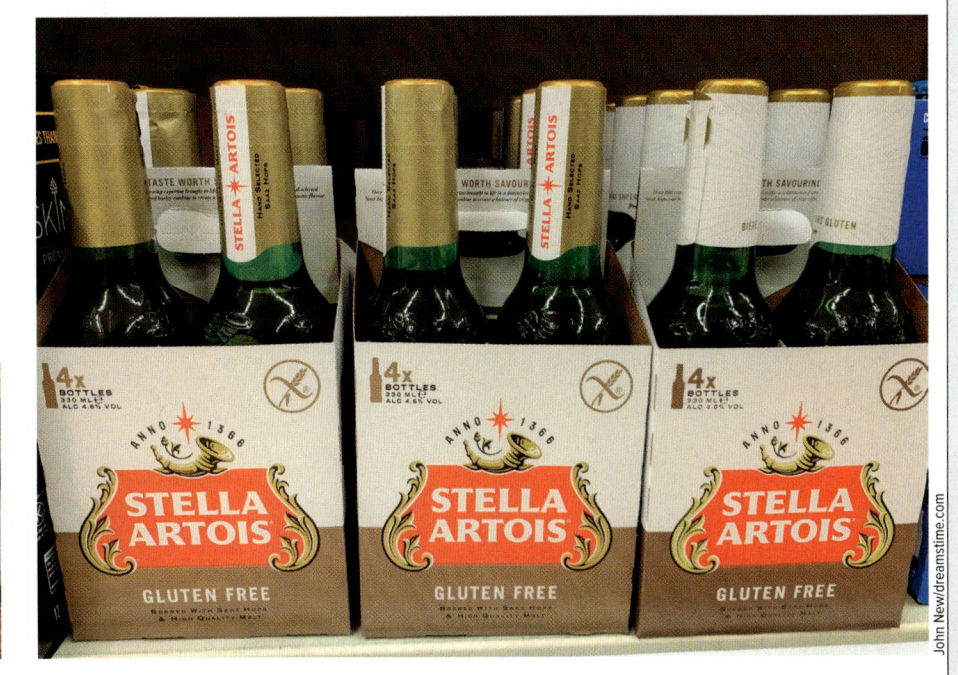

Schnitzer Bräu CC BY-SA 3.0 via Wikimedia Commons

Erin Cadigan/dreamstime.com

John New/dreamstime.com

THE GLUTEN-FREE HANDBOOK

71

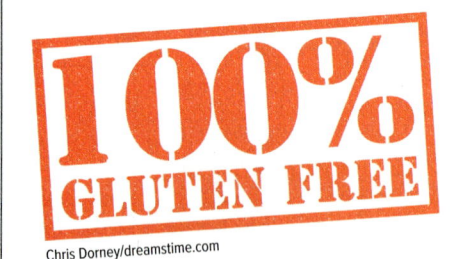

Gluten-free beauty

Most large cosmetic companies cannot guarantee that their products are completely gluten-free because they use a wide range of ingredients from many sources, and they may be processed in a factory that's a gluten environment. In some cases, there are product ingredient cards available at the sales counter or on the company's website and there will be a customer service email or phone number to ask about individual products.

All of the following brands claim some or all of their products are gluten-free, and they are available to customers in most countries, either in store or by mail order direct from the company or from one of the general mail order cosmetic websites.

Alima Pure
www.alimapure.com
Alima Pure makes carbon-neutral, mineral-based makeup that is not tested on animals. The company FAQs state: "All of our products are formulated without gluten-containing ingredients. However, only our loose powder products are created on designated gluten-free equipment."

Gabriel Cosmetics
https://gabrielcosmeticsinc.com
Gabriel and its brands Zuzu Luxe and Clean Kids Naturally have been certified gluten-free by the Gluten Intolerance Group. They are made with natural ingredients with no synthetic chemicals or animal products.

Jane Iredale
https://janeiredale.co.uk
Most of this company's products are gluten-free with a few exceptions that are noted in the Vegan and Gluten Information section of its website. Shipping outside the UK is at the company's discretion but its products are available on other general mail order sites.

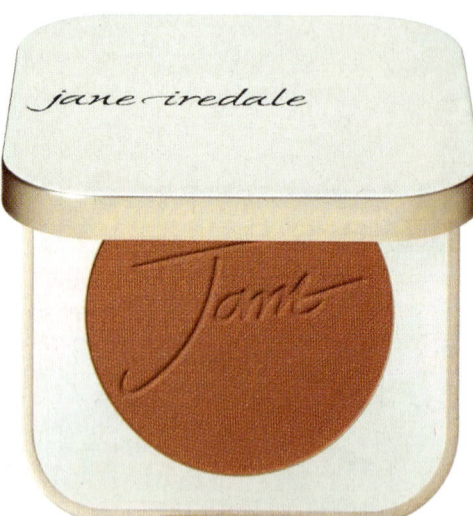

Lily Lolo
www.lilylolo.co.uk
The statement on the Lily Lolo website says: "Not all of our products are gluten-free. The products that are gluten-free are our Lipsticks, Mascara, Concealer, Correctors, Loose eye shadows, Loose Blush, Foundation, Finishing Powder, Bronzers, Lip Glosses, Pressed Eye Shadows, Pressed Blush. All ingredients are listed on our website and packaging if you ever want to check this for yourself too.

With regards to the cross-contamination – the products that are gluten-free are definitely all 100% free from gluten however we cannot guarantee that the environment in which they are developed is completely free from gluten due to our supplier possibly producing products that contain gluten for other brands."

Pangea Organics
https://pangeaorganics.com
A skincare collection that uses plant-based ingredients but confirms in its FAQs that all products are gluten-free. Its website also states: "Pangea offers an open disclosure policy regarding ingredients, so if there is any particular botanical you seek to avoid, you will see it clearly listed in both the Latin and common English names on the ingredient panel or in the Ingredients tab on each product's page."

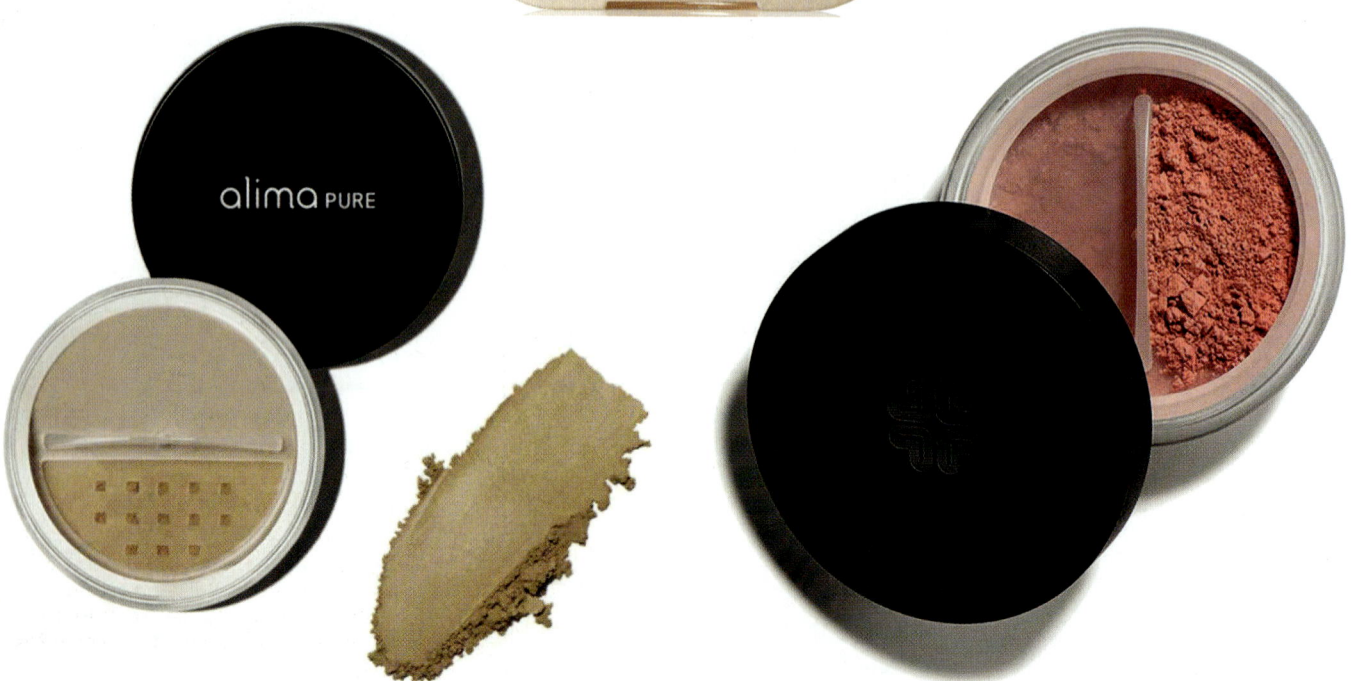

HOW TO LIVE GLUTEN FREE

Red Apple Lipstick
https://redapplelipstick.com
The website states: "Our products are all gluten-free by design and safe from cross contamination. Products are designed and made for persons with Celiac Disease."

Herbal Essences bio:renew shampoos and conditioners
https://herbalessences.com
The bio-renew range is gluten-free in line with the Cosmetics Directive of the European Union Commission, which means they do not contain gluten or any of over 1,300 other ingredients that are excluded by the regulation for personal care and beauty products.

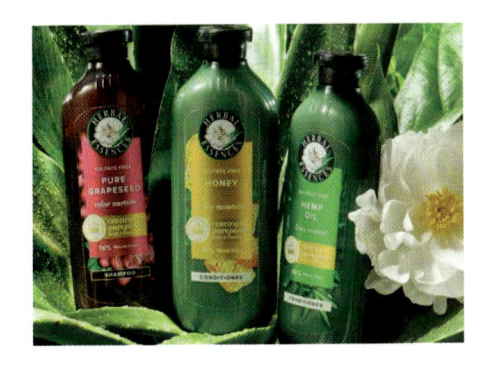

Kirkland Signature shampoo and conditioner
www.costco.co.uk/kirkland-signature; www.costco.com
This is a Costco own brand that is labelled gluten-free and vegan.

Maui Moisture
www.mauimoisture.com
Products do not contain direct sources of gluten, but the items are manufactured in the same facility as other products that do contain gluten.

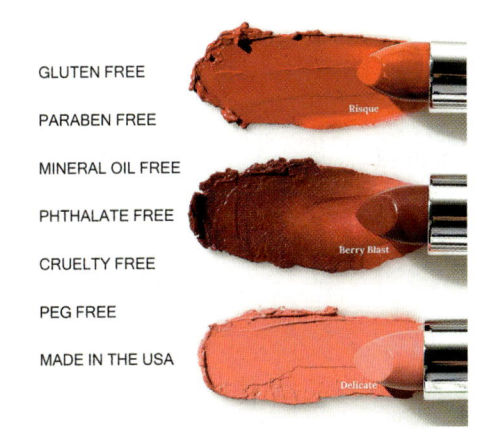

Paul Mitchell
www.paul-mitchell.co.uk/en/gluten-free
Many of this company's hair products are gluten-free. The website can be searched for gluten-free products.

Pravana Truity hair care products
www.pravana.com
Truity is the company's gluten-free range. Others of its products may also be gluten-free, but it cannot guarantee that ingredients have not been touched by gluten in the supply chain.

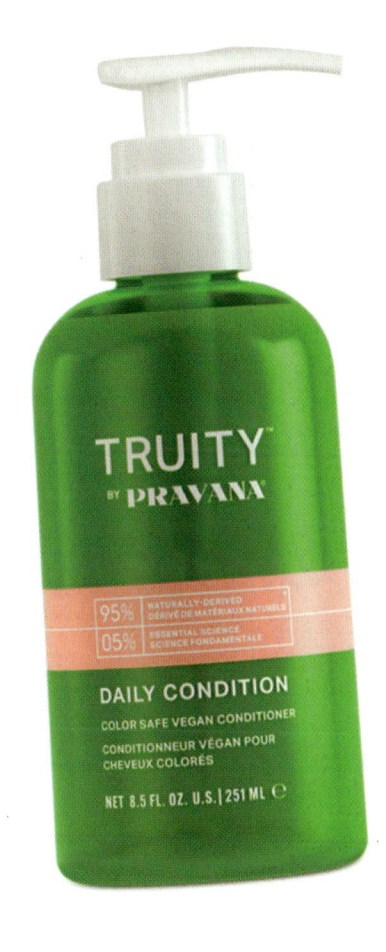

Purezero
www.purezerobeauty.com
The company says that all of its haircare products are gluten-free.

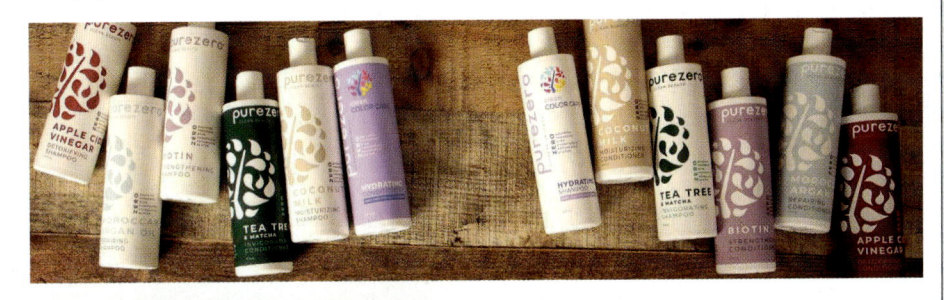

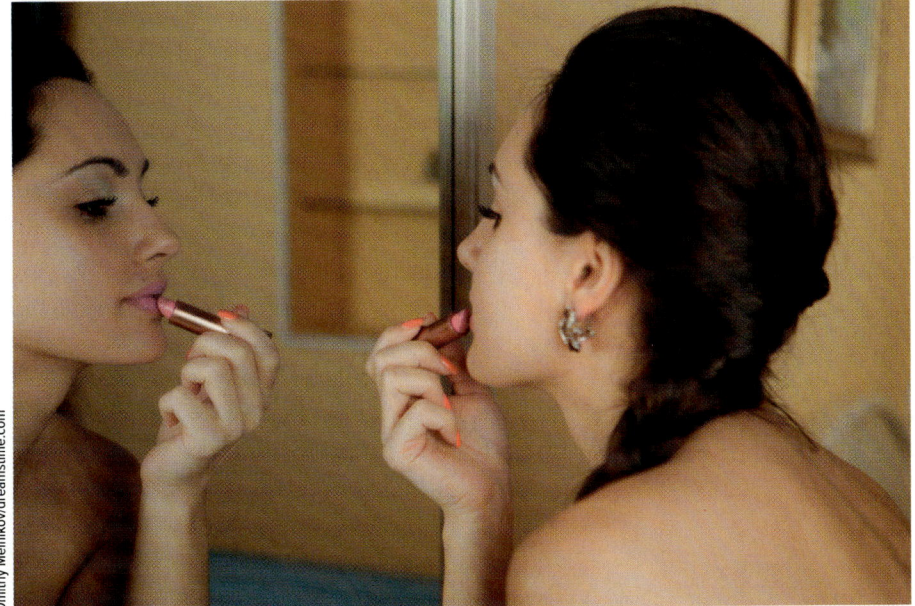

TRESemmé
www.tresemme.com
Some of the company products are gluten-free. A company statement says: "For ingredient labelling our company follows the guidelines of the US Food & Drug Administration (FDA) and uses the International Nomenclature for Cosmetics Ingredients (INCI). If any wheat, rye, barley, or oat-derived raw materials are in our products, they would be listed on the labels."

This is not an exhaustive list. There are many beauty, skin and haircare products that do not contain gluten, so it is best to check packaging and the companies' websites for ingredient information. The list was correct at the time of going to press.

THE GLUTEN-FREE HANDBOOK

Gluten-Free Recipes

Pepperoni and

Prep 20 min
Cook 15-20 min
Makes 2 pizzas

INGREDIENTS

For the base
260g sour cream
250g gluten-free self-raising flour
¼ tsp xanthan gum (can be omitted if the flour contains it)
½ tsp gluten-free baking powder (optional)
½ tsp salt

For the topping
Jar or carton of passata
1 tsp oregano
2 tsp garlic infused oil
Salt and pepper
Grated cheese (mozzarella and cheddar)
Packet of pepperoni slices
Black olives, chopped or sliced
Fresh basil
Mushrooms, thinly sliced

METHOD

1. Mix the base ingredients in a large bowl to form a dough.
2. On a floured board knead the dough briefly until smooth then cut in half and roll out each half quite thinly, to about 25cm across.
3. Heat a frying pan – no oil needed. Carefully lift one of the rolled rounds of dough and place it in the pan. Dry fry on both sides for a few minutes but don't allow to brown too much.
4. Transfer the round to a baking tray. Repeat with the second round.
5. In the meantime, heat oven to 425°F (220°C).
6. Mix together the passata, oregano, garlic infused oil and add salt and pepper to taste. Spread this mixture onto each base. Cover with the mix of grated cheese and top with pepperoni, mushrooms and olive.
7. Bake in the oven until the cheese has melted – about 10 min. Decorate with some fresh basil leaves.

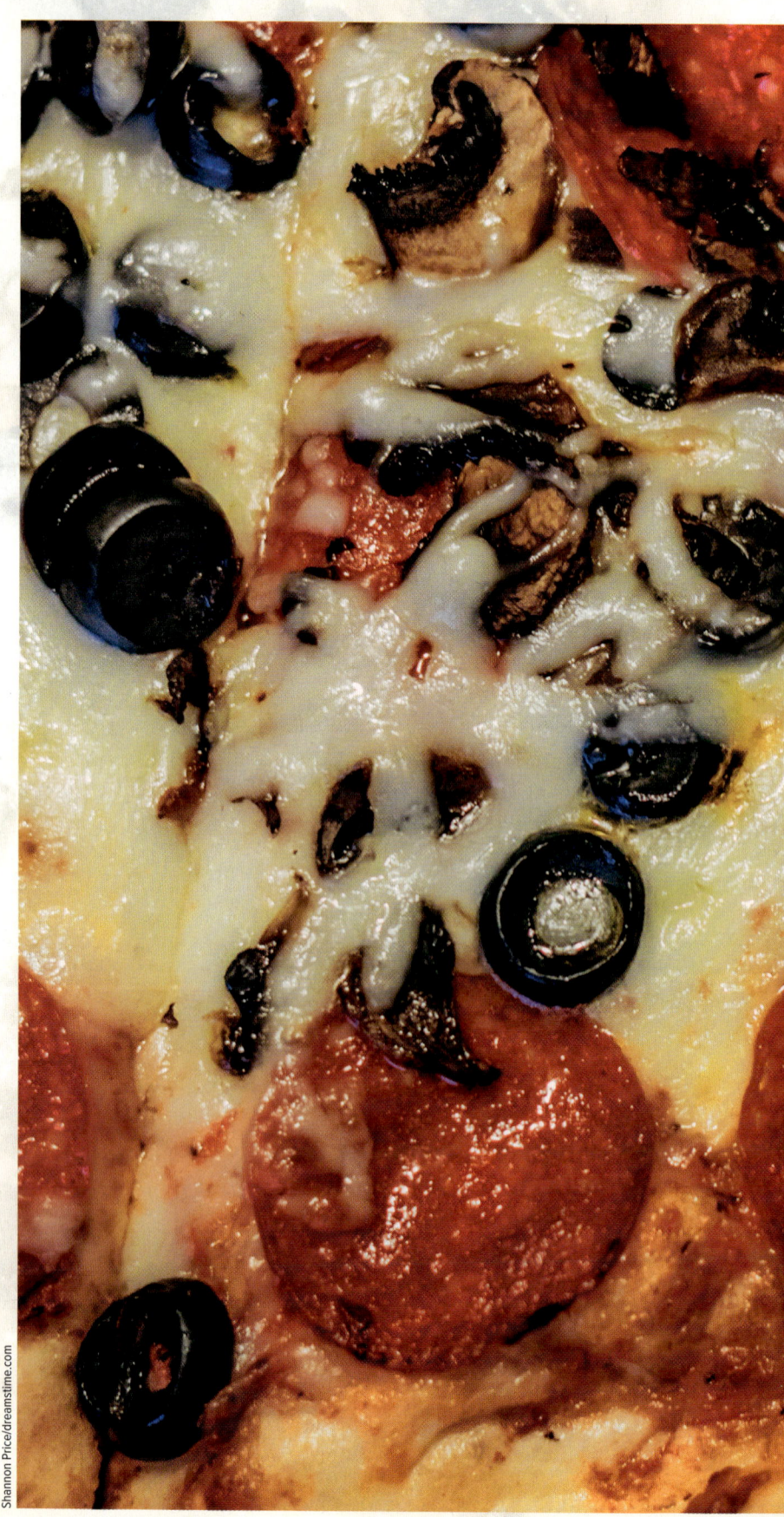

Shannon Price/dreamstime.com

GLUTEN-FREE RECIPES

Olive Pizza

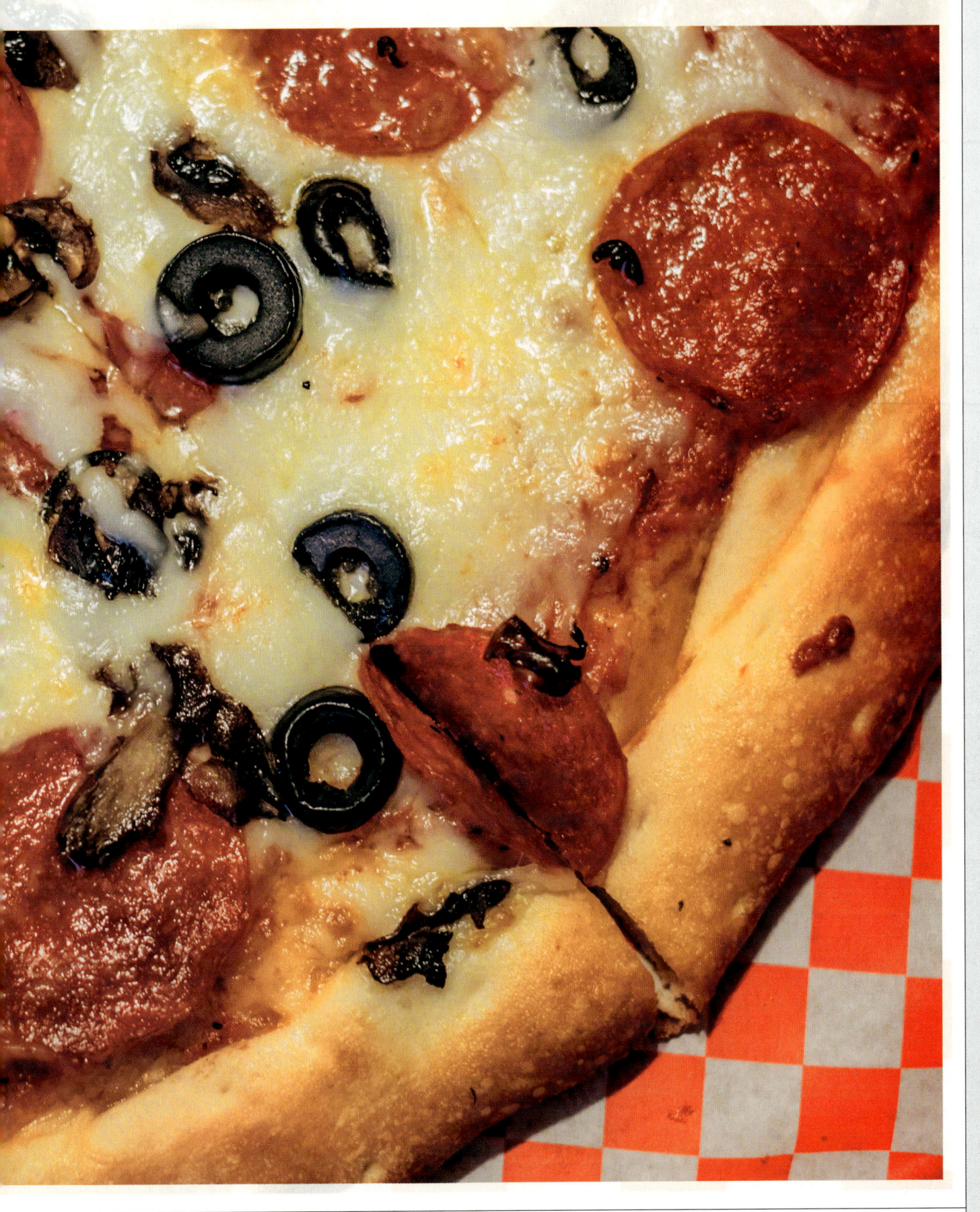

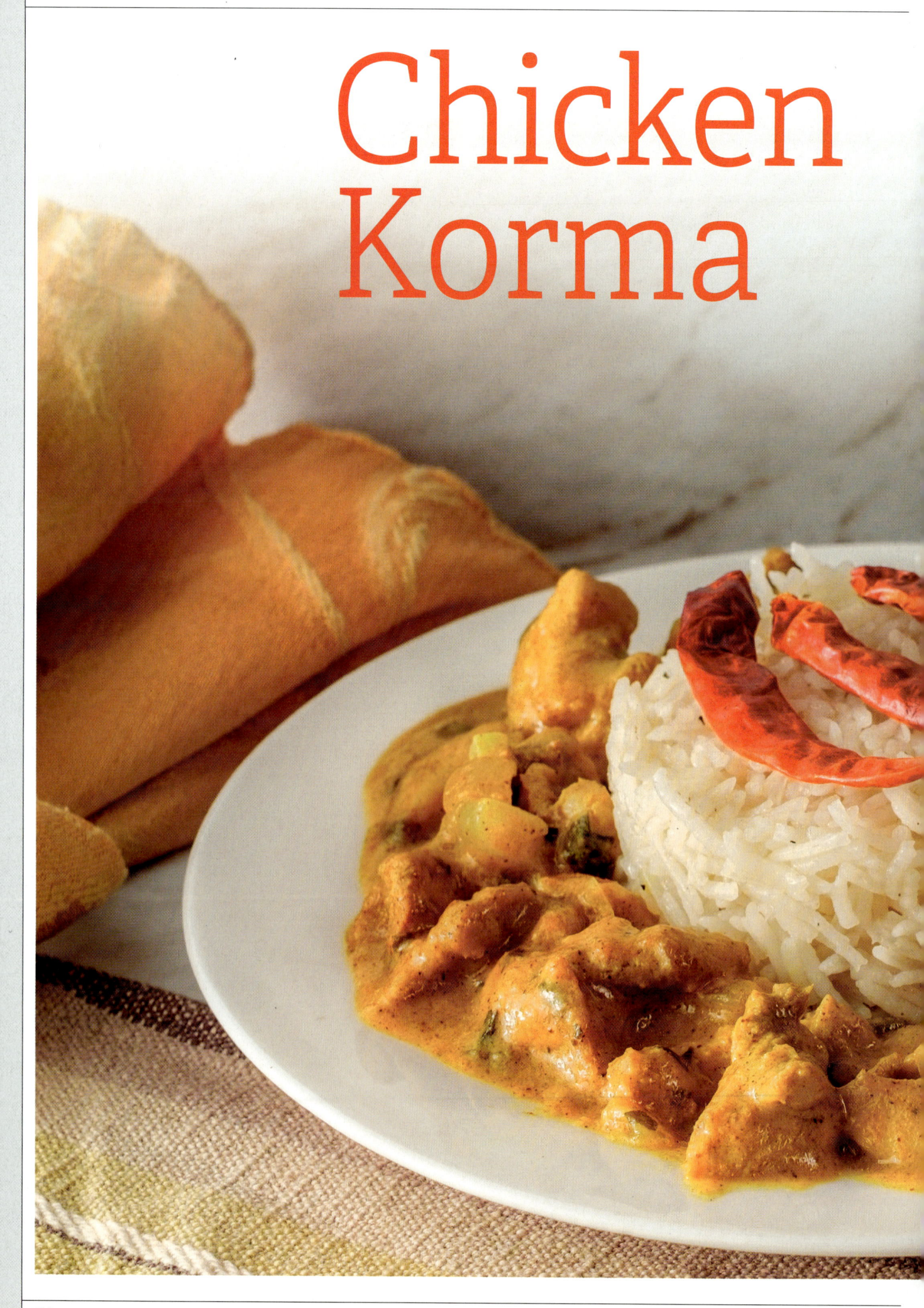

GLUTEN-FREE RECIPES

Chicken Korma

GLUTEN-FREE RECIPES

Prep 15 min plus 12 to 24 hrs for marinading
Slow cook between 3 and 6 hrs
Serves 2

INGREDIENTS
600g chicken breast, cut into good-sized chunks

For the marinade
100g natural yoghurt
1 tbsp mild curry powder
½ tsp turmeric
1 tsp cumin

For the sauce
1 onion
1 tsp chopped ginger
2 tsp chopped garlic
2 tbsp tomato purée
1 tbsp mango chutney
½ tsp salt
45g ground almonds
250ml gluten-free chicken stock
75ml double cream
30g desiccated coconut

To serve
Cooked rice
Chilli peppers to garnish

METHOD
1. Combine marinade ingredients in a bowl and add the chicken breast chunks, mixing to make sure the pieces are well coated. Leave in the fridge overnight or for up to 24 hrs.
2. When ready to cook, remove the chicken chunks from the marinade and place them in a slow cooker along with all sauce ingredients apart from double cream and desiccated coconut.
3. Cook for 3-4 hrs on high or 5-6 hrs on low.
4. At the end of the cooking time add the cream and coconut. For a thicker sauce add a tbsp of cornflour. Cook for another 30 min on high. Serve with boiled rice and decorate with chilli peppers.

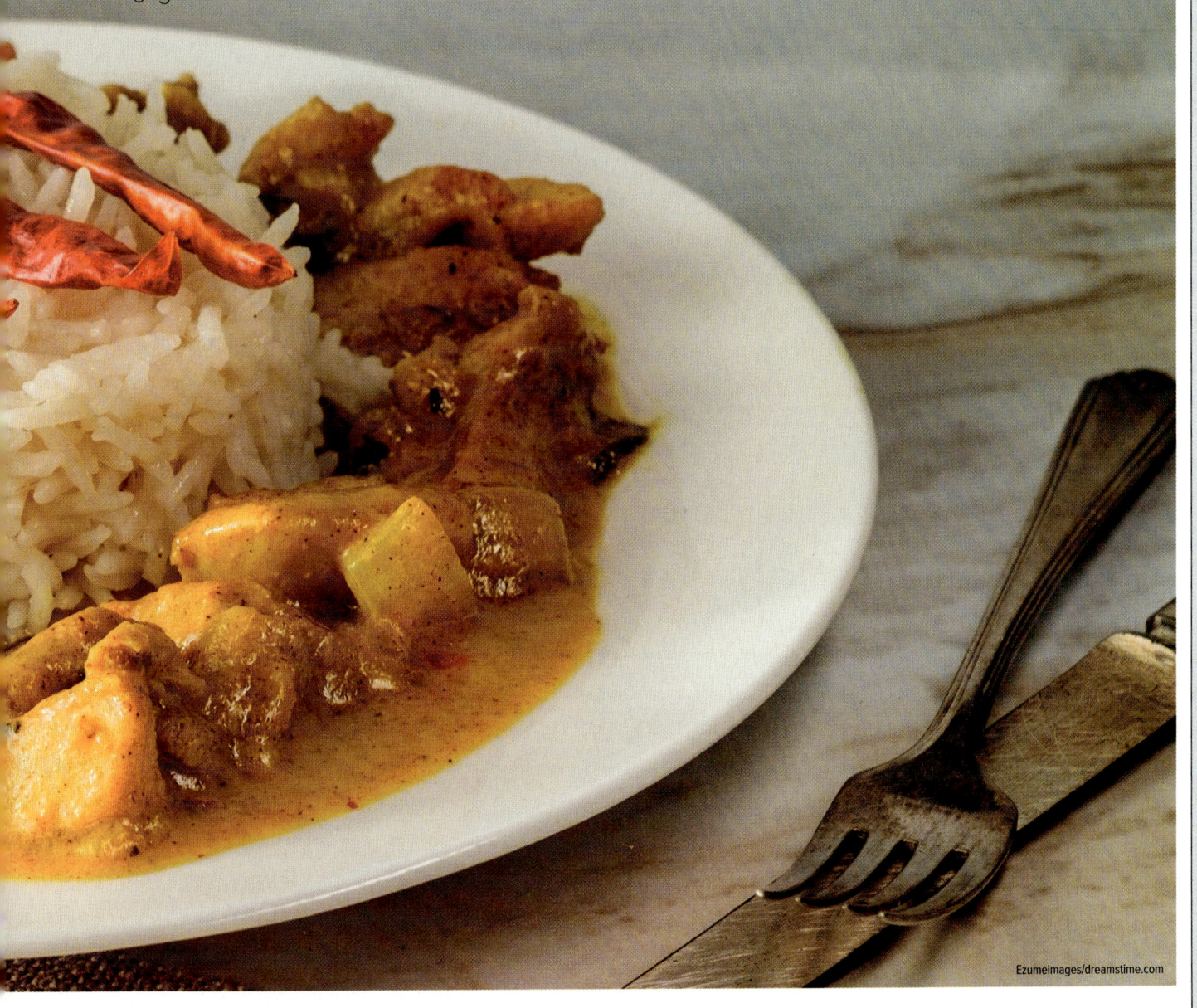

Ezumeimages/dreamstime.com

THE GLUTEN-FREE HANDBOOK

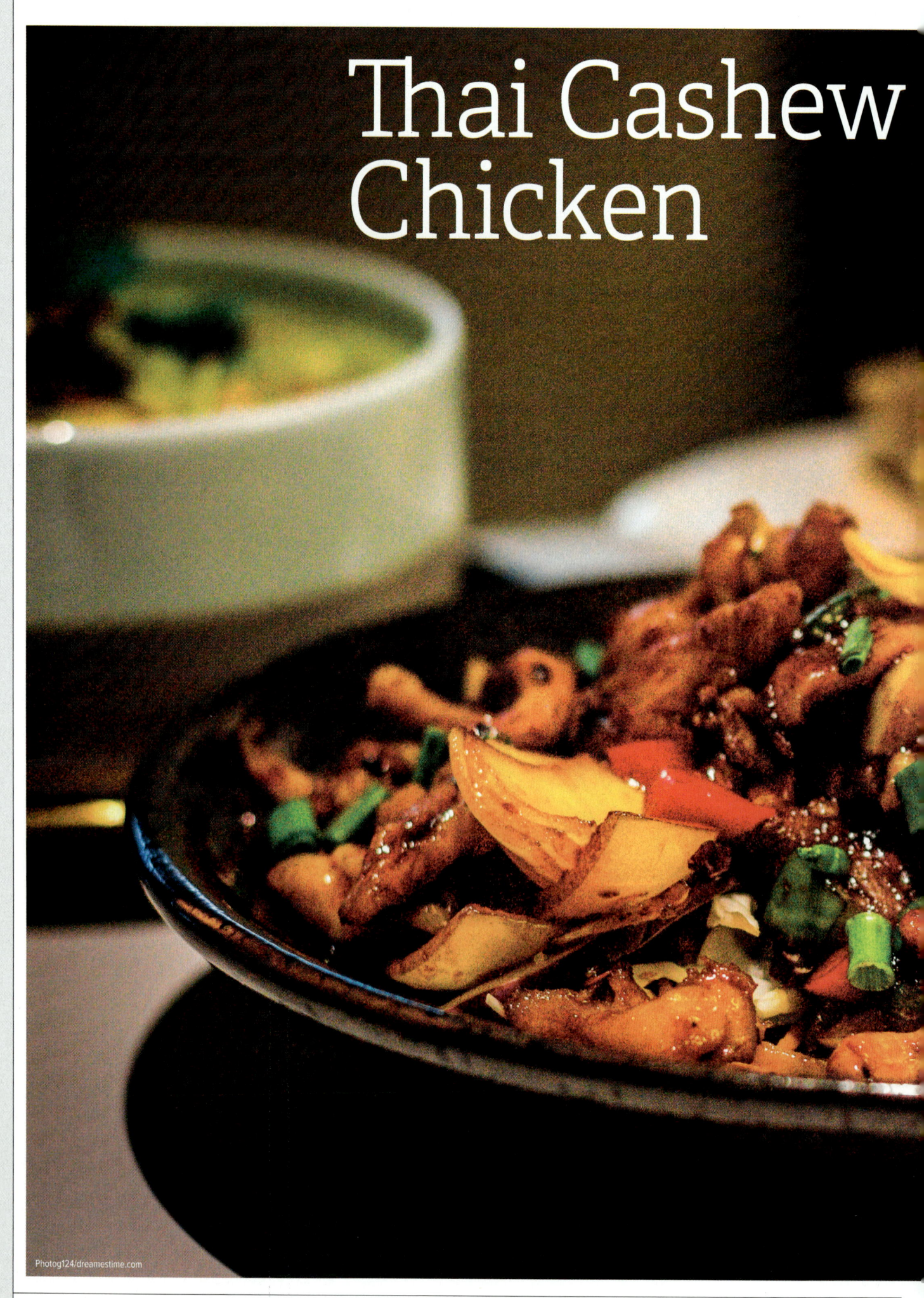

GLUTEN-FREE RECIPES

Thai Cashew Chicken

Prep 15-20 min
Cook 20 min
Serves 4

INGREDIENTS
1.5kg chicken breasts, cubed
3 tbsp cornstarch
⅛ tsp salt
¼ tsp ground black pepper

For the sauce
3 tbsp honey
2 tbsp gluten-free soy sauce or tamari
1 tbsp sriracha sauce
1 tbsp rice vinegar

2 tbsp sesame oil
3 cloves garlic, finely chopped
1 red pepper, cut in strips
1 onion, chopped
2 jalapeño or serrano peppers, diced
2 handfuls of unsalted cashew nuts
Chopped chives or spring onions

METHOD
1. Mix chicken pieces, cornstarch, salt, and pepper together in a large bowl.
2. In a small bowl mix the honey, soy sauce, sriracha and vinegar.
3. Put the oil in a large skillet or wok over a medium-high heat. Add the chicken and sauté until golden brown on all sides.
4. Add the garlic and chopped vegetables. Cook for 3-4 min or until the vegetables are slightly soft.
5. Add the cashews and the sauce and cook for another 1-2 min or until the sauce begins to thicken. Garnish with chopped chives or spring onions.

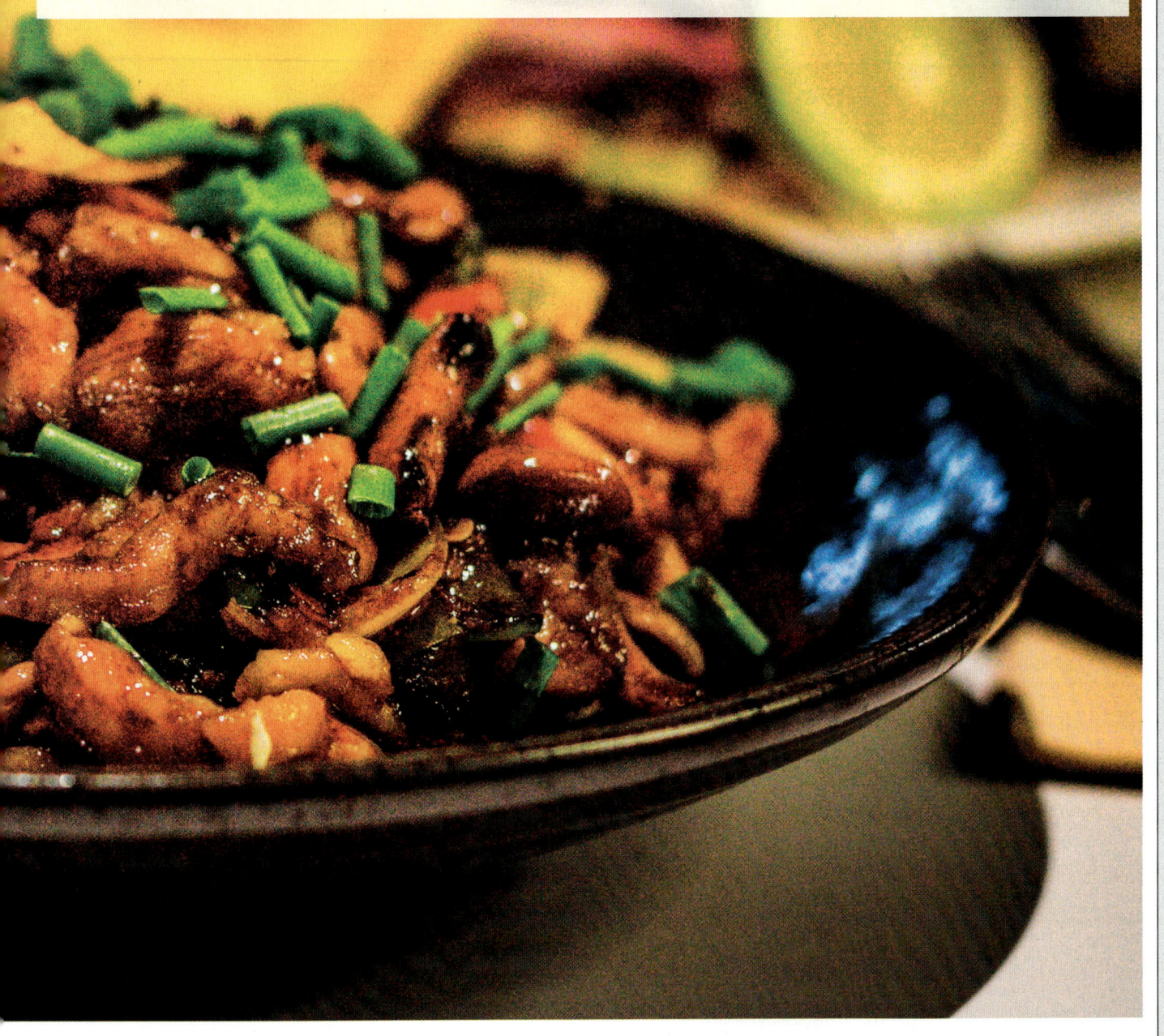

Beef Lo Mein

Prep 10 min
Cook 20 min
Serves 4

INGREDIENTS
For the sauce
8 tbsp gluten-free soy sauce or tamari
1 tbsp arrowroot powder
1 tbsp sesame oil
1 tbsp finely chopped garlic

500g sirloin steak, thinly sliced into strips
1 packet gluten-free spaghetti noodles
Green or red pepper, or a mix of the two, cut into slices
Dozen baby sweetcorn
Handful pak choi or spring greens, chopped
Handful sugar snap peas
225g tinned water chestnuts
2 tbsp vegetable oil
2 tbsp water
Sesame seeds to garnish

METHOD
1. Mix all sauce ingredients together in a small bowl. Once the arrowroot powder is completely dissolved, put half the sauce in a container and add the strips of steak. Mix well and set aside.
2. Bring a pot of water to a boil, break the noodles in half and add to the water. Boil for 3 min then remove from the heat and strain.
3. Heat the oil in a large skillet or wok and add the marinaded steak strips. Fry until the steak is cooked – about 4 min – then remove with a slotted spoon and set aside on a plate.
4. Put the vegetables, minus the water chestnuts, into the wok with the water and cover with a lid. Cook until the vegetables are tender but still crisp.
5. Remove lid and add the noodles, remaining sauce, and water chestnuts. Let everything cook for about 3 min to allow the noodles to begin to crisp up.
6. Add in the steak strips and stir fry for 1 min to mix everything together. Sprinkle with sesame seeds before serving.

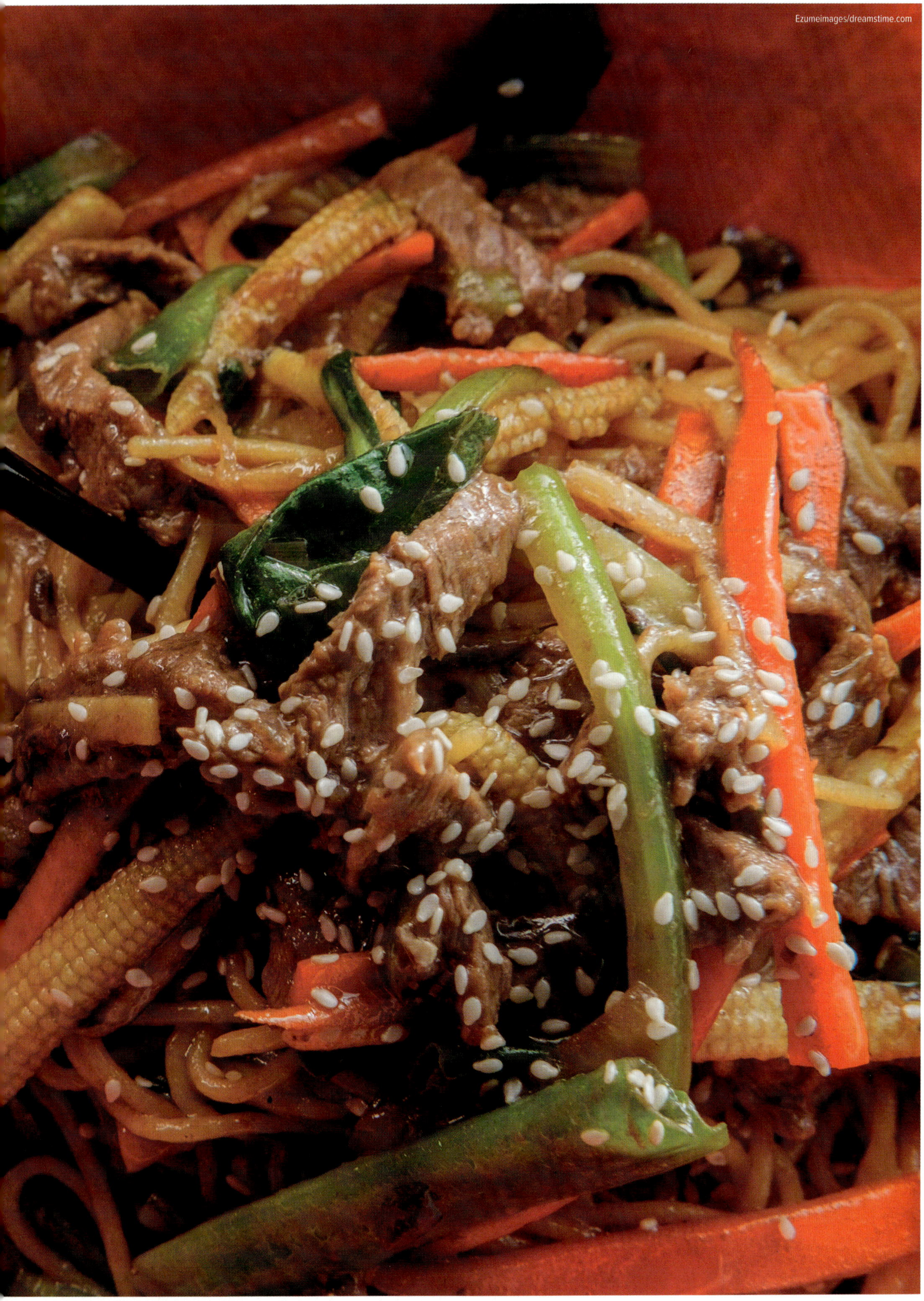
Ezumeimages/dreamstime.com

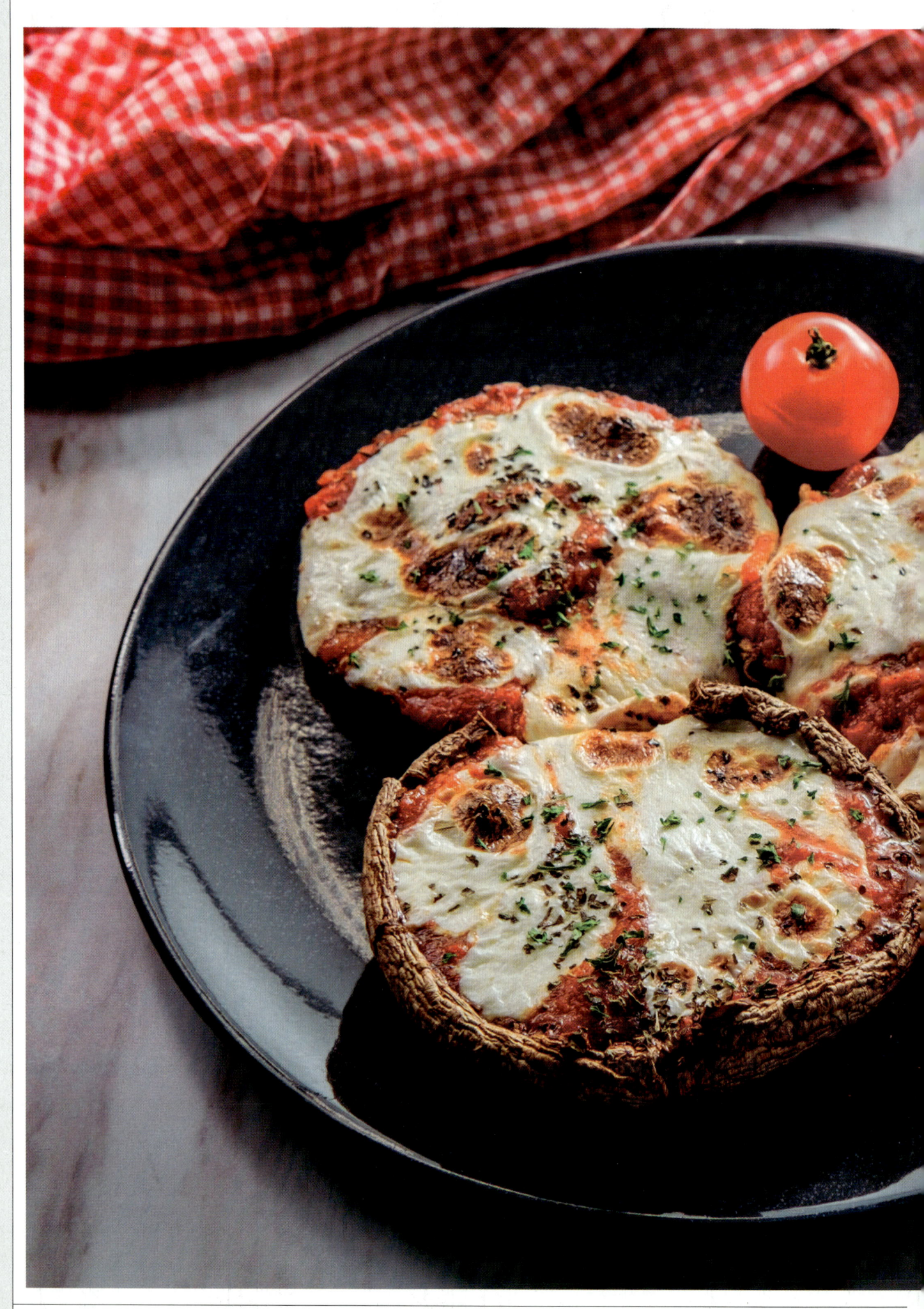

GLUTEN-FREE RECIPES

Pizza Mushrooms

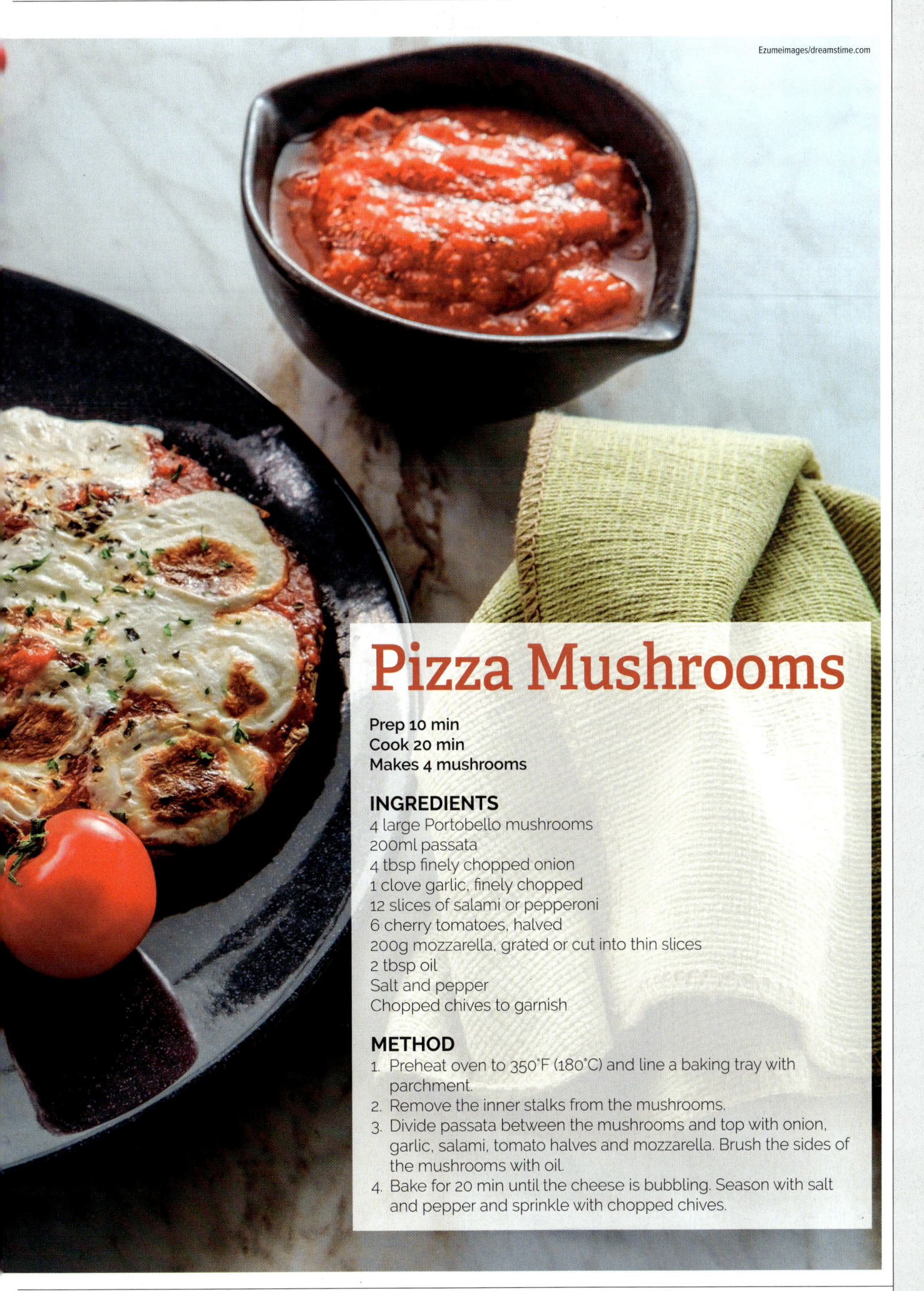

Prep 10 min
Cook 20 min
Makes 4 mushrooms

INGREDIENTS
4 large Portobello mushrooms
200ml passata
4 tbsp finely chopped onion
1 clove garlic, finely chopped
12 slices of salami or pepperoni
6 cherry tomatoes, halved
200g mozzarella, grated or cut into thin slices
2 tbsp oil
Salt and pepper
Chopped chives to garnish

METHOD
1. Preheat oven to 350°F (180°C) and line a baking tray with parchment.
2. Remove the inner stalks from the mushrooms.
3. Divide passata between the mushrooms and top with onion, garlic, salami, tomato halves and mozzarella. Brush the sides of the mushrooms with oil.
4. Bake for 20 min until the cheese is bubbling. Season with salt and pepper and sprinkle with chopped chives.

Soba Noodle Salad

Prep 25 min
Serves 6

INGREDIENTS

Salad
225g buckwheat noodles (or any whole grain noodle)
½ small bunch coriander, chopped
½ yellow pepper, chopped
1 carrot, grated
Handful broccoli florets
1 small cucumber, chopped
¼ red or white cabbage, shredded
2 spring onions, sliced
4 radishes, sliced
Sesame seeds
Peanuts, chopped
Mint leaves
Chilli flakes and/or nigella (optional)

Dressing
3 tbsp gluten-free soy sauce or tamari
55g peanut butter or almond butter
1 tsp sesame oil (optional)
1 tbsp fresh grated ginger
2 tbsp rice vinegar
1 tbsp maple syrup
Juice ½ lime

METHOD
1. Cook the noodles according to directions on packaging. Drain and let cool.
2. Stir dressing ingredients together in a small bowl or jar.
3. Chop the salad vegetables.
4. Toss the salad with the dressing and top with sesame seeds, chopped peanuts, mint leaves and chilli flakes, if desired.

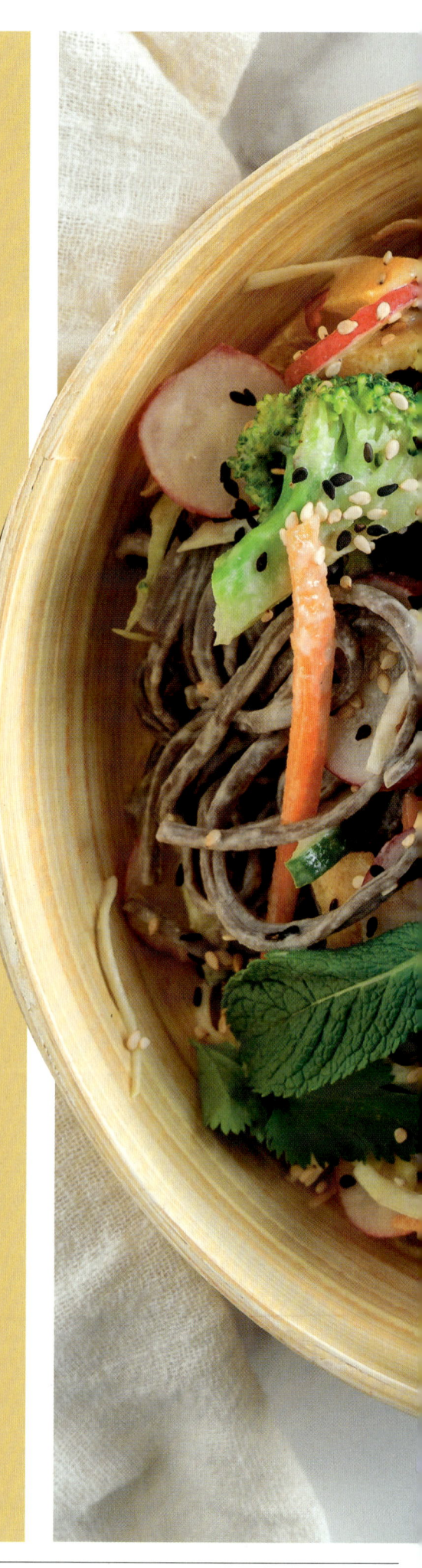

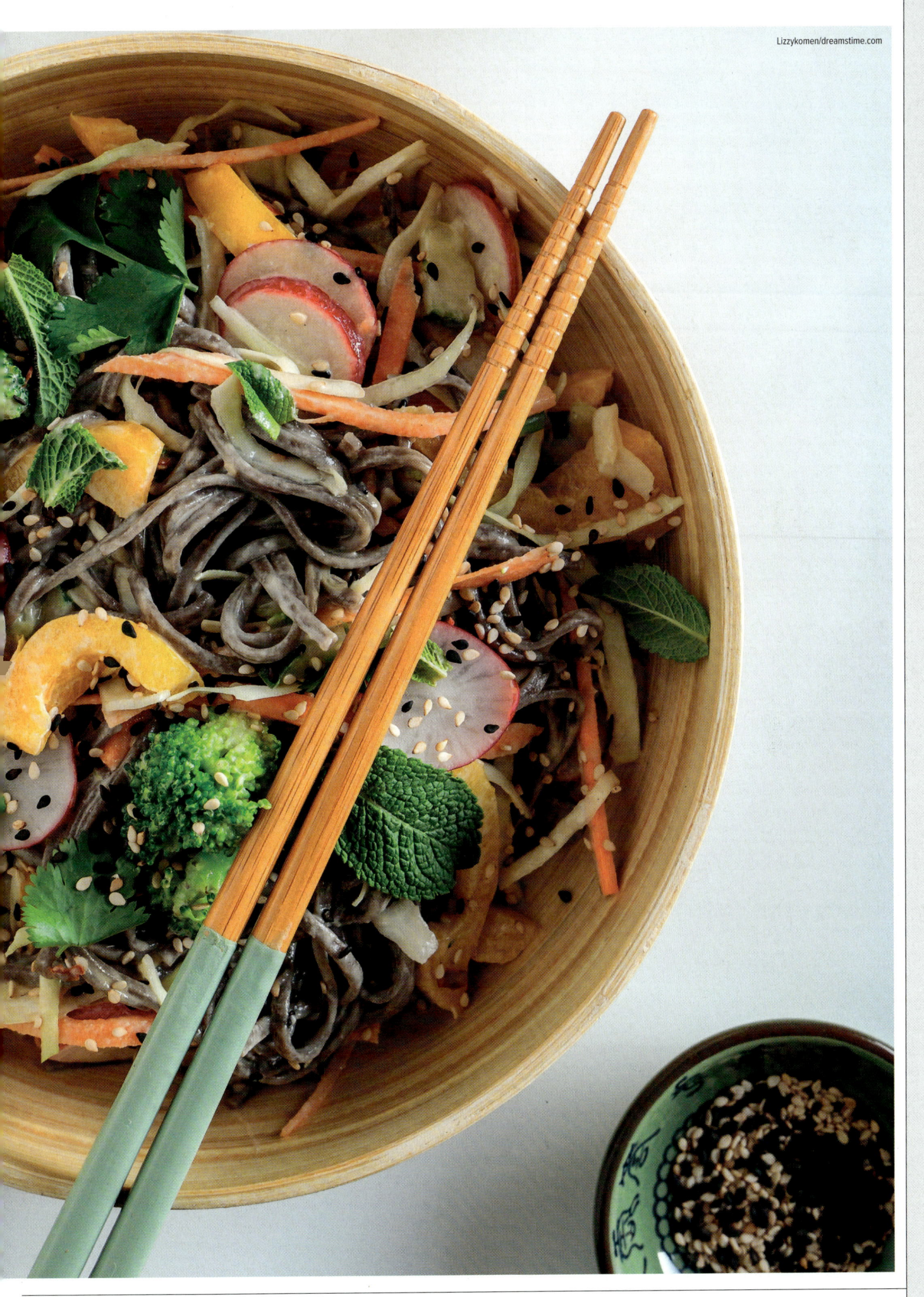

GLUTEN-FREE RECIPES

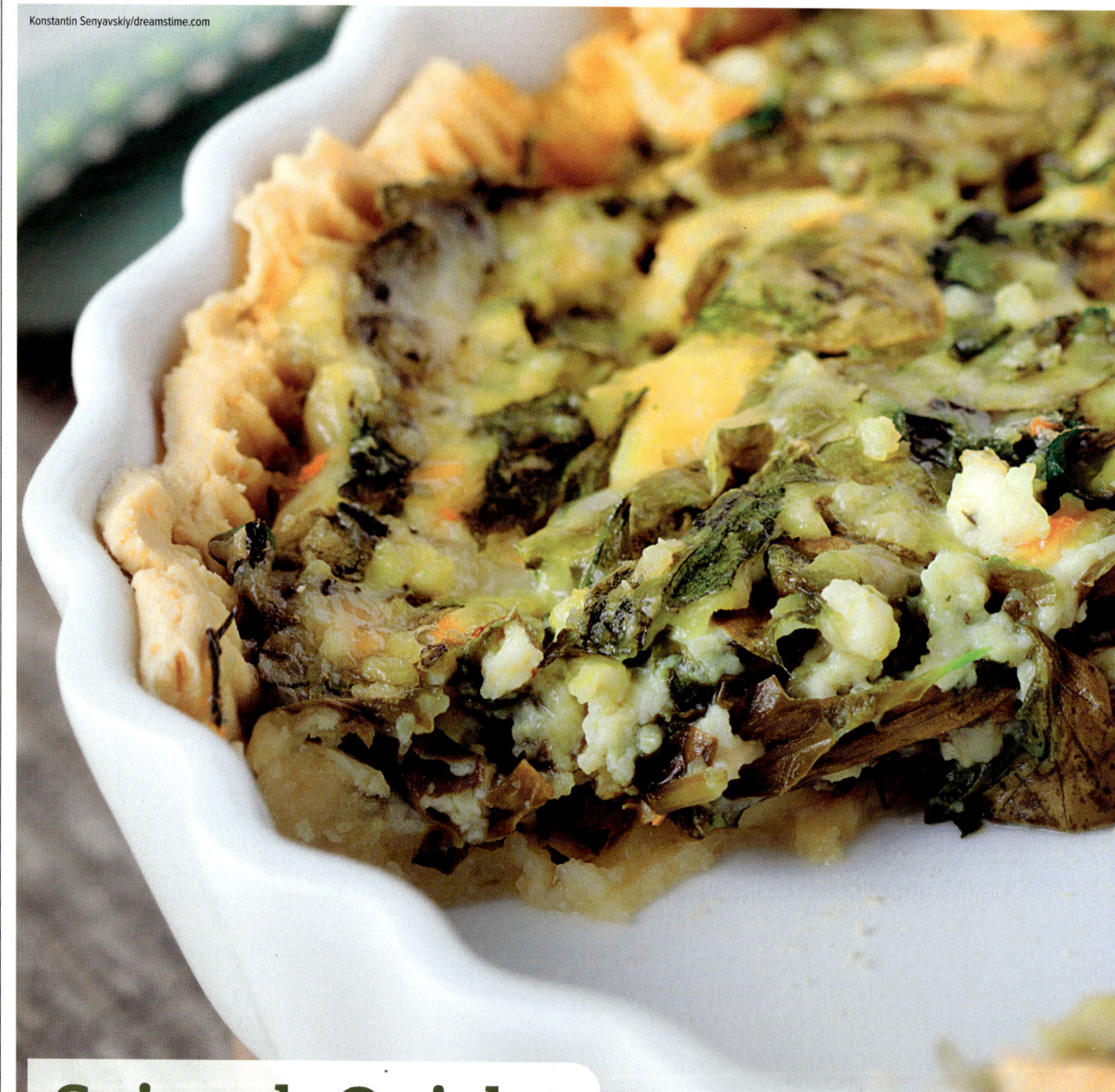

Spinach Quiche

Prep 30 min
Cook 45 min
Serves 6

You will need a 20 or 22cm quiche tin, preferably with a removable bottom and fluted edges

INGREDIENTS
For the pastry
100g unsalted butter cut into small pieces
½ tsp salt
1 large egg
1 tbsp cold water
50g almond meal (ground almond)
50g gluten-free flour
170g light buckwheat flour, or sorghum flour

For the filling
3 large eggs
250ml thick cream
1 tsp salt
½ tsp ground nutmeg
170g grated Emmental cheese
225g fresh spinach leaves, rinsed, dried, and roughly chopped

GLUTEN-FREE RECIPES

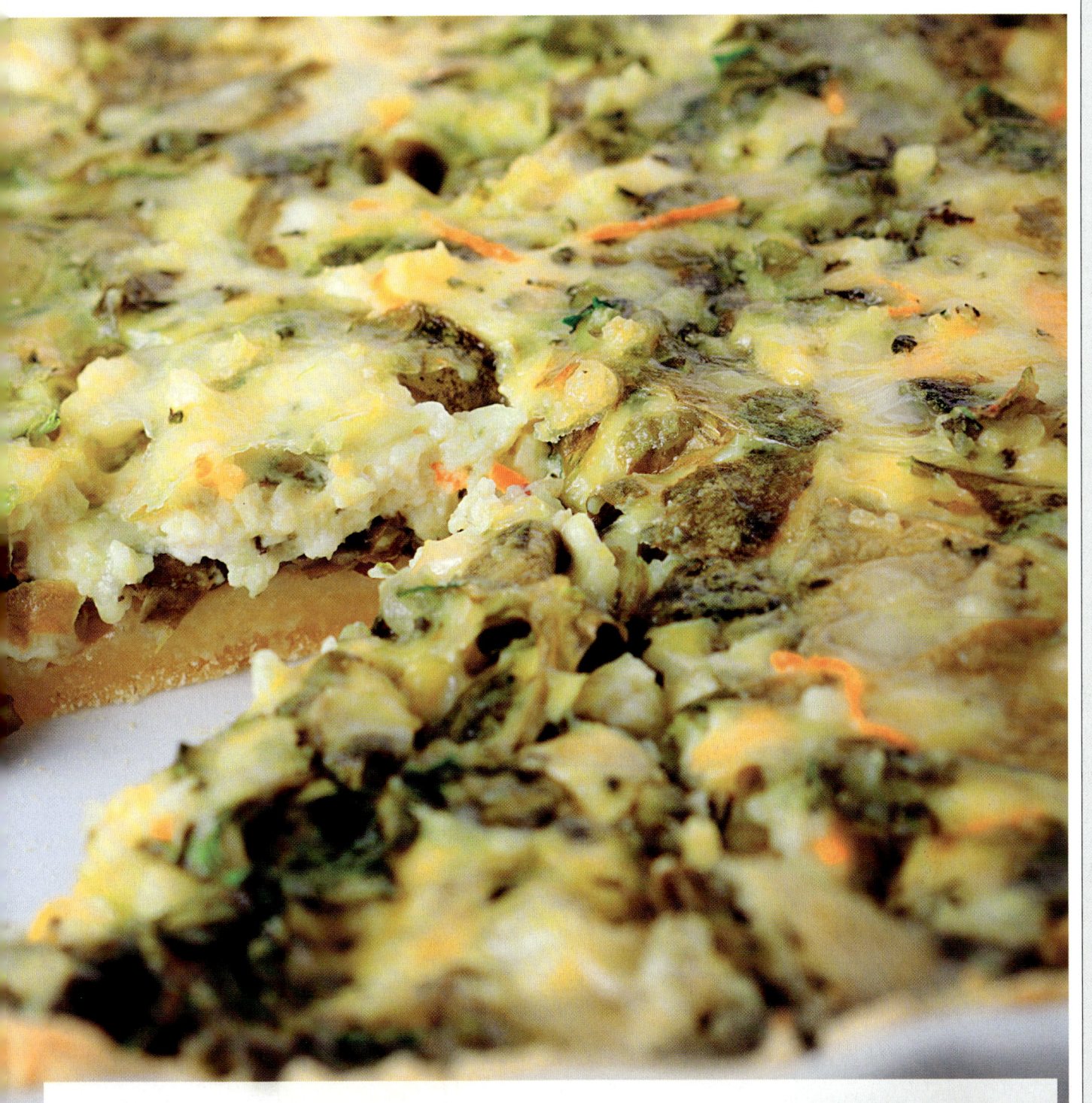

METHOD
1. Preheat oven to 375°F (190°C).
2. Put butter pieces and salt in a bowl and beat until smooth.
3. Add the egg, cold water, almond meal, and gluten-free flour and mix until smooth.
4. Add the buckwheat flour (or sorghum flour) and beat until the mixture forms a ball.
5. Use a spatula to scrape the soft dough onto lightly floured wax paper. Lightly dust the ball with flour and shape into a flat round.
6. Wrap the dough in the wax paper and refrigerate for at least 1 hr.
7. Roll out the dough between two sheets of lightly floured wax paper. Remove the top sheet of paper and gently turn out the pastry into the quiche tin.
8. Bake in the oven for 15 min or until the crust is light golden brown.
9. While the pastry is cooking, whisk the eggs, cream, salt, and nutmeg.
10. Sprinkle half the cheese over the cooked pastry, then scatter half of the spinach leaves over the cheese. Pour in about ¾ of the egg mixture.
11. Sprinkle over the remaining cheese and spinach then top with the remaining egg mixture.
12. Place the quiche tin on a large baking sheet to prevent dripping and bake in the oven for 30 min or until the filling is set and the top is golden.

THE GLUTEN-FREE HANDBOOK

GLUTEN-FREE RECIPES

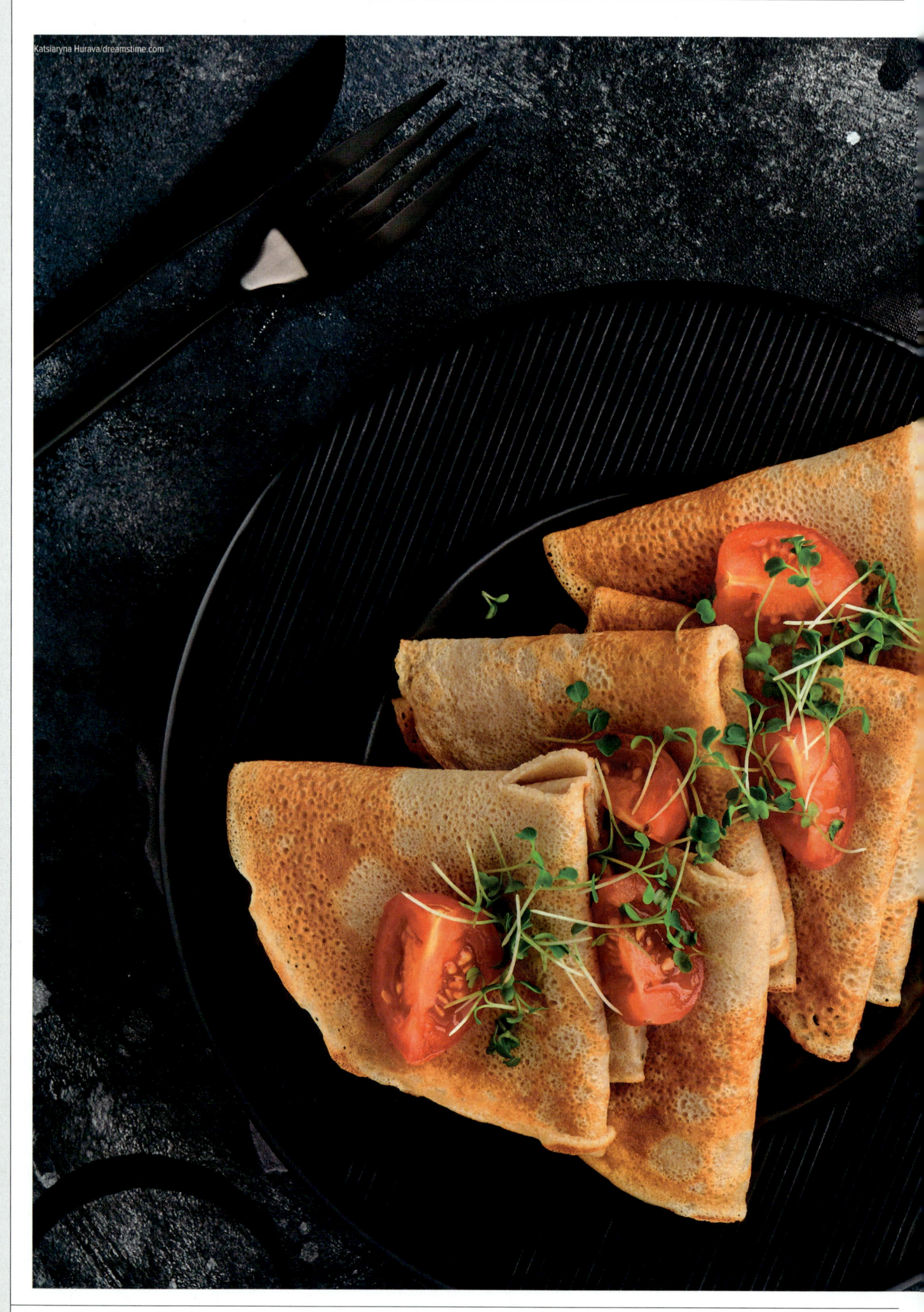

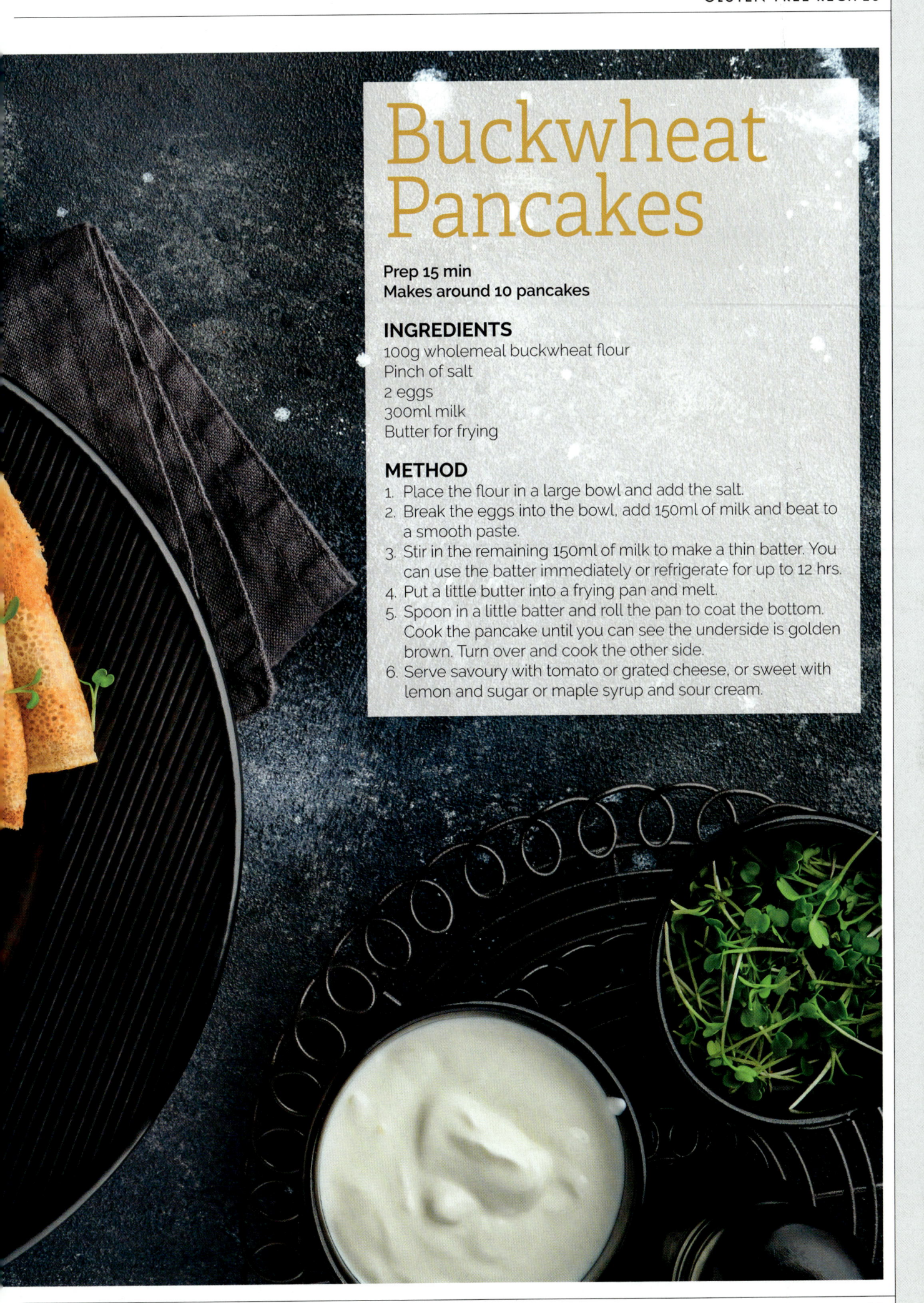

Buckwheat Pancakes

Prep 15 min
Makes around 10 pancakes

INGREDIENTS
100g wholemeal buckwheat flour
Pinch of salt
2 eggs
300ml milk
Butter for frying

METHOD
1. Place the flour in a large bowl and add the salt.
2. Break the eggs into the bowl, add 150ml of milk and beat to a smooth paste.
3. Stir in the remaining 150ml of milk to make a thin batter. You can use the batter immediately or refrigerate for up to 12 hrs.
4. Put a little butter into a frying pan and melt.
5. Spoon in a little batter and roll the pan to coat the bottom. Cook the pancake until you can see the underside is golden brown. Turn over and cook the other side.
6. Serve savoury with tomato or grated cheese, or sweet with lemon and sugar or maple syrup and sour cream.

Quinoa Frittata

Prep 10 min
Cook 40 min
Serves 4

INGREDIENTS
60g quinoa (uncooked)
6 eggs
40g feta cheese (crumbled)
Handful baby spinach
100g bacon (ham or chicken)
1 tsp butter

METHOD
1. Cook the quinoa in your preferred way.
2. Whisk the eggs and add in the cooked quinoa, feta cheese, spinach and bacon, ham, or chicken.
3. Heat an ovenproof frying pan and melt the butter. Pour the egg mixture into the pan and cook for 2 min on a high heat.
4. Transfer the pan to the oven and bake at 350°F (180°C) for 15 min or until the middle is firm.

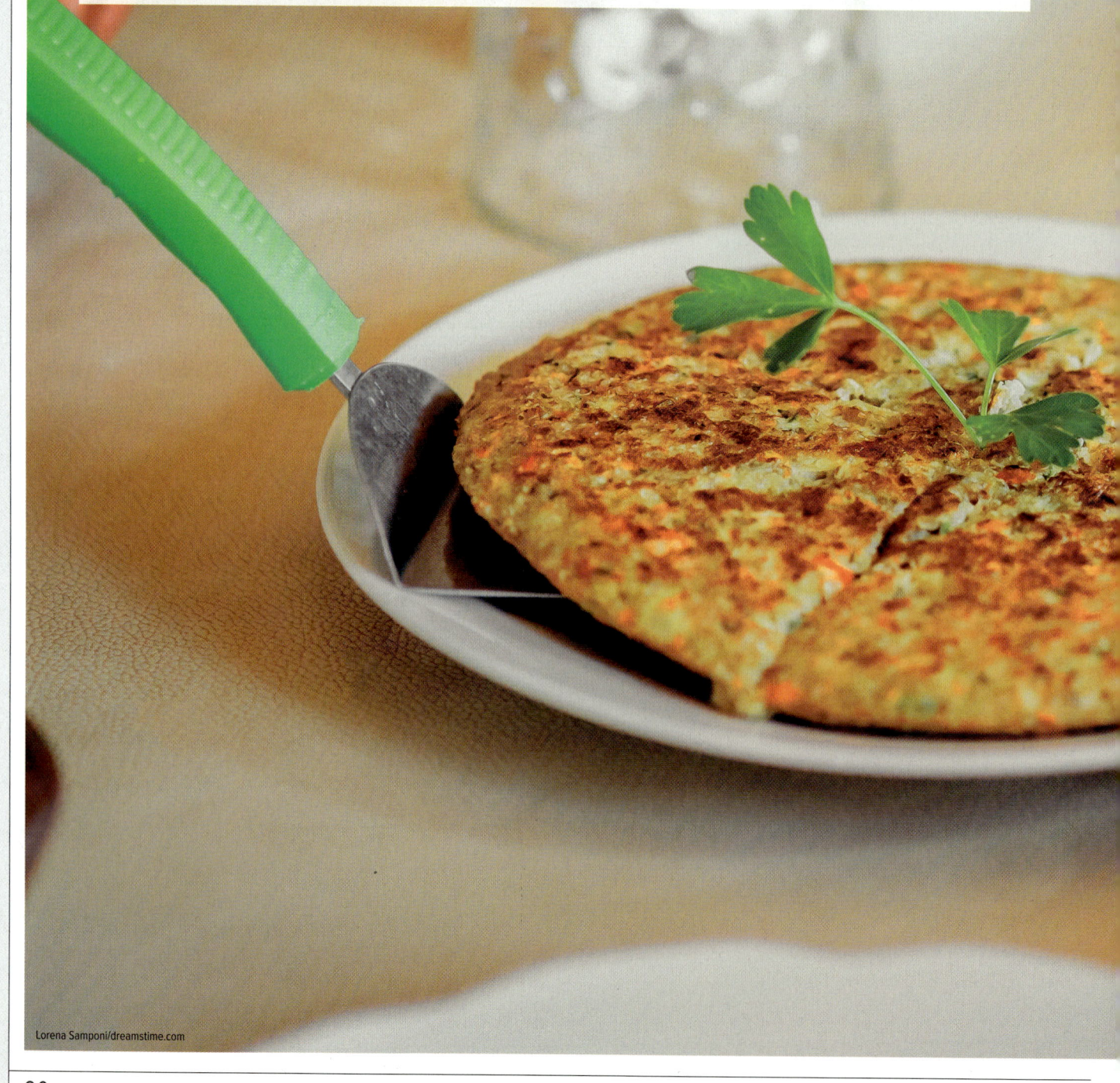

Lorena Samponi/dreamstime.com

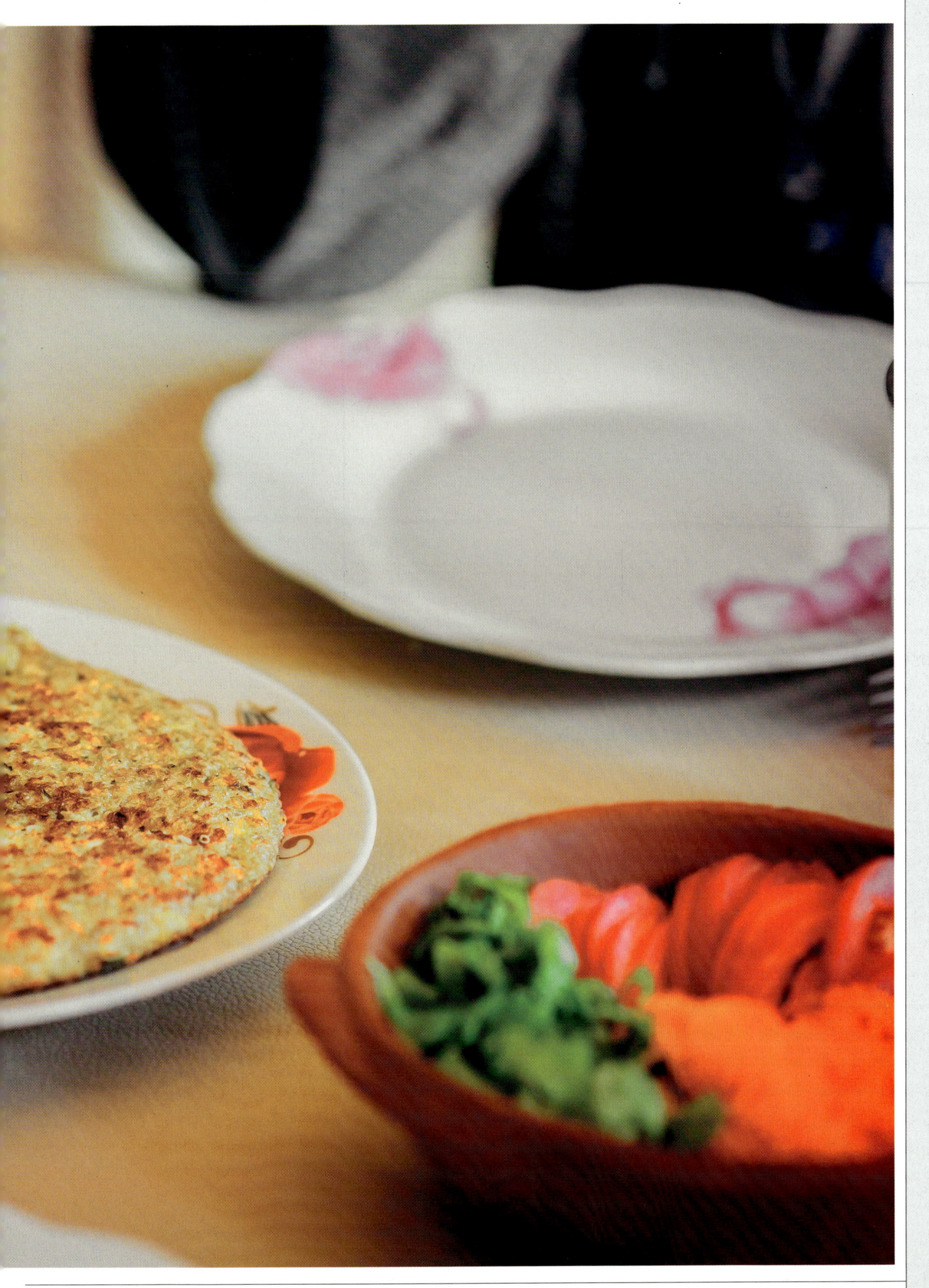

Gluten-Free Recipes

Apple, Almond, and

Prep 25 min
Cook 65 min
Makes around 20 servings

INGREDIENTS
For the syrup
200g sugar
325ml unsweetened apple juice
2in piece ginger, unpeeled, cut in half lengthwise and crushed
Zest from 1 medium lemon
1 tbsp fresh lemon juice
4 tbsp brandy

For the cake
4 large eggs
160g sugar
1 tsp salt
220ml vegetable oil
2 tbsp freshly grated ginger
230g almond flour
175g finely chopped walnuts
2 tsp ground cinnamon
¼ tsp freshly grated nutmeg
350g grated apple

METHOD
1. Preheat oven to 350°F (180°C). Line a 22x33cm baking tray with parchment paper and lightly grease.
2. Simmer together sugar, apple juice, ginger and lemon zest until the syrup reaches 234°F (112°C). Remove from heat and add lemon juice and brandy. Set aside to cool.
3. Combine eggs, sugar, and salt in a mixing bowl. Whisk until the eggs become thick, and pale. Slowly add the oil until it is fully incorporated and thick. Whisk in the grated ginger.
4. Fold in the almond flour, walnuts, cinnamon, and nutmeg. Add the grated apple. Pour the mixture into the prepared pan. Bake in the lower middle of the oven for about 50 min, until golden brown and the top of the cake springs back to the touch.
5. While the cake is still warm, loosen the sides and cut the cake into diamond shapes. Strain the syrup over the cake using a fine-mesh strainer, then leave for an hour to allow cake to absorb the syrup.

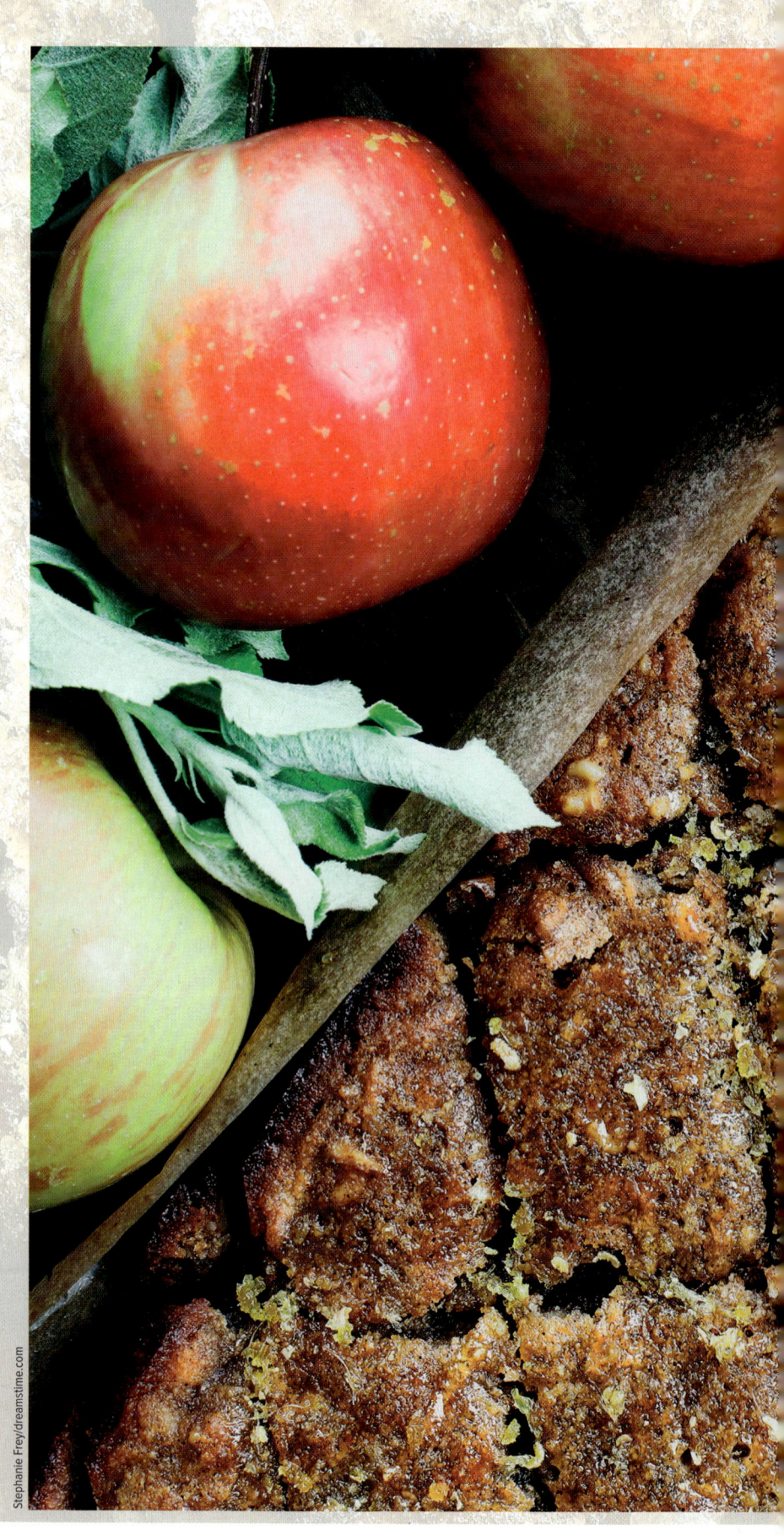

Stephanie Frey/dreamstime.com

GLUTEN-FREE RECIPES

Ginger Tray Bake

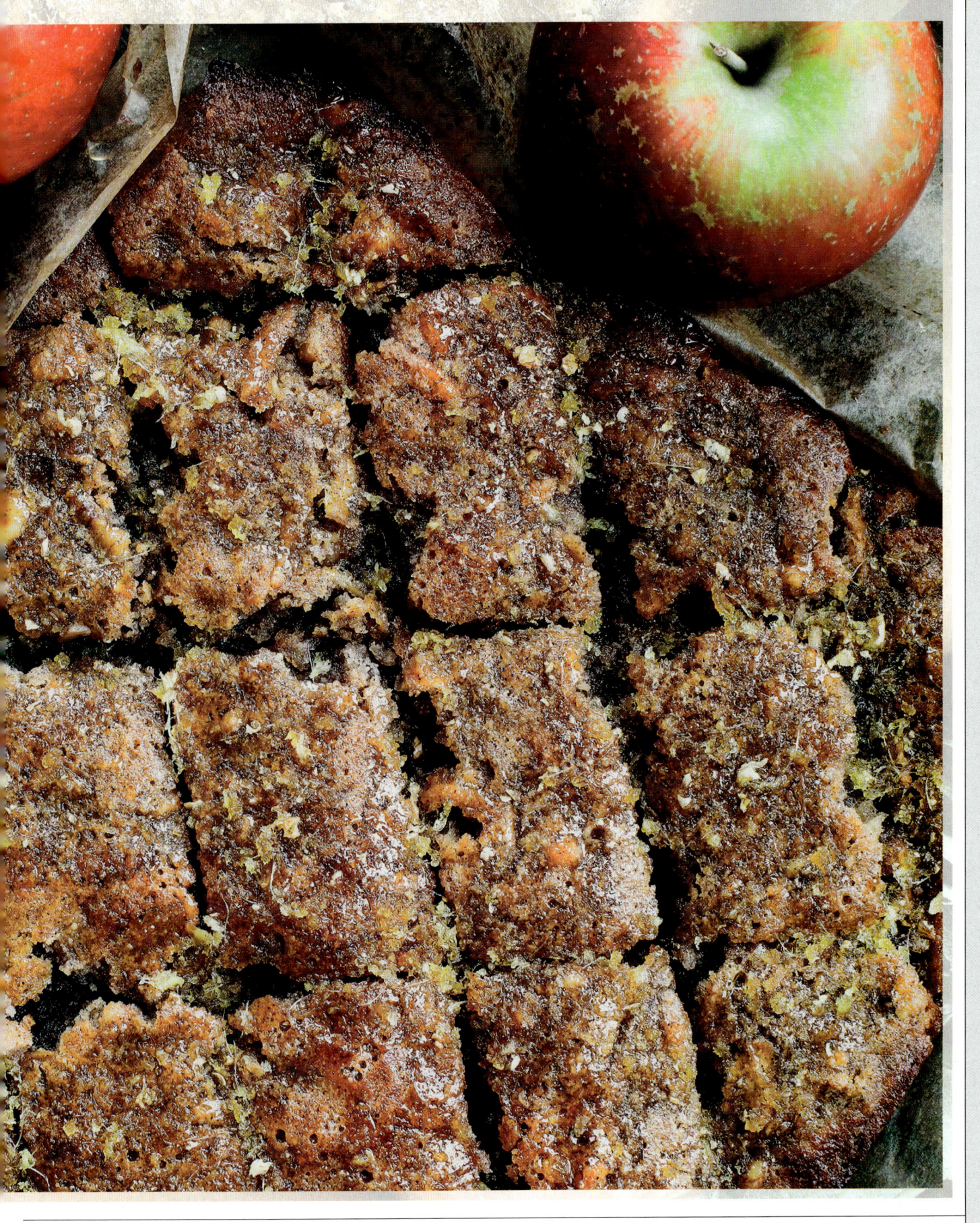

THE GLUTEN-FREE HANDBOOK

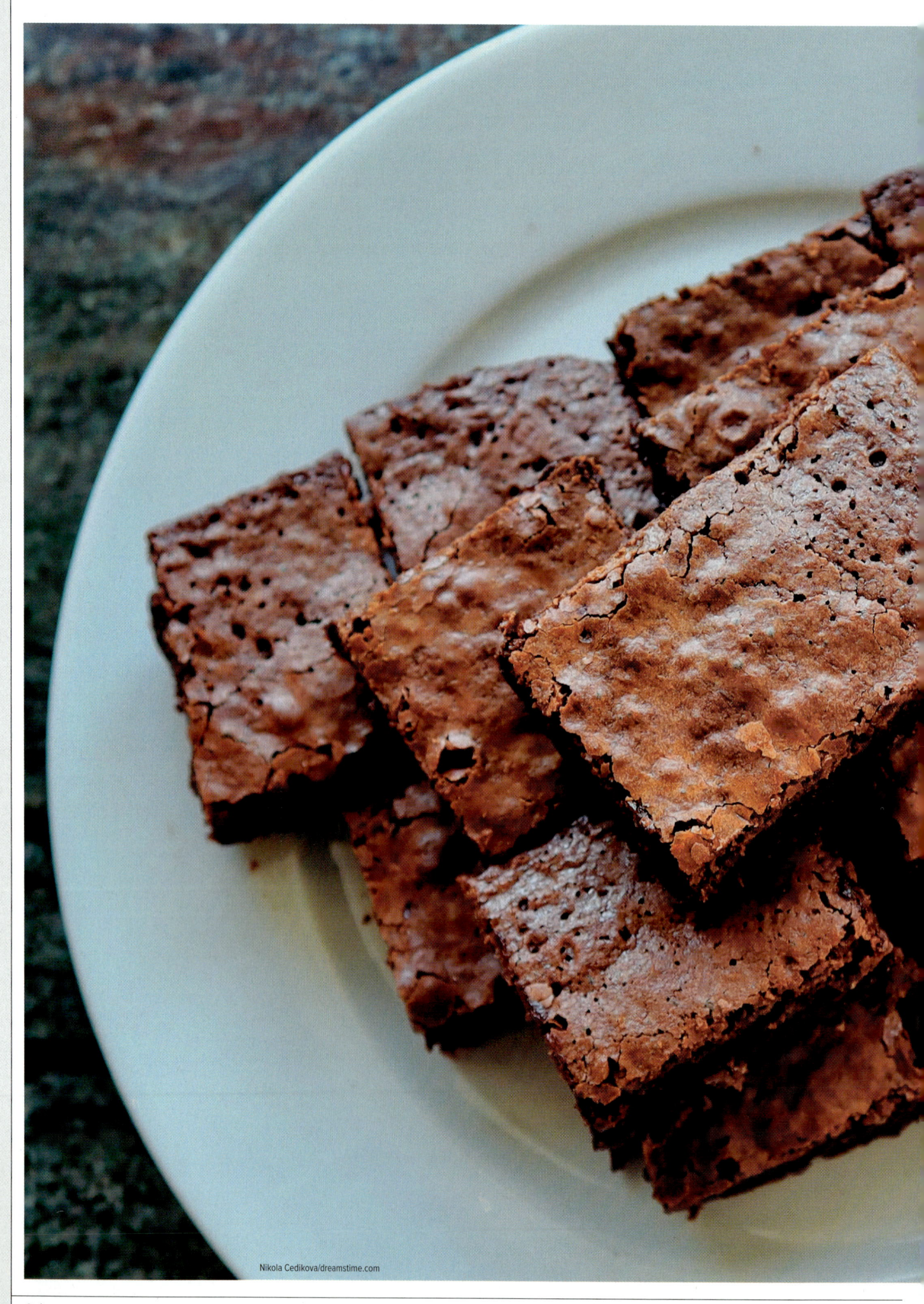

GLUTEN-FREE RECIPES

Nikola Cedikova/dreamstime.com

Brownies

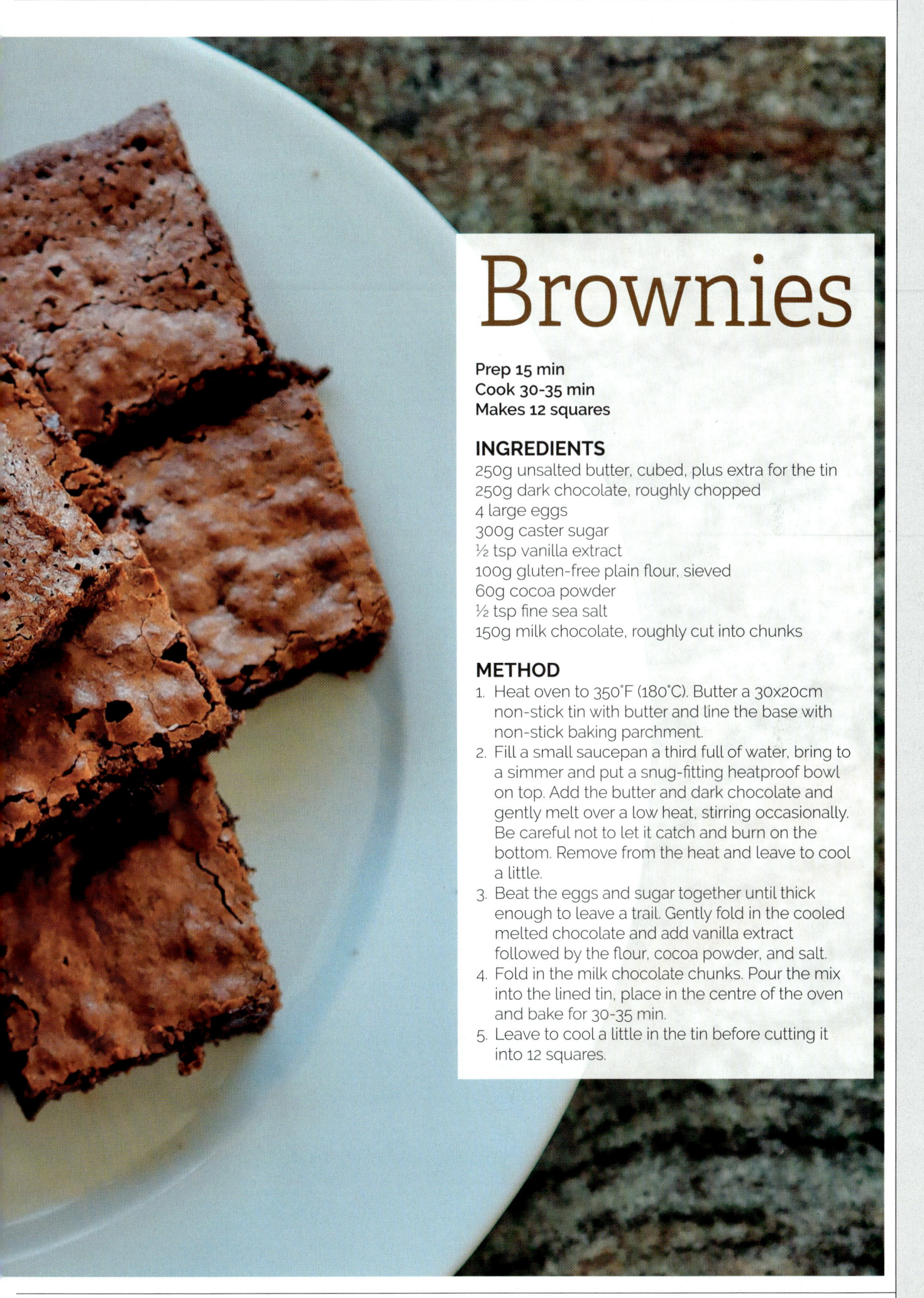

Prep 15 min
Cook 30-35 min
Makes 12 squares

INGREDIENTS
250g unsalted butter, cubed, plus extra for the tin
250g dark chocolate, roughly chopped
4 large eggs
300g caster sugar
½ tsp vanilla extract
100g gluten-free plain flour, sieved
60g cocoa powder
½ tsp fine sea salt
150g milk chocolate, roughly cut into chunks

METHOD
1. Heat oven to 350°F (180°C). Butter a 30x20cm non-stick tin with butter and line the base with non-stick baking parchment.
2. Fill a small saucepan a third full of water, bring to a simmer and put a snug-fitting heatproof bowl on top. Add the butter and dark chocolate and gently melt over a low heat, stirring occasionally. Be careful not to let it catch and burn on the bottom. Remove from the heat and leave to cool a little.
3. Beat the eggs and sugar together until thick enough to leave a trail. Gently fold in the cooled melted chocolate and add vanilla extract followed by the flour, cocoa powder, and salt.
4. Fold in the milk chocolate chunks. Pour the mix into the lined tin, place in the centre of the oven and bake for 30-35 min.
5. Leave to cool a little in the tin before cutting it into 12 squares.

GLUTEN-FREE RECIPES

Chocolate Chip Cookies

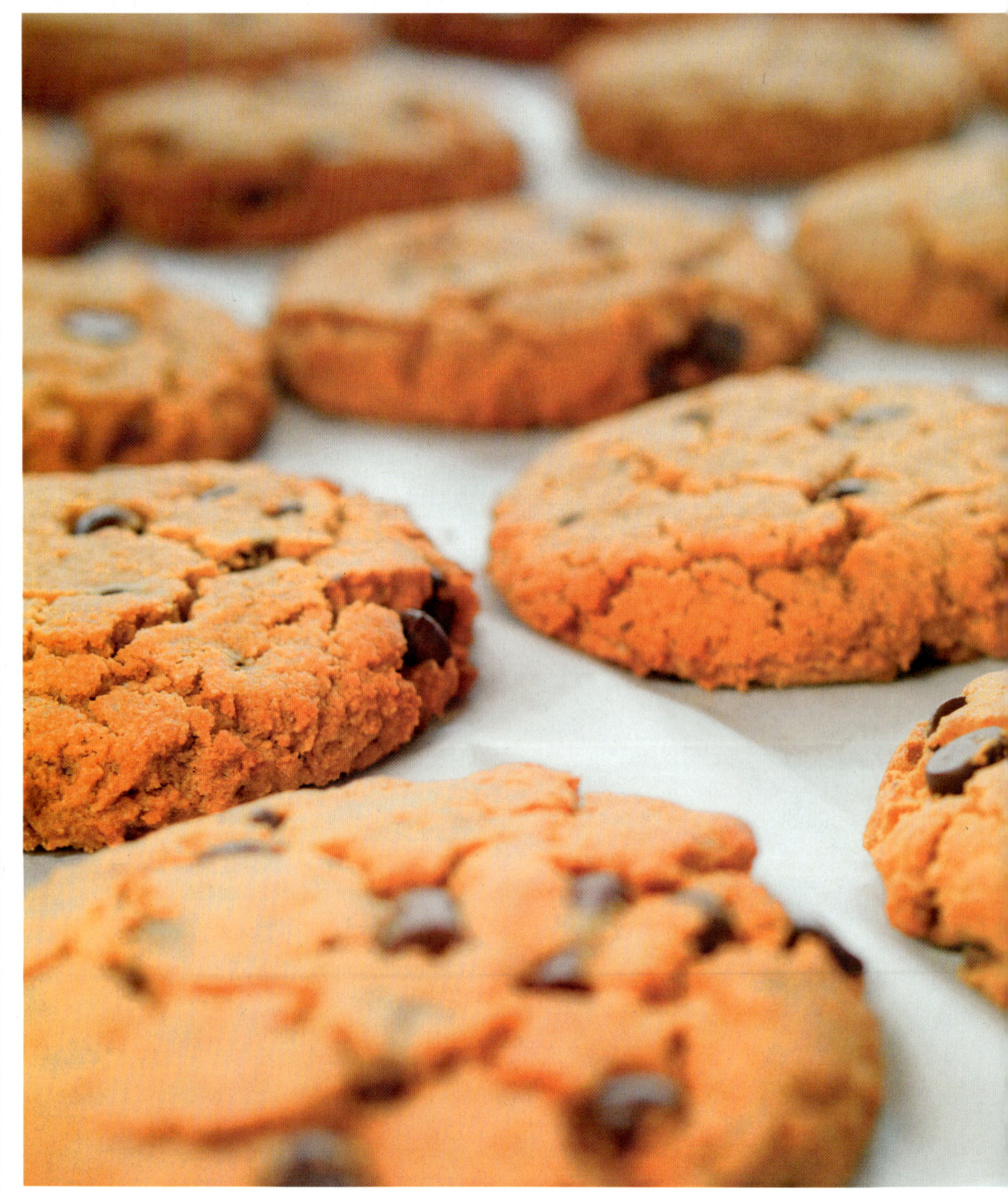

Gluten-Free Recipes

Prep 1 hr
Cook 15 min
Makes 10-20 depending on your preferred size

INGREDIENTS
100g caster sugar
100g light brown sugar
120g hard margarine, melted
1 large egg
½ tsp vanilla extract
300g gluten-free plain flour
½ tsp salt
½ tsp bicarbonate of soda
160g chocolate chips

METHOD
1. In a large bowl, mix caster sugar and light brown sugar with the melted margarine.
2. Add the egg and vanilla extract and continue to mix.
3. In a separate bowl, combine the flour, salt, and bicarbonate of soda.
4. Add the flour mix to the original bowl and combine.
5. Add the chocolate chips, spreading them evenly through the mix. Cover the bowl with clingfilm and chill in the fridge for about 45 min.
6. Meanwhile, heat the oven to 325°F (170°C) and prepare a couple of baking trays with good quality, non-stick baking parchment.
7. Remove the cookie dough from the fridge and roll it into balls (about the size of a golf ball for smaller cookies). Place them on the trays, well-spaced to allow for spreading.
8. Pop the trays into the oven for 15 min or until golden brown. Remove from the oven and leave to cool on the baking trays.

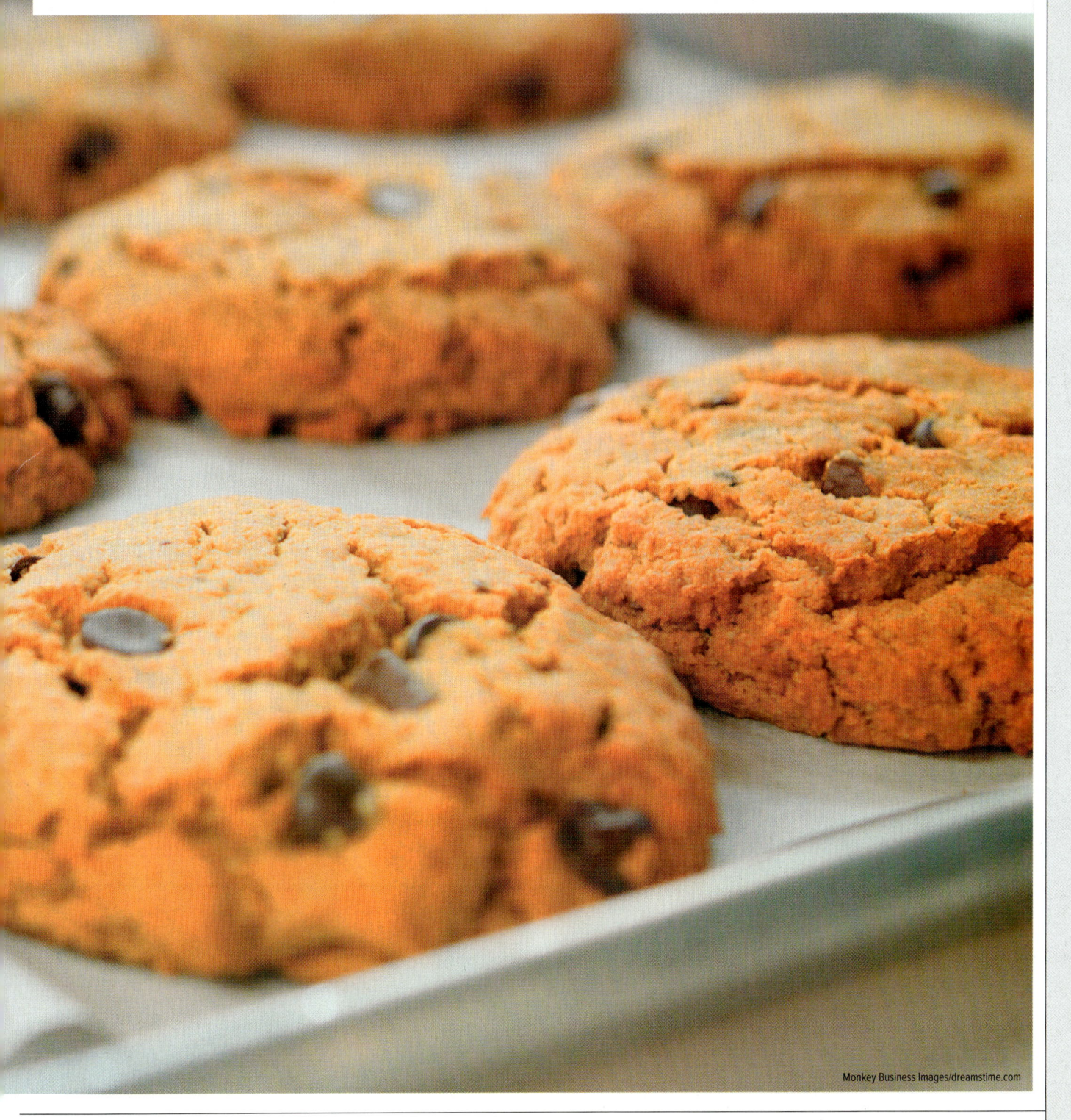

Monkey Business Images/dreamstime.com

Gluten-Free Recipes

Pumpkin

Prep 1 hr
Cook 1 hr 50 min
Serves 12

INGREDIENTS
Vegetable oil
1.5kg pumpkin

For the pastry
250g gluten-free plain flour
½ tsp xanthan gum
50g soft light brown sugar
Pinch of ground cinnamon
125g unsalted butter, cold
1 large egg
Semi-skimmed milk

50g unsalted butter
125g golden caster sugar
4 level tbsp gluten-free plain flour
¼ tsp ground nutmeg
½ tsp ground cinnamon
2 tsp vanilla extract
3 large eggs
Icing sugar

METHOD
1. Preheat the oven to 350°F (180°C). Lightly grease a 25cm non-stick loose-bottomed pie tin with vegetable oil.
2. Cut the pumpkin into wedges, discarding the seeds. Place on a baking tray and cover with foil. Bake in the oven for around 50 min, then remove the foil and cook for a further 10 min. Take out of the oven and leave to cool.
3. Sieve the flour and xanthan gum into a large bowl and stir in the brown sugar and cinnamon.
4. Chop the butter into cubes and rub it into the flour mixture with your fingers until the mixture resembles fine breadcrumbs. Beat the egg in a separate bowl, then add it to the flour mix.
5. Work together into a rough dough, adding milk if necessary to stop it being too dry and crumbly. Shape the dough into a flat round, wrap in clingfilm and place in the fridge for at least 30 min.
6. Remove the pumpkin flesh from the skin with a spoon and rub through a sieve or use a food processor to create a purée.
7. Melt the butter over a low heat until it turns brown. Add the brown butter to the puréed pumpkin with the caster sugar, flour, nutmeg, cinnamon, and the vanilla extract. Whisk 2 of the eggs in a separate bowl, add to the pumpkin mix and blend well.
8. Take the pastry out of the fridge and roll it out to about 1cm thick. Transfer it to the prepared pie tin and press it round the sides. Trim away any overhanging pastry, prick the base with a fork, then place in the fridge to chill for another 10 min.
9. Place a round of baking parchment over the pastry and cover with baking beans or rice. Bake blind for 10 to 12 min then remove the paper and beans and cook for a further 5 min until golden. Remove from the oven and allow to cool completely.
10. Spoon the pumpkin mixture into the cooled pastry case and spread evenly.
11. Roll out the pastry trimmings and cut into shapes to decorate the top of the pie. Beat the remaining egg and brush it over the pastry.
12. Place the pie in the oven for 45 to 50 min until golden. Dust with icing sugar and cinnamon, if desired, and serve.
13. As an alternative, create smaller pies with the pastry, divide the pumpkin mix between them and cook as above. Decorate them with whipped cream and brown sugar.

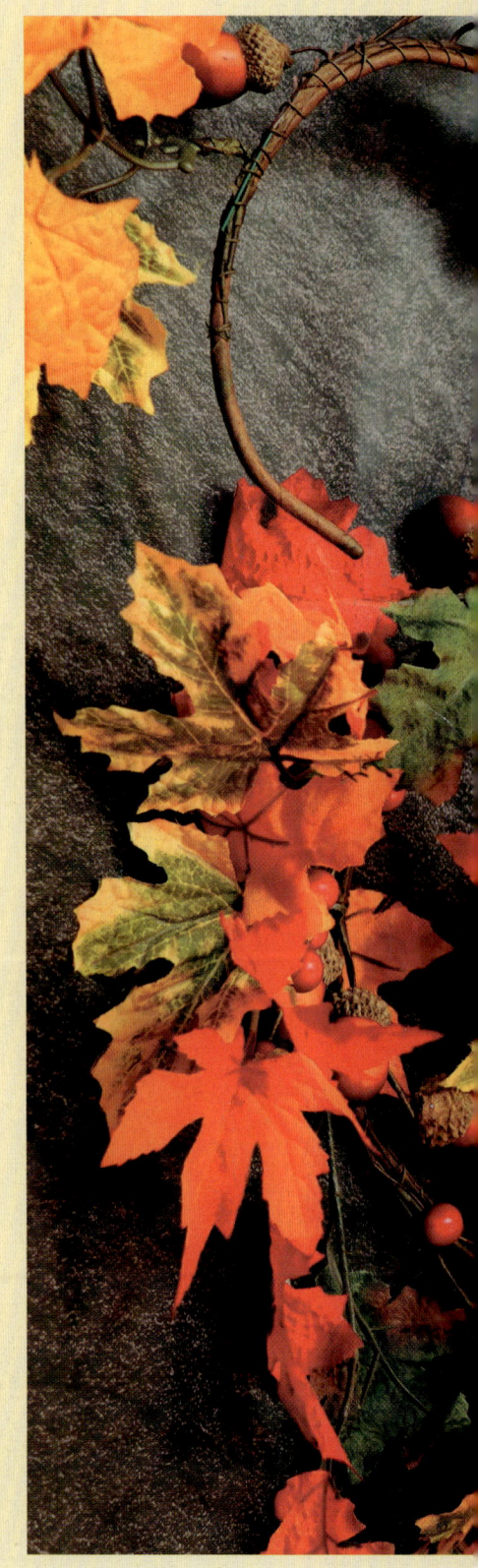

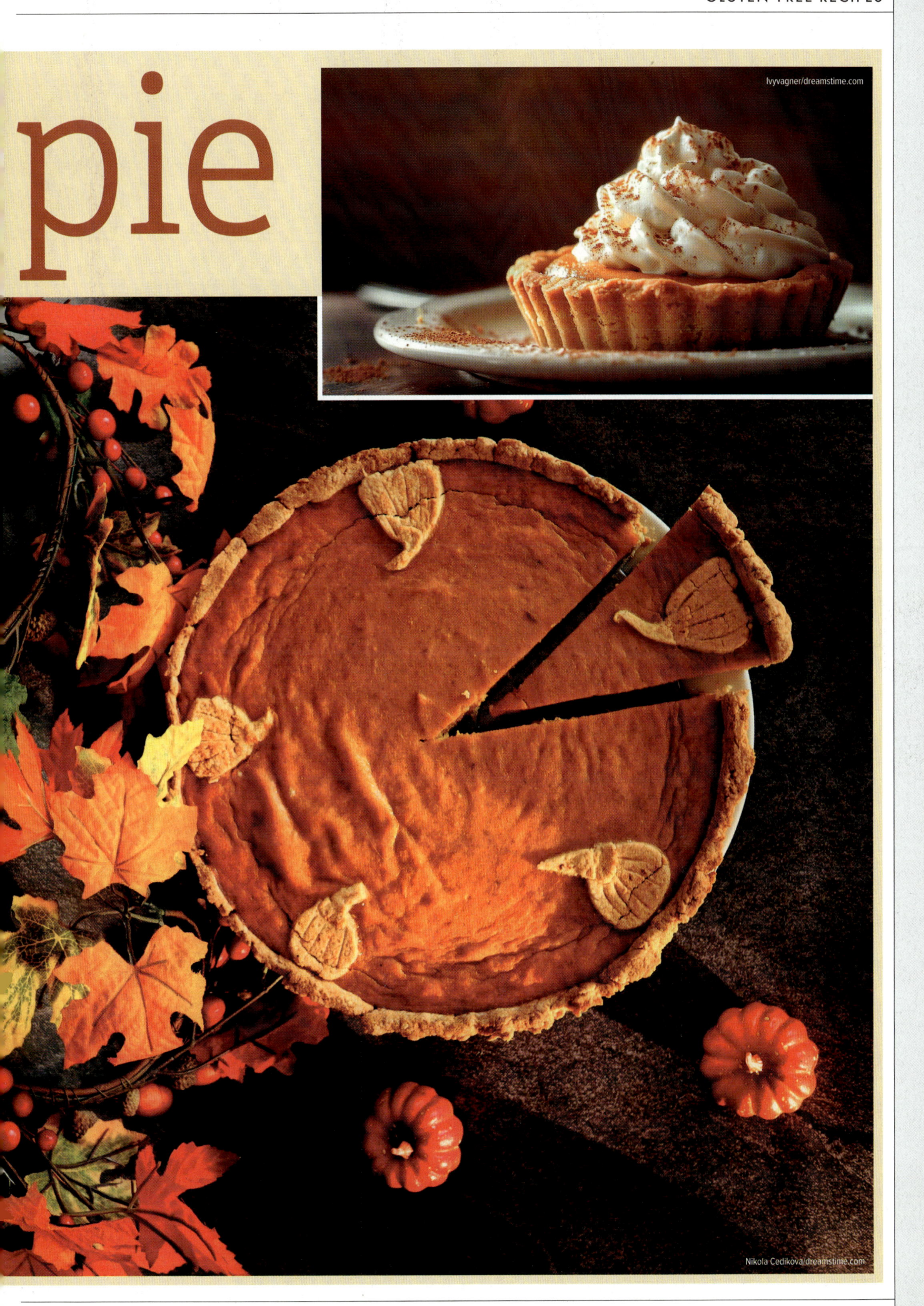

GLUTEN-FREE RECIPES

pie

THE GLUTEN-FREE HANDBOOK

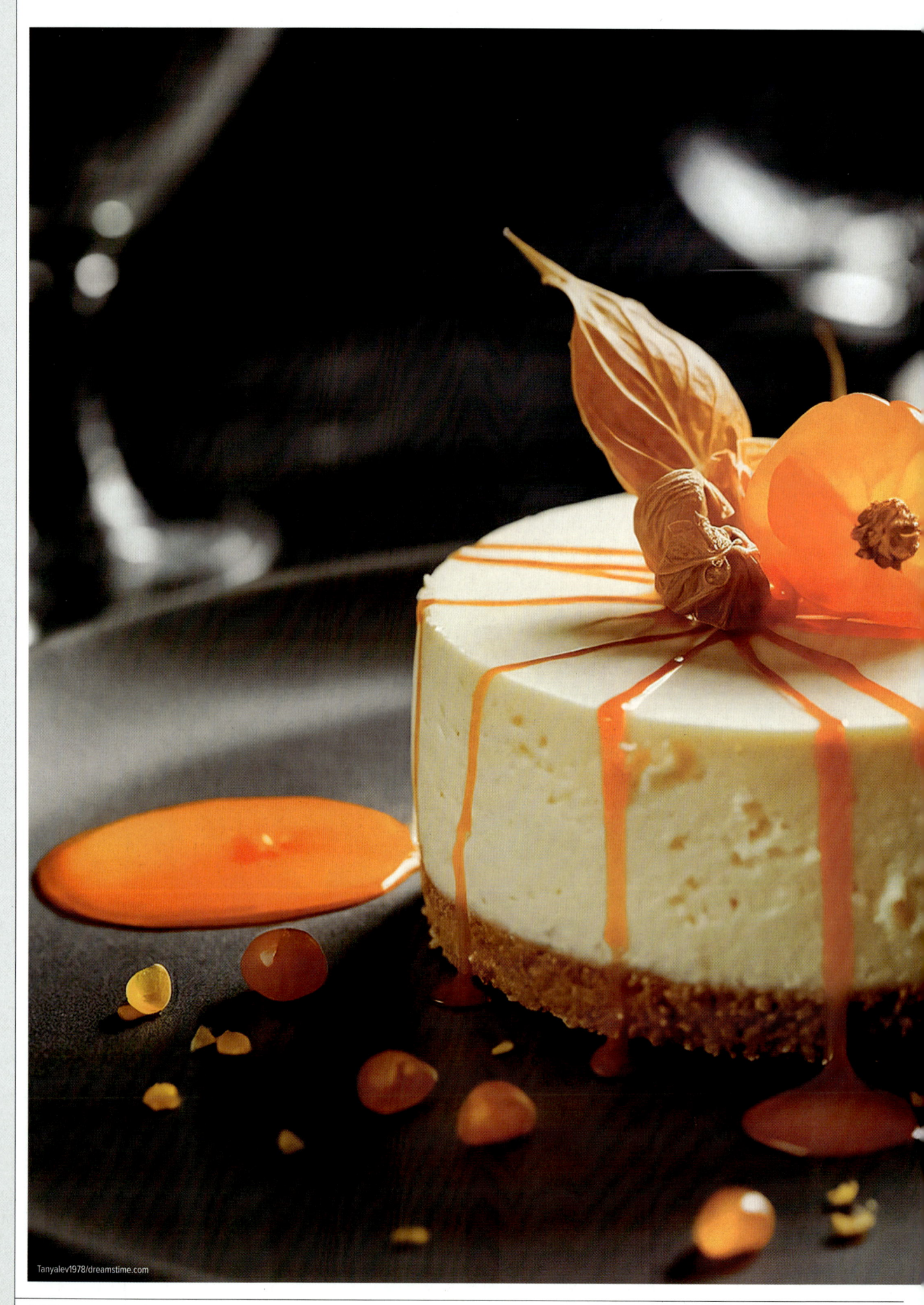

GLUTEN-FREE RECIPES

Orange Cheesecake

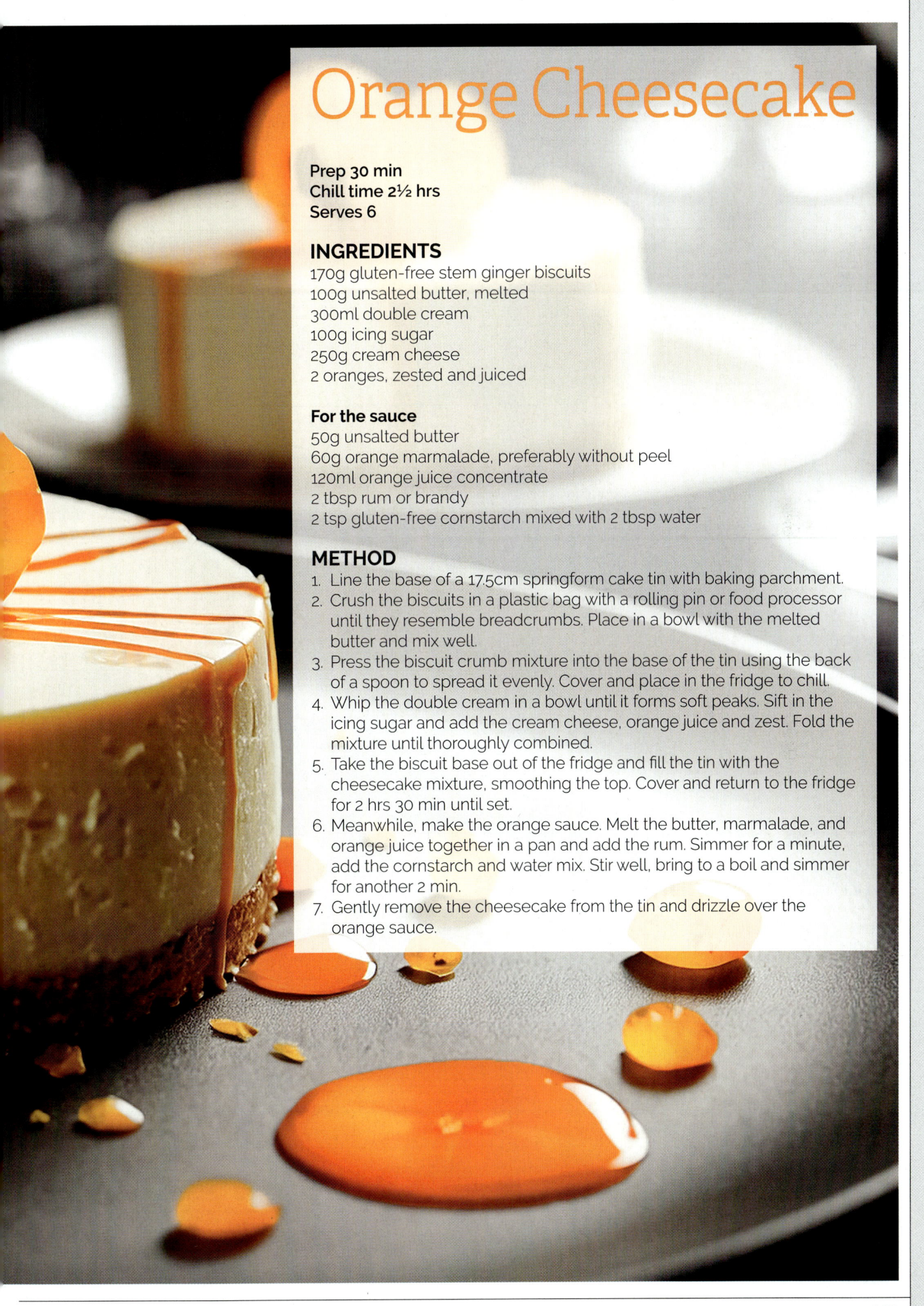

Prep 30 min
Chill time 2½ hrs
Serves 6

INGREDIENTS
170g gluten-free stem ginger biscuits
100g unsalted butter, melted
300ml double cream
100g icing sugar
250g cream cheese
2 oranges, zested and juiced

For the sauce
50g unsalted butter
60g orange marmalade, preferably without peel
120ml orange juice concentrate
2 tbsp rum or brandy
2 tsp gluten-free cornstarch mixed with 2 tbsp water

METHOD
1. Line the base of a 17.5cm springform cake tin with baking parchment.
2. Crush the biscuits in a plastic bag with a rolling pin or food processor until they resemble breadcrumbs. Place in a bowl with the melted butter and mix well.
3. Press the biscuit crumb mixture into the base of the tin using the back of a spoon to spread it evenly. Cover and place in the fridge to chill.
4. Whip the double cream in a bowl until it forms soft peaks. Sift in the icing sugar and add the cream cheese, orange juice and zest. Fold the mixture until thoroughly combined.
5. Take the biscuit base out of the fridge and fill the tin with the cheesecake mixture, smoothing the top. Cover and return to the fridge for 2 hrs 30 min until set.
6. Meanwhile, make the orange sauce. Melt the butter, marmalade, and orange juice together in a pan and add the rum. Simmer for a minute, add the cornstarch and water mix. Stir well, bring to a boil and simmer for another 2 min.
7. Gently remove the cheesecake from the tin and drizzle over the orange sauce.

Eating out gluten-free

Socialising shouldn't pose a challenge or lead to embarrassment for anyone who needs to avoid gluten.

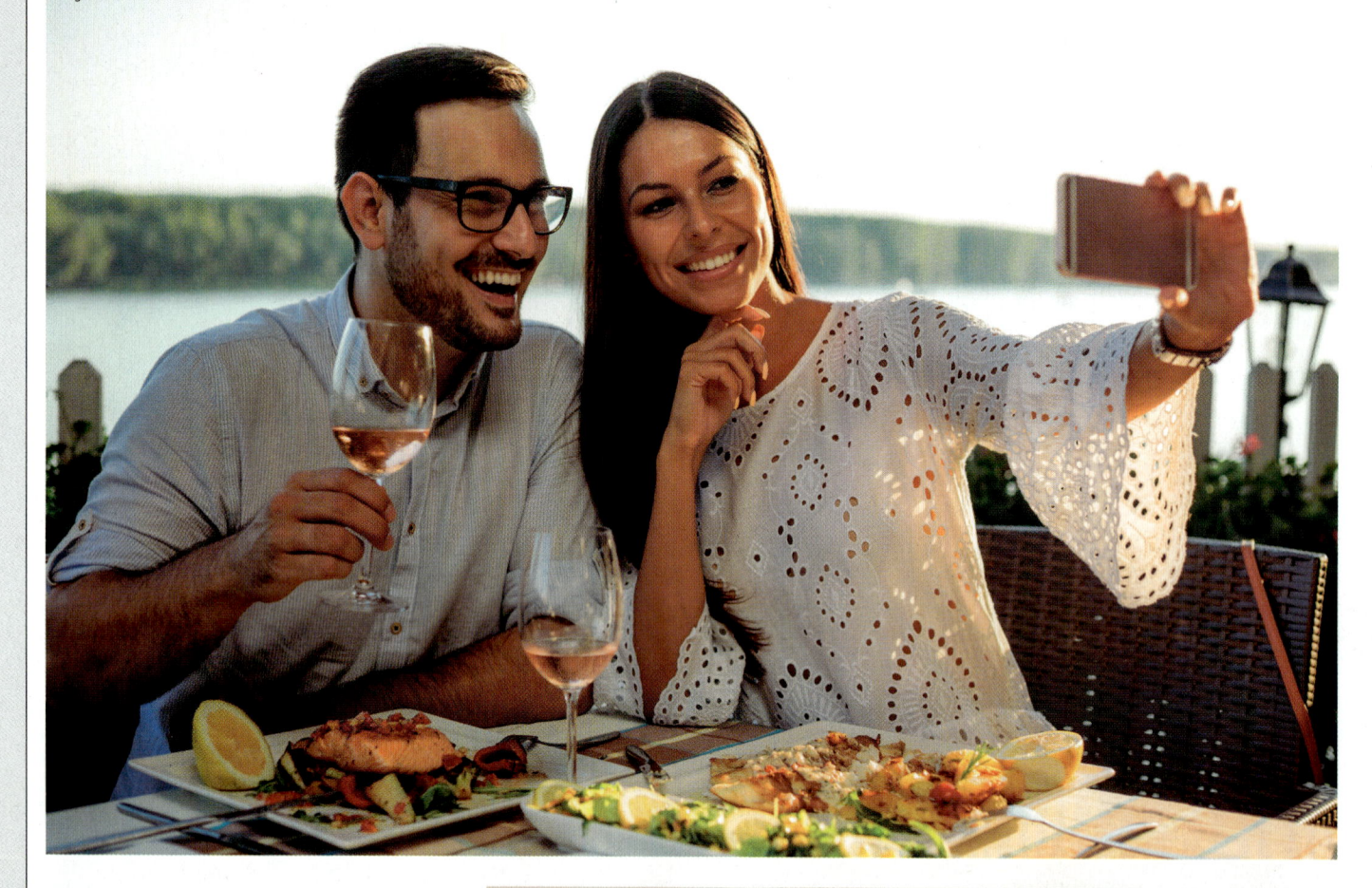

Eating out with friends and family is one of the great pleasures in life and it's wrong if it leads to awkwardness for anyone in the party. For a person who needs to take care over gluten, or anyone who wants to invite a gluten-free friend to join them for a meal, there are a few things that can be done to ensure you all have an enjoyable time.

The main thing to bear in mind is that everyone has the right to question the food they are about to eat, so there should be no embarrassment in quizzing the restaurant owners or staff about their

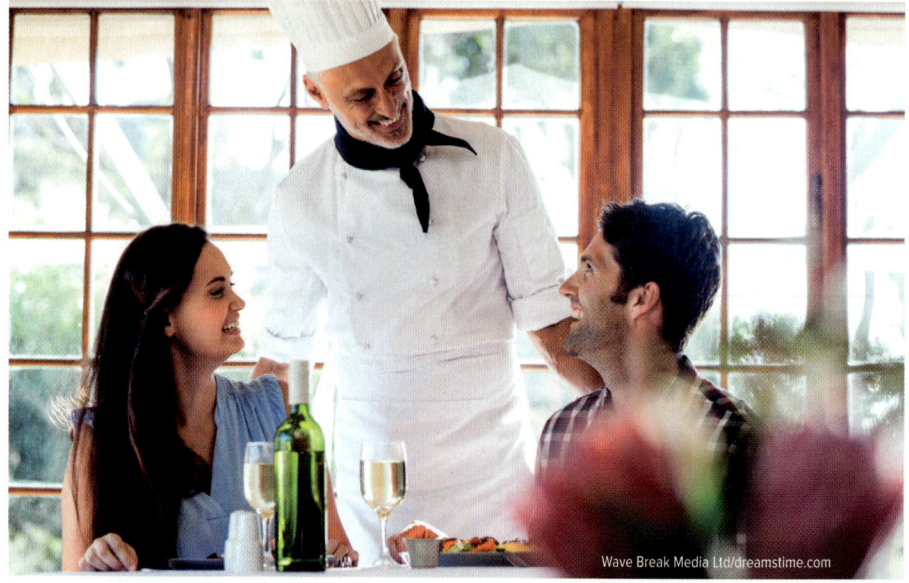

EATING OUT GLUTEN-FREE

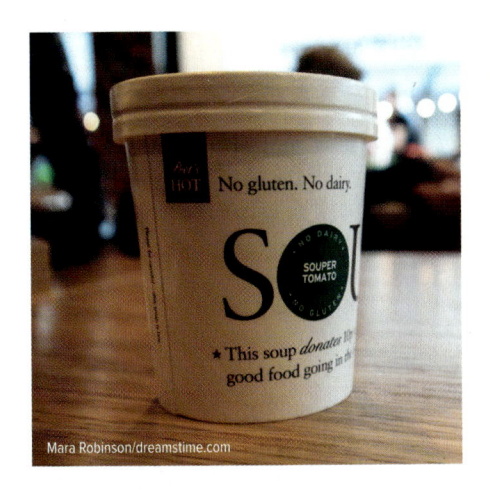

gluten policies. There is far more awareness and many more choices of restaurants and cafes that serve gluten-free menu items today than there has been in the past. Gluten-free is not the gastronomic desert it once was and there are a number of restaurants that provide only gluten-free food. Even some lunchtime sandwich shops, and fast-food establishments now offer a few suitable menu items.

Although, if you are very sensitive you must bear in mind cross-contamination in preparation and serving areas, and multi-food uses of deep fat fryers and ovens. Happily, there is a growing consciousness of possible contamination in restaurants and cafes, and they approach the subject openly. The Pizza Express chain, for example, provides a colour-coded pizza slicer to accompany its gluten-free pizzas to ensure there's no transfer of wheat traces.

Although you may have to accept that not every establishment will be willing, or able, to accommodate gluten-free eating, these days there is a very good chance of finding a good one that will.

Planning your meal out

Do some research beforehand on restaurant websites. They often have sample online menus that will give you a clue as to whether they offer a good range of gluten-free dishes. And you should be able to read their allergy policies there as well.

Coeliac UK, the National Celiac Association in the US and Coeliac Australia all have lists of accredited restaurants. Online review websites can help you find a local establishment offering gluten-free, as diners often leave comments on gf food they have enjoyed. Lots of gluten-free bloggers also offer their opinions on places they have visited.

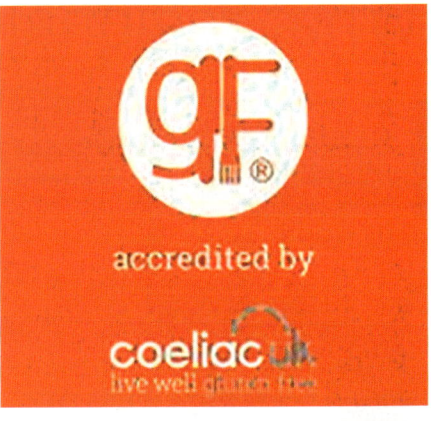

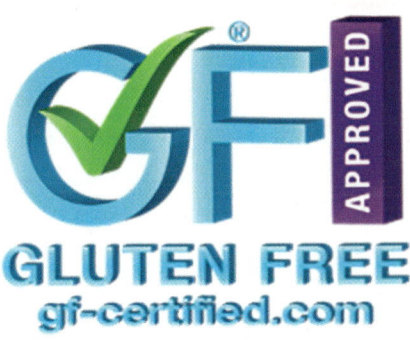

Once the restaurant or café has been chosen and booked, it's a good idea to phone ahead to warn them that your food has to be strictly gluten-free. Ask to speak to the manager and/or the head chef so you know the message has been received by someone in authority. Mention cross-contamination if you know this could be an issue.

Speak to your server when you sit down at the table and make sure that they, and the manager, appreciate that your gluten-free status is a serious health issue and not just a healthy eating choice.

When your food arrives, get the waiting staff to confirm it is definitely gluten-free. If you sense any hesitation, politely ask them to fetch the manager. If you're still not reassured, then don't eat the food. If you have made your requirements plain from the outset there should be no question of having to pay for it.

If you enjoy a really good gluten-free meal out it is helpful to leave a positive review of the restaurant for others to use as a guide.

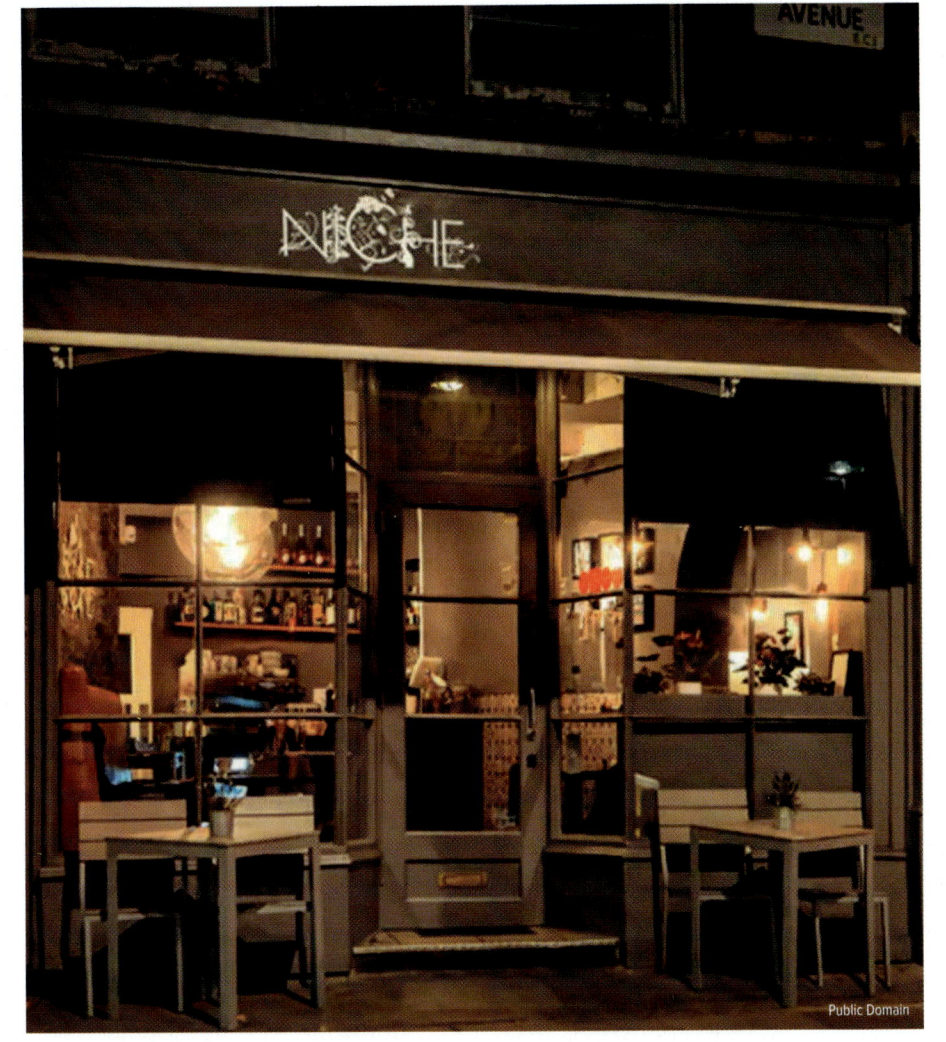

THE GLUTEN-FREE HANDBOOK

EATING OUT GLUTEN-FREE

What regional foods are best for gluten-free?

If you like experiencing food from other countries, either eating in at restaurants or having a takeaway, there are some cuisines that offer a lot of gluten-free choice.

Thai
The base ingredients for many Thai dishes are rice, rice noodles, bean thread noodles, coconut milk and fresh vegetables and meats – all of which should be safe for gluten-free eating. However, watch out for fish sauce as it may be wheat based. Check on whether wheat flour has been used to thicken curry sauces, satay and coconut or green tea ice cream. Avoid teriyaki sauce, oyster sauce, soy sauce, soba noodles and deep-fried foods.

Mexican
Much of Mexican cuisine is based on corn, rice and beans and so should be safe. Go for corn tortillas, quesadillas, tacos, fajitas, refried beans, and salsas. Avoid flour tortillas and dishes such as burritos. Check sauces haven't been thickened with wheat flour and that cheese has been freshly grated, as some pre-packed grated cheese has flour dusted through it to prevent clogging.

Spanish
Classic Spanish dishes use a lot of rice, potatoes, fresh meat, fish, and shellfish. Cured hams like serrano and iberico are fine as they are dry cured without any coatings. Watch out for sauces, though, that might contain wheat flour thickeners, and snack foods such as tapas – pintxos, cosas de picar and cazuelas. Pintxos consist of rounds of crostini with toppings. Other tapas to avoid are meat balls that may contain wheat flour or breadcrumbs as a binder, croquettes fried in breadcrumbs, and small dishes in sauce that could contain wheat thickeners.

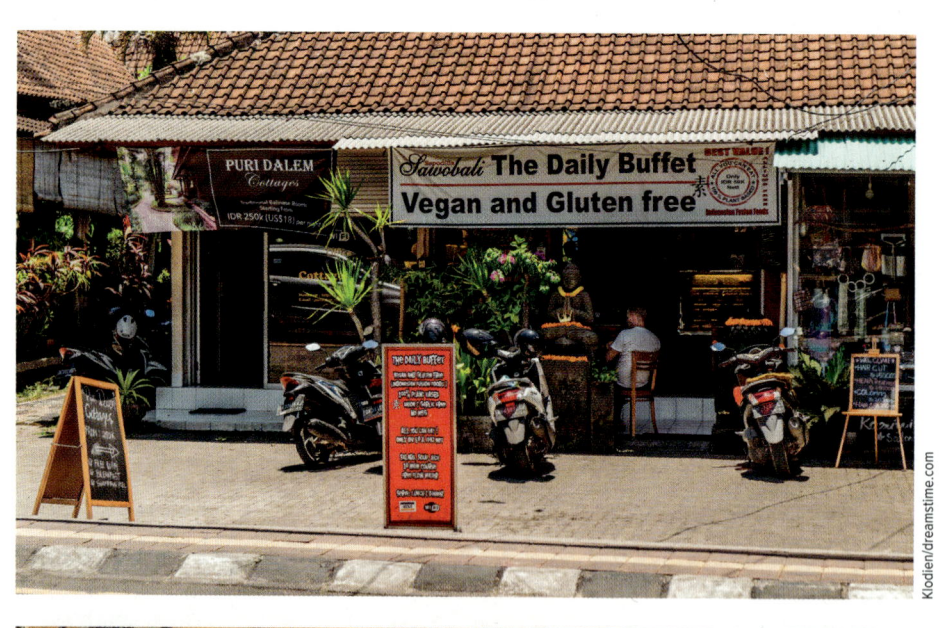

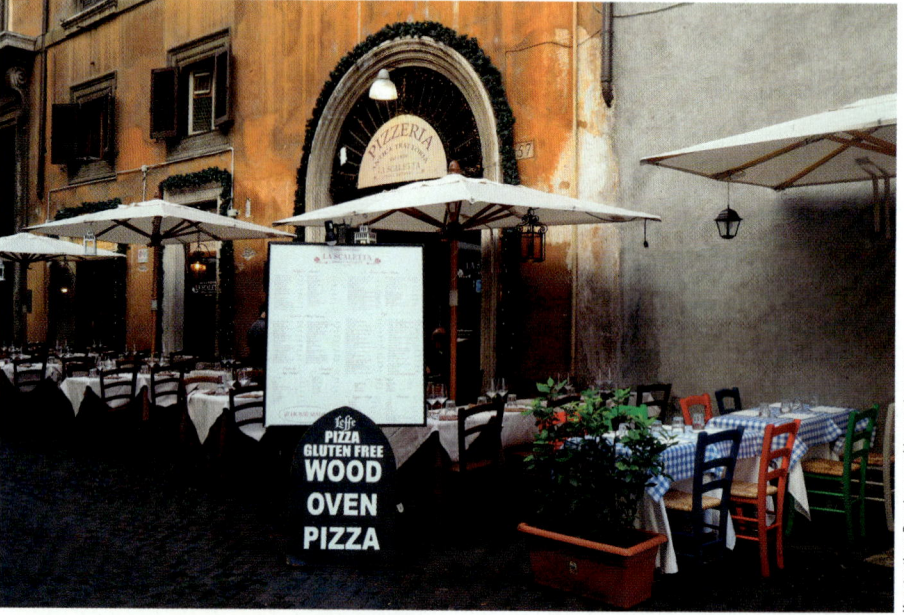

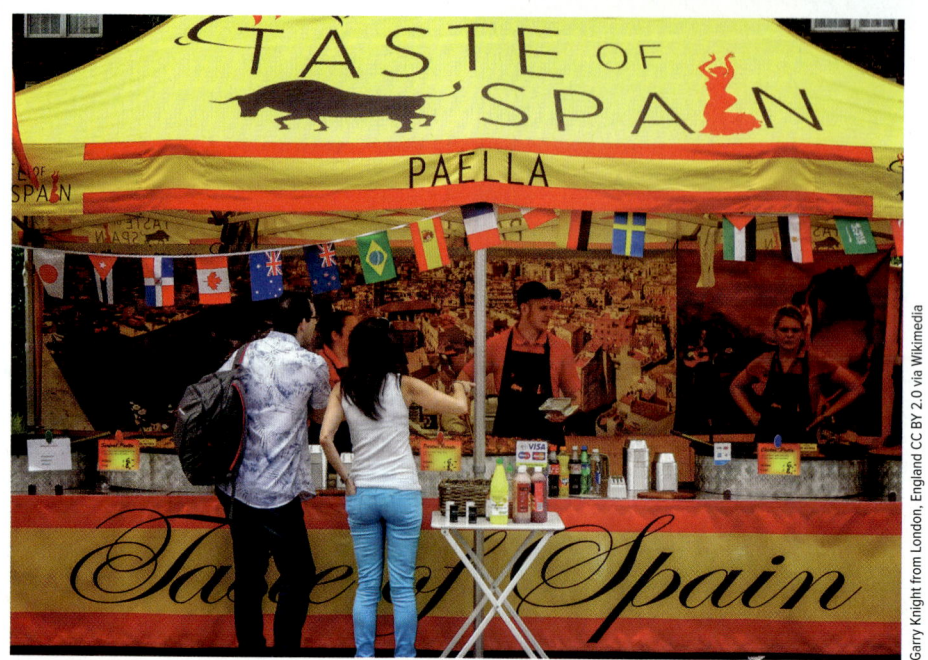

Indian
Mostly rice-based dishes with curries that are thickened using onion and gram flour. The same goes for onion bhajis and poppadoms, which use lentil or rice

EATING OUT GLUTEN-FREE

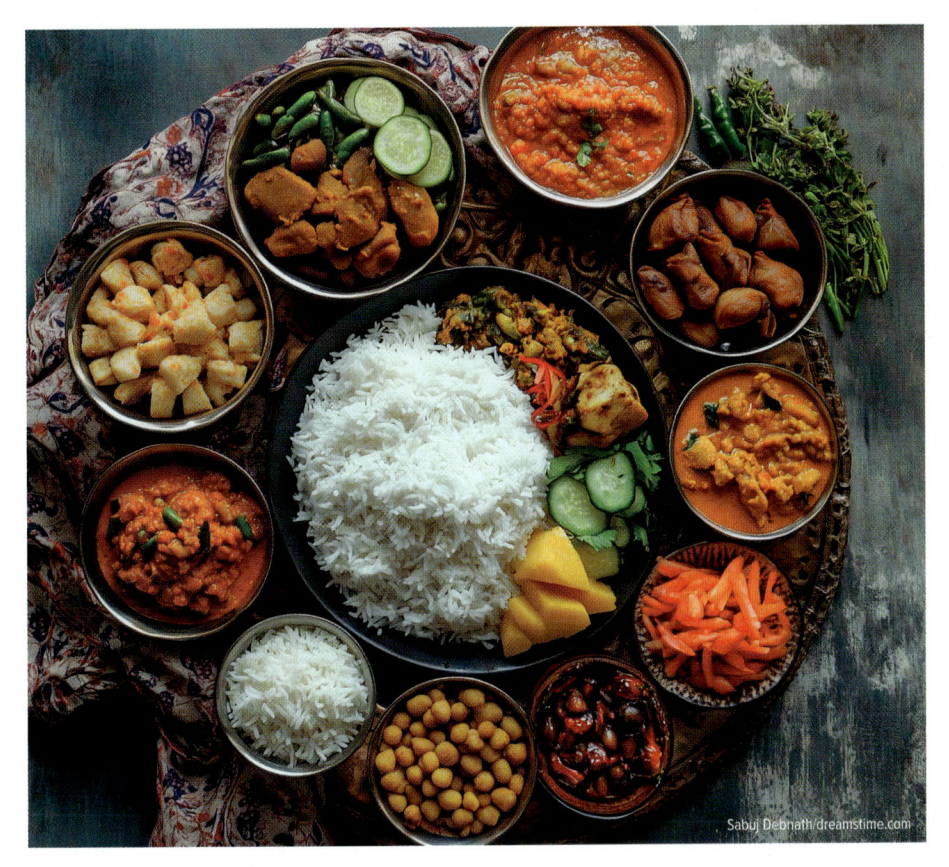

flour. Avoid samosas and any of the breads – naan, roti, chapati, etc – as they are usually made with wheat flour, and check with the restaurant about cross-contamination with the oil used for the poppadoms.

Greek
The fresh grilled meat, seafood and salads served in Greek restaurants lend themselves to gluten-free eating. Dolmades, stuffed tomatoes and peppers all use rice. Most of the hearty stews will be thickened with tomato paste but check that this is the case.

Avoid pita bread and taramasalata, which can contain bread to bulk out the fish roe. Hummus should be fine but it's wise to check this one as well for added extras.

Italian
By its nature, Italian food is laden with wheat products. However, there are many restaurants that do offer gluten-free pasta and pizzas on their menus. The important thing to check is that they are aware of, and deal with, any issues of cross-contamination before you book to visit them.

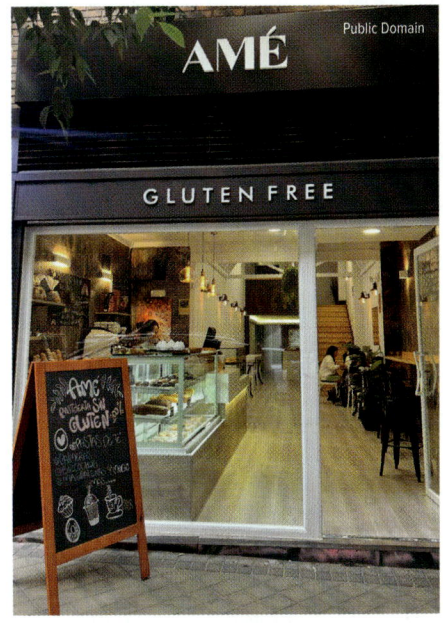

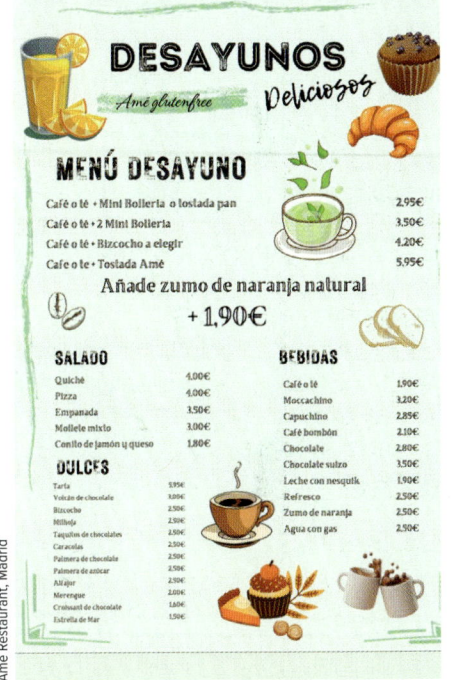

Gluten Free Menu
All Gluten Free Items are made in a Gluten Environment. Only you know your tolerance level. Please use your best judgment.

11" Cheese Pizza	$16.95
11" 1 Topping Pizza	$18.50
Each additional topping	$2.50
11" Fit For A King Pizza	$22.95
Cheese, Pepperoni, Sausage, Mushrooms, Black Olives, Bell Peppers, and Onion	
11" The Works Pizza	$20.75
Cheese, Pepperoni, Sausage, Mushrooms & Onion or Anchovy	
11" Vegetarian Pizza	$20.75
Cheese, Mushrooms, Black Olives, Bell Pepper & Onion	

All Gluten Free Pastas are served a la carte

Pasta Primavera	$18.95
Gluten free mostaccioli with garlic & fresh vegetables	
Shrimp Filippi	$22.70
Our own shrimp dish served with Gluten free mostaccioli	
Mostaccioli Marinara	$15.50
Gluten free mostaccioli with marinara	
Mostaccioli With Pesto	$18.95
A Gluten free mostaccioli with fresh basil pesto or pesto cream	
Chicken Parmigiana	$20.75
A Gluten free version of our house favorite	

Sandwiches???
All of our sandwiches can be made on a plate without the bread!

Filippo's Restaurant, California

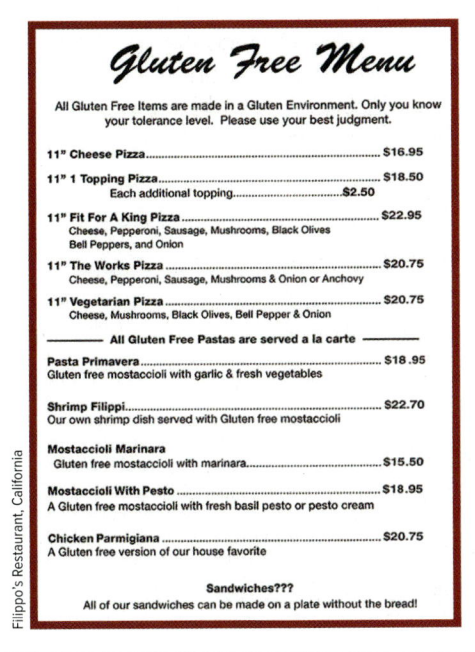

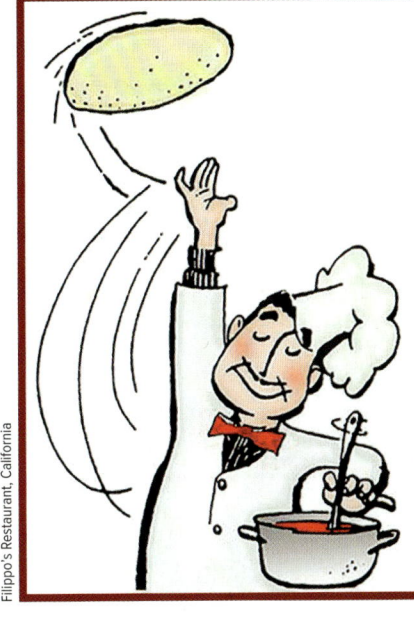

GLUTEN FREE PIZZA DOUGH

Whole Grain Brown Rice Flour, Whole Grain Millet Flour, Potato Flour, Tapioca Flour, Sorghum, Guaram Gum, Olive Oil, Cake Yeast, Whole Eggs, Salt, Sugar

We make our Dough in a "Gluten Environment" but in a separate area of the kitchen. The shells are par cooked and individually frozen. We then cook them on screens in our brick ovens. Every effort is made to keep our Gluten Free items separate from other items. *"Only you know your tolerance level."* We hope you enjoy our efforts!! Thank you,
Tom & The Crew

THE GLUTEN-FREE HANDBOOK

105

TRAVEL GLUTEN-FREE

Enjoying a happy gluten-free holiday

If you know that eating is going to be restricted it can be daunting organising a holiday to an unfamiliar place, but that shouldn't hold you back.

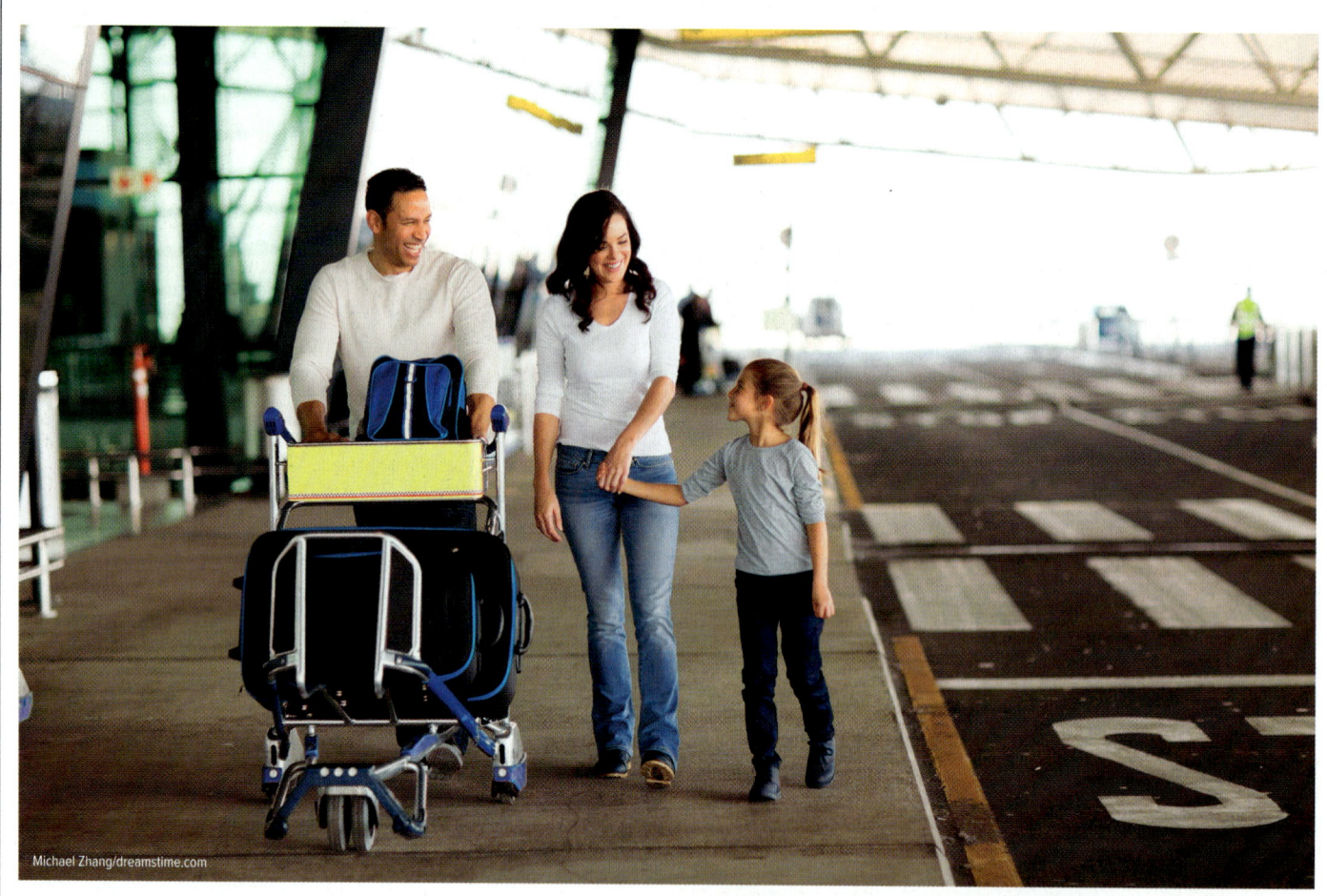

Michael Zhang/dreamstime.com

Prykhodov/dreamstime.com

Planning a getaway
Book early! Most holiday providers prefer, and sometimes require, a reasonable amount of time to prepare, so aim to begin the process at least three months before you want to go away.

DIY booking
If you are doing all the organising yourself, do some initial research on the internet. Overall, it's a good idea to find out how accommodating the country you are thinking of visiting is to those requiring gluten-free.

Specifically, even in your home country, have a look at your chosen

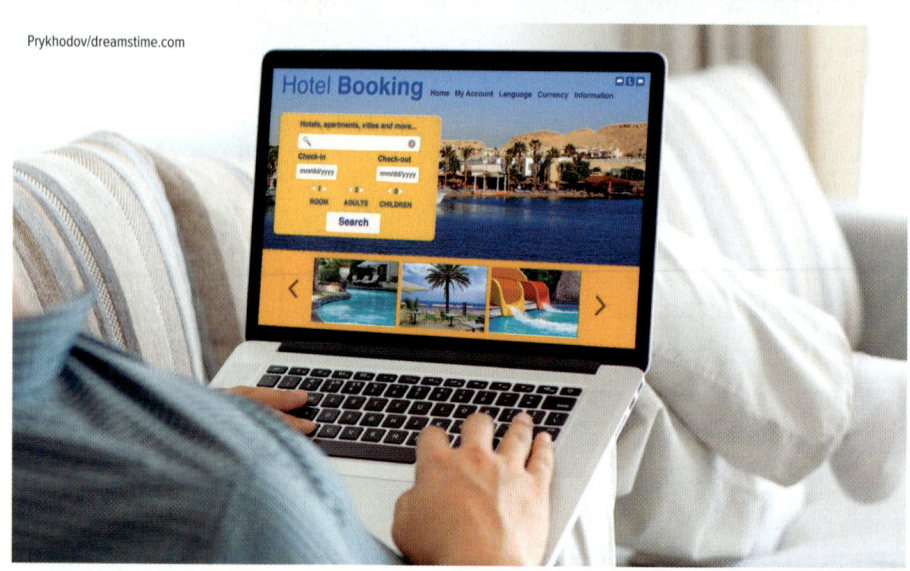

TRAVEL GLUTEN-FREE

FINDING GLUTEN-FREE GOODIES ALL OVER THE WORLD
Alexandra from London

Alexandra Chapman is a journalist and food devotee. "To tell you the truth, I thought the world had ended when I discovered I couldn't eat gluten. My body had told me this since the age of 15 but I ignored it, no matter how bad the symptoms. From skin problems to a permanently upset stomach, to headaches and hair loss, I continued to dismiss what I deep down knew was the root of my problem. I gave in after a work trip to Italy, where I was so ill after eating that I missed meetings and deadlines – no pizza or pasta was worth that pain and upset.

After initially receiving some confusing medical advice at a time when coeliac awareness was seemingly limited, I made a huge life change and have been following a strict gluten-free diet for almost 12 years now. My skin is clear, my stomach happy, my headaches have gone, and I have full, healthy hair.

As someone who was literally sick and tired of getting unexpectedly 'glutenated', I set up an Instagram account and blog to help my fellow members of the gluten-free community who want to relax when doing one of the best things in life: eating.

From a US/UK/Lat Am family, I seek out tested gluten-free options wherever I am lucky enough to go in the world. The further you get from home the harder it can be, but the more worthwhile it is. Some of the best gluten-free food I've ever eaten has been in the places I would least expect.

Nothing gets me more excited than a foreign supermarket filled with new gluten free treats. In fact, I have zero restraint and so on return come back through UK Customs with a suitcase packed to breaking, hence the title of my blog and Instagram account: The Gluten Free Suitcase."

Visit Alex's Insta page for more information www.instagram.com/theglutenfreesuitcase

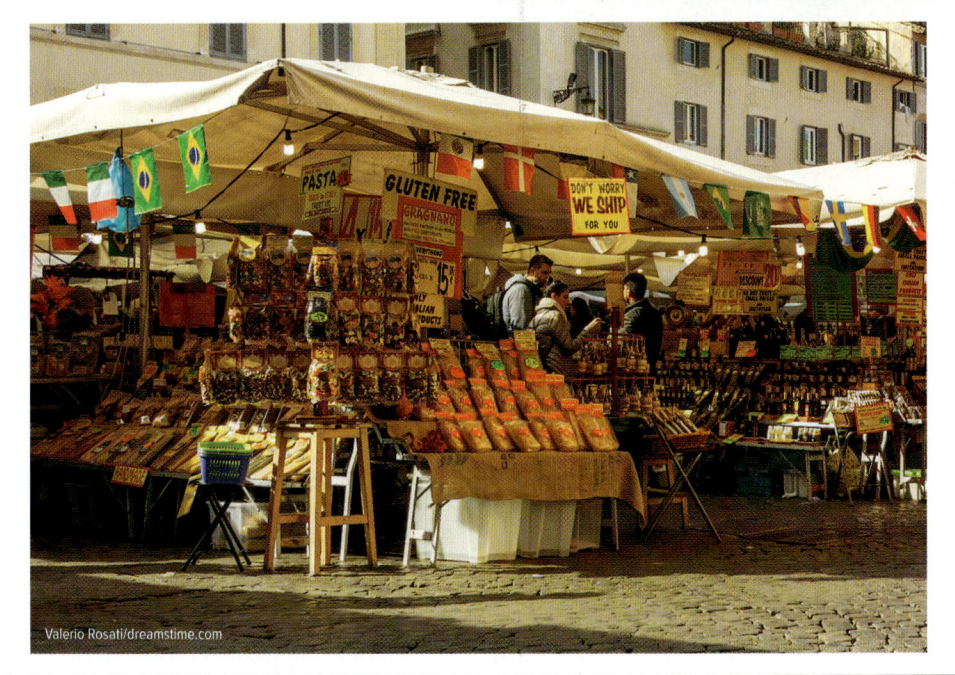

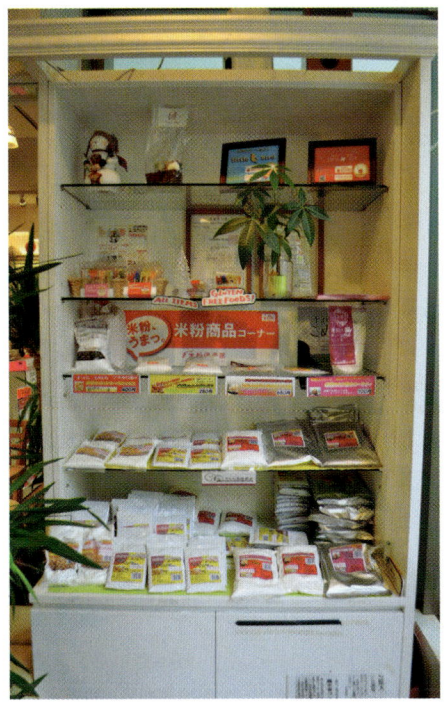

hotel, B&B, cruise company, airline, or train operator's website to see if they have a Dietary Restrictions page or a Policy on Allergens page. That should give you an indication of their awareness, commitment, and responsibility. Be aware that most operators will state that they cannot guarantee the absence of cross-contamination.

Once you are happy that you have found what you're looking for, make contact directly with the hotel, tour provider, airline, etc, to alert them to your requirements. Don't rely on a comment on the booking form. Preferably, email them so that you get a written reply and have a name to quote and proof of what you have requested in case you need to show this as confirmation or authorisation at a later date.

Travel Agents

If you are booking through a travel agency or a specific tour operator, then mention the importance of being gluten-free in the very first conversation or correspondence. This will help them to focus your choices on the most appropriate locations, hotels, camp sites, cruise ship options, etc, and put you in touch with their Allergen Department, if they have one. Then do your own research along the lines of the DIY Booking advice before you finally commit.

THE GLUTEN-FREE HANDBOOK

TRAVEL GLUTEN-FREE

Things to consider

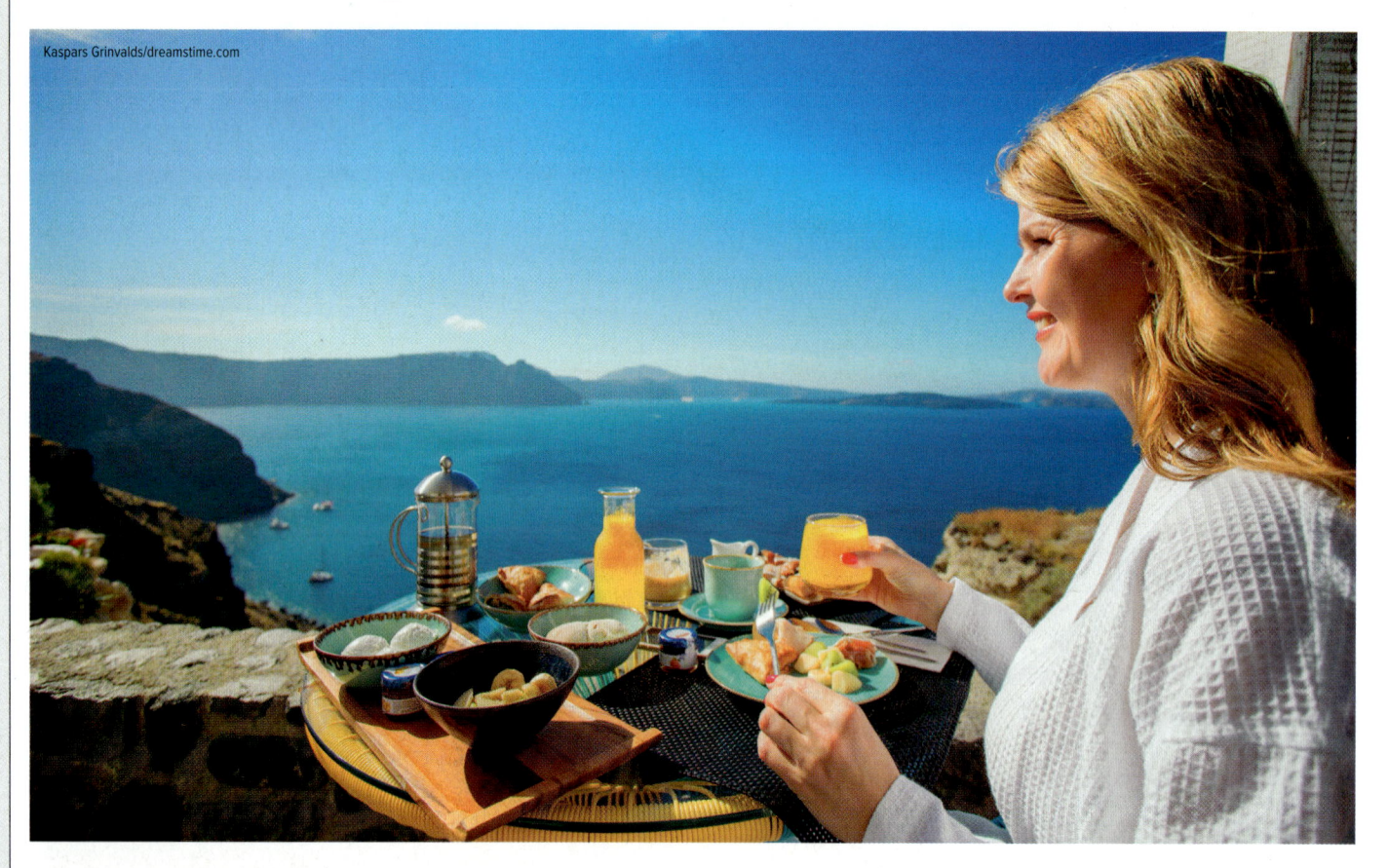

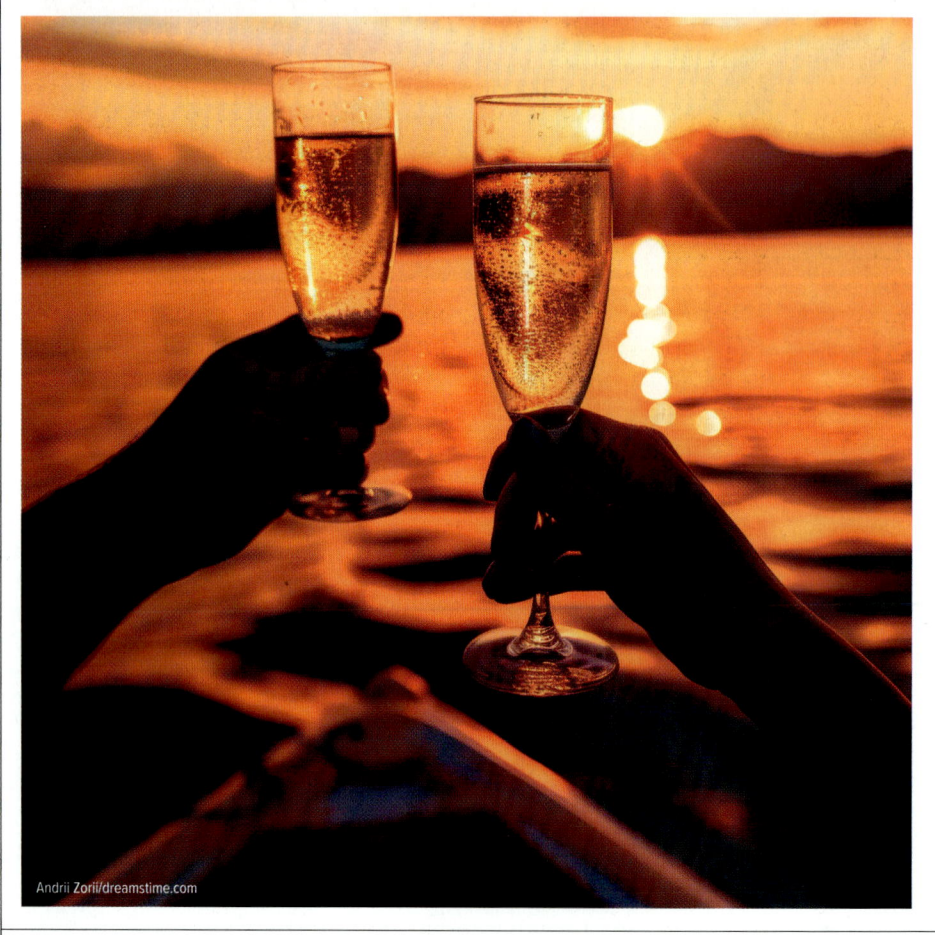

Importing food
If you are unsure about the availability of gluten-free products where you are going you may want to bring supplies of your own. Some countries, however, have strict rules on bringing in plant-based foods. Find out the rules from the customs agency of the country you want to visit. You should be able to find a contact through the relevant embassy or consulate website.

A doctor's letter
If you have a diagnosed gluten condition, it could be useful to have a note from your doctor to that effect. If you want to carry gluten-free food with you it would be helpful proof if you are questioned by immigration or an airline.

Travel insurance
It's important that you declare your gluten status on your travel insurance form in case you are unfortunate to fall seriously ill on holiday.

TRAVEL GLUTEN-FREE

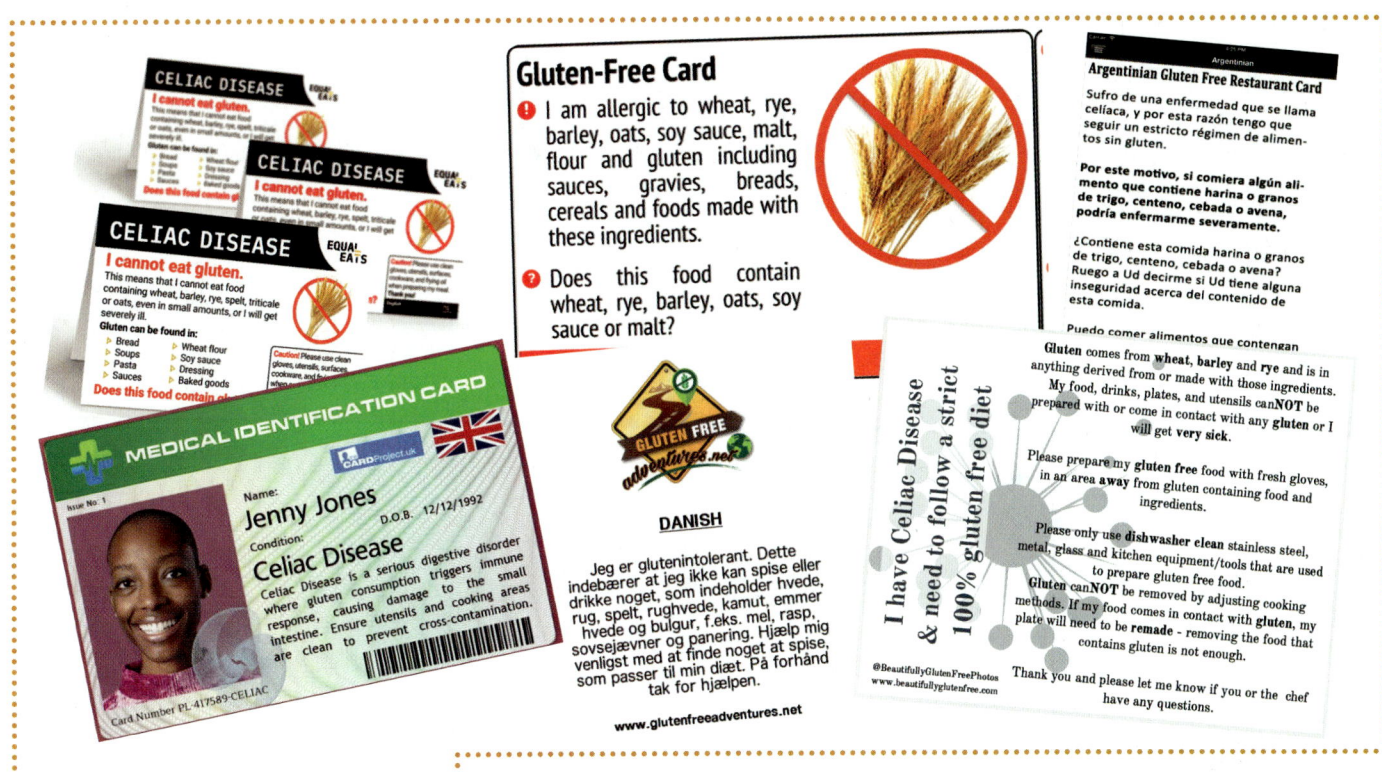

A medical alert card
It is a good idea to carry a card stating that you are coeliac or have a wheat allergy in case you have to be taken to hospital for any reason. In European Union countries you should also have a Global Health Insurance card.

Restaurant bookings
Eating out abroad is the same as in your own country. Advice is given on page 102.

Restaurant cards
It is a good idea to have a card or sheet that translates your gluten status and requirements in the language of the country you are visiting. You can either do that yourself with the help of a translation app or look online for one of the many companies that provide both free and paid-for ones.

Finding restaurants
Research places to eat before you go and mark them on a local map or pin them on Google Maps on your phone to make them easy to find once you get there. Don't forget to download the map to your phone so you can still use it even if you don't have access to wi-fi. There are restaurant finder websites listed in the chapter starting on page 110.

Translation apps
Download a translation app to your phone so you can communicate that you have an issue with gluten or to ask if gluten-free foods are available in shops, etc. Many of the apps provide verbal translations as well as written.

Buffets
Not every guest is careful with the use of serving spoons at a buffet so it might be useful to take a couple of your own serving spoons with you to avoid cross-contamination.

Airline meals
Book these well ahead of taking your flight and get something in writing to confirm that they have been ordered. Then ask when you check in to make sure the airline has definitely allocated you a gluten-free meal on that flight. Belt and braces, check with the cabin staff as you board. If you wait until you're in your seat, you'll have no chance to get something to replace the missing meal. And don't forget to check your return flight as well!

Carry your own snacks for the journey
Often airports, ferry terminals, train stations, roadside cafes and petrol stops are gluten-free wastelands!

Medicines and beauty products
Wherever possible, take enough supplies of known safe medicinal products – painkillers, Imodium, insect bite cream – and sunscreen, moisturiser, shampoo, etc, to last for the duration of the holiday. Labelling on local products cannot be guaranteed to include information on whether wheat starch, etc, has been used in their manufacture.

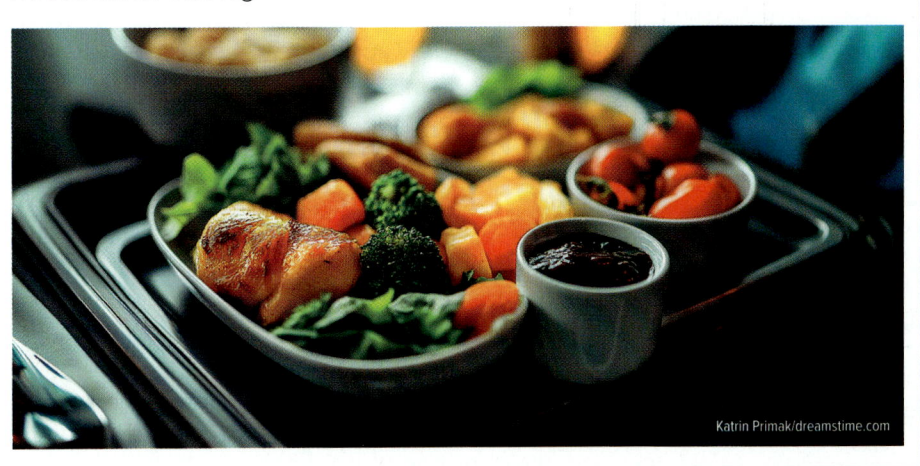

THE GLUTEN-FREE HANDBOOK

BOOKS APPS WEBSITES

Books, apps, and websites

There is a wealth of information and practical advice available in books and online. These lists are by no means exhaustive, but they will hopefully point out some of the places to look.

Mail-order meals
United Kingdom
Baked to Taste
https://bakedtotaste.co.uk
From their base in Devon this company supplies cakes, scones and pastries, savoury pies, quiches, and snacks, all gluten-free. They also have a range of vegan and vegetarian dishes.

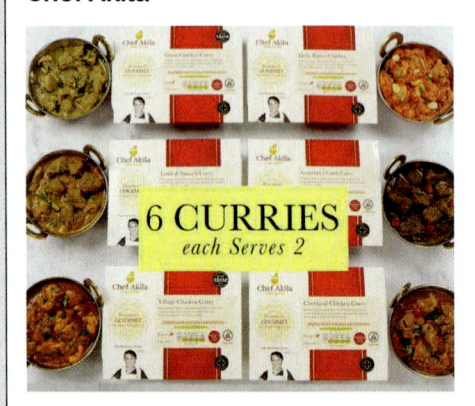

Chef Akila
www.chefakila.com
A wide range of hand-cooked, gluten-free Indian meals, as well as curry selection boxes for six chicken, meat, vegetarian, or low carb meals. Select gluten-free from the By Diet menu listing on the home page.

Field Doctor
www.fielddoctor.co.uk
Personalised meals delivered frozen in batches on a subscription basis. The nutritionists at Field Doctor design a gluten-free and other allergens menu from their 60+ different meals to suit the customer's needs. You decide how many meals and how often you want them delivered.

Wildcraft
https://wildcraftbakery.com
A specialist gluten-free bakery that also has a cafe in Leeds and a Really Wild Club loyalty programme. The online shop sells breads, doughnuts, scones, pies, and biscuits.

Sue's Free From Kitchen
www.theglutenfreekitchen.co.uk
A bakery in North Yorkshire that produces gluten-free cakes and tarts, crumbles, cheesecakes, and cupcakes as well as savoury tarts and ready-to-roll pastry.

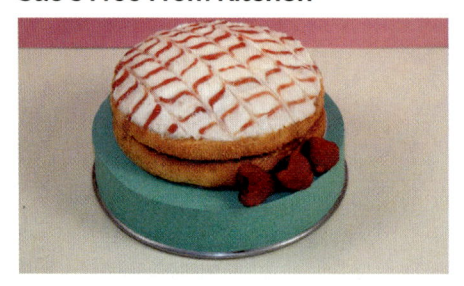

Wheat Free Bakery Direct
www.wheat-freebakerydirect.co.uk
A family business based in Scotland that supplies choux pastry goods, baguettes, naans, bagels, cupcakes, cookies, rolls and pizza bases.

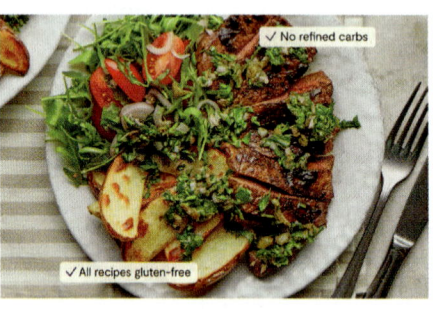

Mindful Chef
www.mindfulchef.com
Recipe boxes with the ingredients to make up to five gluten-free meals, delivered weekly. The company makes the point in the FAQs on its website that its ingredients are gluten-free, but its prepared ranges (breakfast, frozen meals) are made in factories that also handle gluten. It has strict rules and procedures in place to mitigate against cross-contamination and those products that may be affected are labelled as such.

Real Food Hub
www.realfoodhub.co.uk
Suppliers of meat, fish, cheese, etc, direct from the farmers and makers.

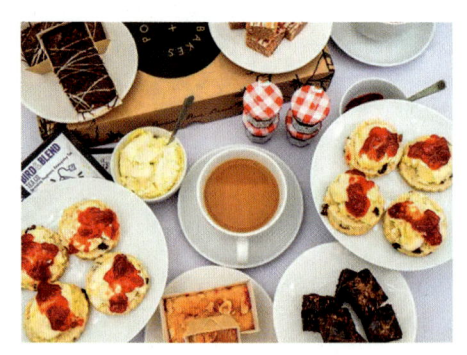

It has an extensive gluten-free range listed on a separate tab from its home page that includes gift boxes and hampers, sauces, jams, a charcuterie selection, and gluten-free beers, among other items.

United States
Metabolic Meals
https://mymetabolicmeals.com
A subscription service that delivers meals each week from a rotating menu. In its Nutrition FAQs the company says all its meals are gluten-free and made in a dedicated gluten-free facility.

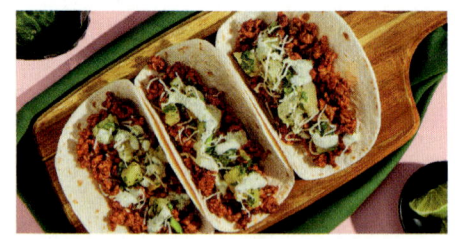

Green Chef
www.greenchef.com
Meal kits that provide pre-measured and prepared ingredients and step-by-step instructions for cooking them. The company says it has been made a validated Gluten Free Safe Spot by the Gluten Free Food Service, which is a food safety programme of the US Gluten Intolerance Group.

Epicured
https://epicured.getprado.com
A selection of medically tailored meals delivered on either a one-off order basis or a subscription plan. There are menu items for every sort

BOOKS APPS WEBSITES

of main meal, including breakfast, as well as small plates, snacks, sides, beverages, dressings, and sauces.

Modify Health

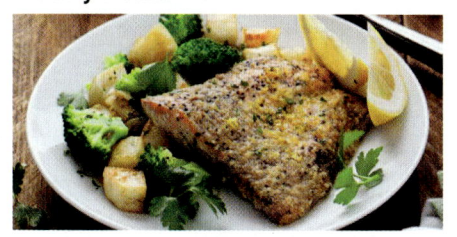

https://modifyhealth.com
Meals to cover a variety of dietary needs, including gluten-free, ordered on a weekly basis, and delivered with free shipping. You can also opt to join a Gluten-free FIT Quickstart Program, designed to get you on a path to healthier eating with the help of a dietician.

Mom's Meals

www.momsmeals.com
Ready-made meals that cater for gluten-free as well as diabetic, vegetarian, and low sodium diets along with other requirements such as food for those who have difficulty chewing or swallowing.

Gold Belly

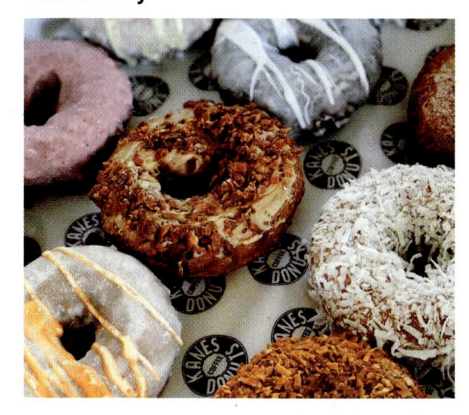

www.goldbelly.com/collections/gluten-free
Gluten-free meals kits, ready meals, desserts, sides, and appetizers. The company supplies favourites such as mac and cheese, pizza, and donuts, among many other tempting treats. Also ships to Canada.

BistroMD

www.bistromd.com
More than 120 gluten-free meals that you can select as part of a meal delivery program that provides breakfast, lunch, and dinner for either five or seven days a week.

Australia
Activate Foods

https://www.activatefoods.com.au
Gluten-free meals delivered to the Central Coast, Sydney, and Newcastle areas. You choose your meal preference from categories such as calorie-controlled, fresh, frozen, diabetic-friendly and family meals.

A Life Plus

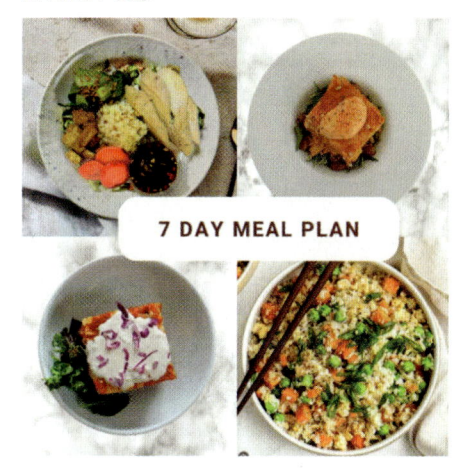

https://alifeplus.com.au/pages/healthy-meals-delivered-to-your-door-1
Chef-made, ready-to-eat, gluten-free, and healthy meals. You state your preferences, and the chef will create meals that suit your taste. Choose from a three-day, five-day, or seven-day meal plan.

nourish'd

https://nourishd.com.au
Delivered all over Australia, this company offers gluten-free choices from a rotating menu in three different meal sizes – regular, large, and extra-large.

Délidoor

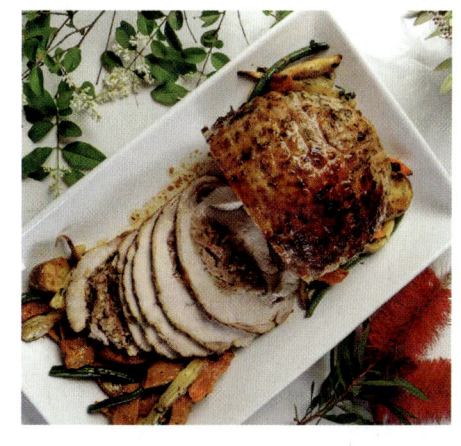

https://delidoor.com.au
Supplier of everyday meals for one, two or four people. It also offers various sauces to add to your own ingredients – carbonara, napolitana, and Bolognese are some examples. You can order on an individual basis or join a meal plan.

Wilding Foods

https://wildingfoods.com.au
All the company's meals are gluten-free using natural organic ingredients. Meals are currently delivered to Victoria and New South Wales.

Online cookery courses
Ûdemy

www.udemy.com/topic/gluten-free-cooking-and-baking
UK-based courses with lots of topics covering gluten-free cookery as well as courses on adapting to a gluten-free lifestyle.

Naomi Devlin

www.naomidevlin.co.uk/online-gluten-free-cookery-school
UK-based cookery school with online courses on making gluten-free noodles, bao and dumplings, sourdough starter, flaky pastry, and interesting breads.

Smart Raspberry

www.smartraspberry.com/classes-clubs/onlinecoeliac
UK-based cookery school specialising in training young people to cater for a gluten-free life.

Robyn's Gluten-free Baking Courses

www.glutenfreebakingcourses.com
US-based five courses including The Bread Course, The Flatbread Course and The Holidays Course.

America's Test Kitchen

www.onlinecookingschool.com/courses/gluten-free-baking
US-based course that includes an overview on gluten-free ingredients and lessons in baking and with three recipes to make.

Bake Club

https://bakeclub.com.au/products/gluten-free-baking-online-course
Australian-based gluten-free baking course with lots of recipes included.

THE GLUTEN-FREE HANDBOOK

BOOKS APPS WEBSITES

Recipe books

A selection of recently published cookery books, many of which also contain guidance to living gluten-free.

Eat and Enjoy Gluten Free
Laura Strange

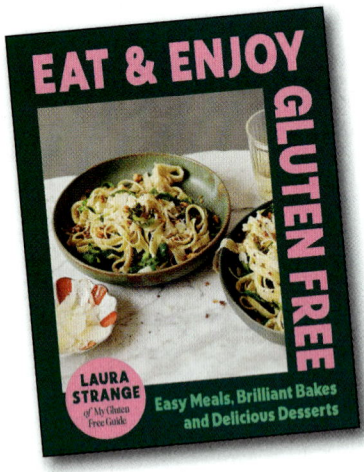

This book is split into two sections – Meals for Everyone and Baking Up a Storm. It covers midweek meals that can be ready in 30 minutes to international dishes and delicious pasta, as well as some yummy desserts.
Hardie Grant Publishing

Budget Gluten Free
Gluten Free Air Fryer
Becky Excell

These books showcase how you can make the most of your weekly shop and live gluten-free for less as well as making good use of your air fryer.
Quadrille Publishing

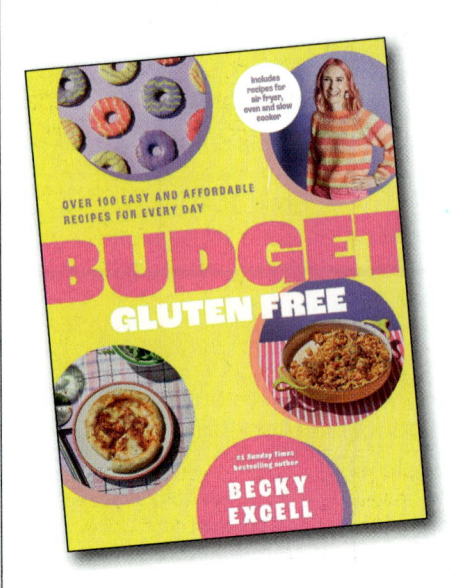

The Gluten-Free Family Cookbook
Lindsay Cotter

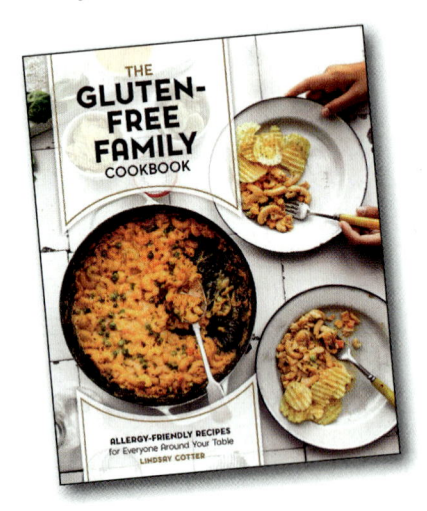

With 75-plus allergy-friendly recipes, many customisable for other specialty diets as well.
Fair Winds Press

The Big Gluten-Free Cookbook for Beginners
Gigi Stewart

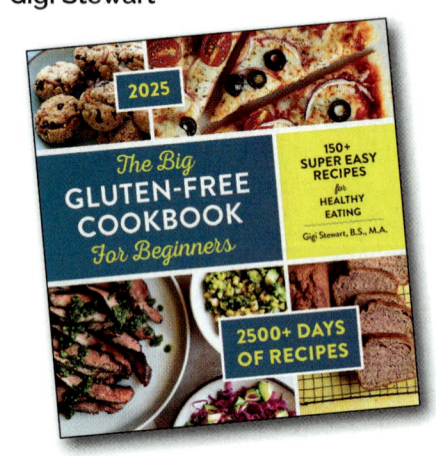

160 recipes for healthy eating, plus tips on organising your kitchen, checking labels and preparing your own gluten-free staples.
Callisto Publishing

The Ultimate Gluten-Free Cookbook
Sophia Matthews

Quick recipes with simple, everyday ingredients and including access to an interactive app to make cooking easier. From baking your own bread and pancakes to family recipes you could serve to guests, too, without breaking the bank.
Independently published

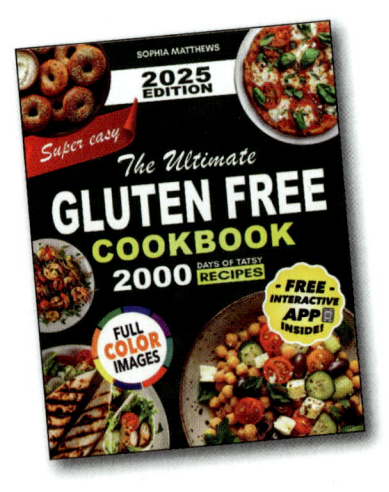

Gluten-Free Baking Cookbook
Doris Beasley

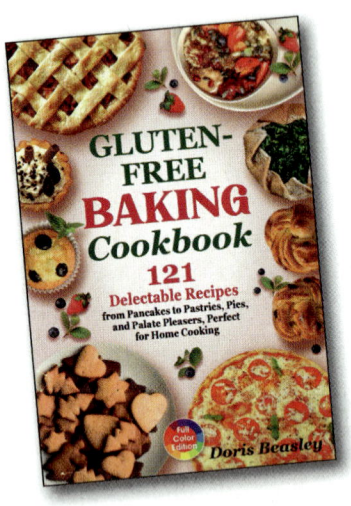

121 recipes for tempting baked goods, from tarts to cupcakes, pies to muffins, plus some fun facts to enjoy.
Independently published

Gluten Free Air Fryer Cookbook
Joan V Barnes

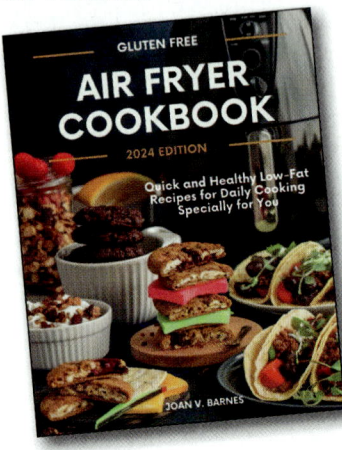

Crispy and delicious air fryer meals – appetisers, main meals, and desserts for family and for special occasions.
Independently published

BOOKS APPS WEBSITES

The Complete Low FODMAP Gluten-free Cookbook
Jennifer Simon

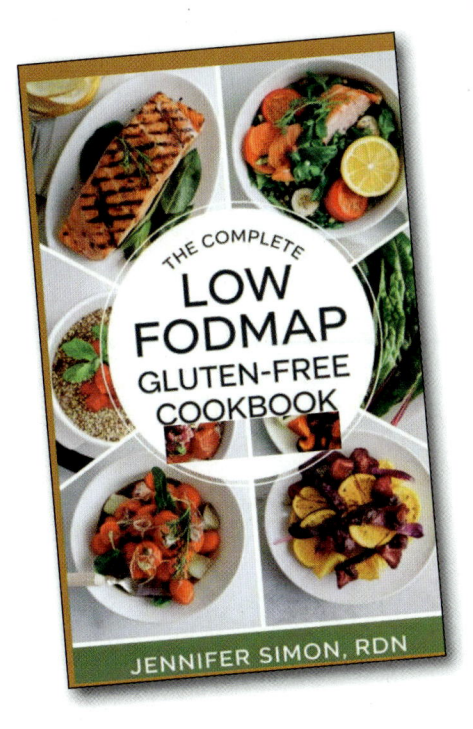

A guide to managing your diet by eliminating gluten and increasing your intake of low FODMAP foods.
Independently published

Gluten Free Cookbook UK
Diane Romano

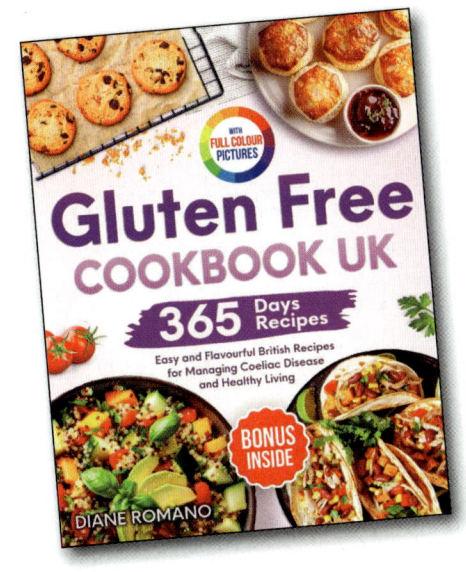

Recipes for every day of the year plus two bonus e-books on gluten-free bread and cooking with an air fryer.
Independently published

Love Gluten Free
Megan McKenna

80 recipes from the *Celebrity Masterchef* finalist that can be enjoyed by the whole family, regardless of their dietary requirements.
Hamlyn

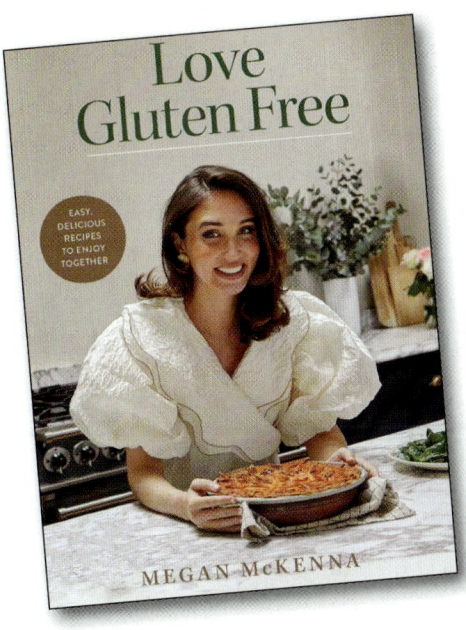

Travel

UK travel agencies
www.thecoeliactravelconsultant.com
https://thehealthyholidaycompany.co.uk/gluten-free-holidays

US travel agencies
www.glutenfreevacations.com
www.artisansofleisure.com/tour/Food_Restrictions_tours_luxury_travel_Gluten_Free_Travel.php

Australia travel agencies
www.travelleaders.com/agents?slctInterest=Gluten-Free%20

Canada travel agencies
https://celiaccruise.com

Apps
All of these apps are available for iOS and Android

Coeliac UK Living Well Gluten Free
www.coeliac.org.uk/information-and-support/your-gluten-free-hub/food-and-drink-information/live-well-gluten-free-app
To save typing the long URL, look under the Food and Drink Information tab on coeliac.org.uk The app has a product scanner, the option to set your dietary preferences in searches, and around 3,000 accredited venues around the UK and recommendations from the coeliac community.

Find Me Gluten Free
www.findmeglutenfree.com
A restaurant search app that helps you find a good place to eat all over the world.

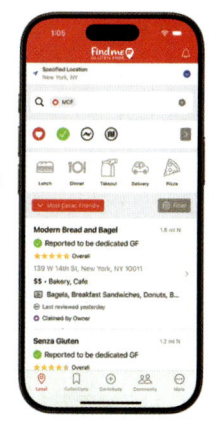

Gluten Free Restaurant Cards
www.celiactravel.com/cards
Contains cards covering 63 countries that can be shown to restaurant staff to confirm your gluten status and advise what you can and can't eat in their own language.

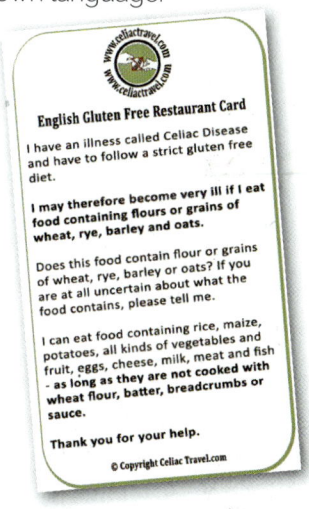

The Gluten Free Scanner
www.scanglutenfree.com
Use this app to scan barcodes on more than 500,000 products to find out whether they are gluten-free.

Spokin.com
www.spokin.com
A food allergy app where you can look up restaurants and grocery shops, allergy-friendly venues, and products around the world for a range of conditions, including gluten issues.

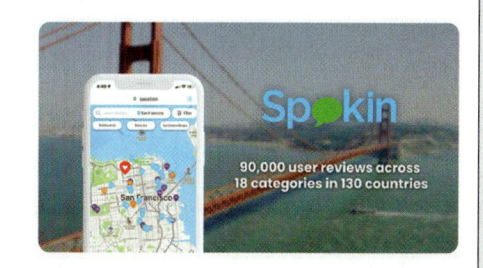

Information correct at time of going to press. Key Publishing does not endorse any of the companies or products seen here. Other suppliers are available.

THE GLUTEN-FREE HANDBOOK   113

Helpful organisations

There are a number of official places you can go for more information about gluten-related matters.

Practical Help
Communities of people who can give advice on all aspects of managing and living well with a gluten sensitivity.

Coeliac UK
www.coeliac.org.uk/
An independent UK charity with expertise in Coeliac Disease and the gluten-free diet. You can access a lot of information online or become a member for a small annual fee and increase the range of information and receive newsletters and updates. It provides trustworthy advice and support to members, funds research and fights for better availability of gluten-free food. There are local volunteer groups and a helpline on 0333 332 2033 (Monday to Friday 10.00am to 4.00pm) to speak to a team of food advisors and dietitians if you are unsure about any foods while shopping or eating out.

Celiac Disease Foundation
https://celiac.org/
From its base in California, CDF operates a global organisation committed to speeding up diagnosis and treatments for Coeliac Disease. Its aim is to improve the health and well-being of the millions of individuals around the world affected by the autoimmune disease, through investments in research, advocacy and education.

National Celiac Association
https://nationalceliac.org/
US-based non-profit organisation dedicated to educating and advocating for individuals with Celiac Disease and Non-celiac Gluten Sensitivities, their families, and communities throughout the country. A membership is not a requirement to access most of its information but having one offers newsletters, a regular magazine, educational programs and other benefits.

Coeliac Australia
https://coeliac.org.au/
A registered charity offering membership, support, education and credible information to Australians with Coeliac Disease and associated conditions requiring a gluten-free diet. It works in partnership with lead researchers and institutions in the search for prevention and cure for the disease.

Celiac Canada
www.celiac.ca/
A national charity giving everyone with Celiac Disease support, advice and lifelong tools to help them manage a gluten-free lifestyle. It offers a product finder, information about reading labels and runs events.

Anaphylaxis UK
www.anaphylaxis.org.uk/
A UK charity supporting people living with serious allergies and the possibility of experiencing anaphylactic shock, as well as their families and businesses, schools and other educational establishments.

Asthma and Allergy Foundation of America
https://aafa.org/get-involved/community-get-support/
A non-profit organisation supporting people with allergies to help them to manage their conditions.

Allergy and Anaphylaxis Australia
https://allergyfacts.org.au/
A registered charity dedicated to providing credible, evidence-based information, resources and services to support Australians with allergic disease and those who care for them.

Certification Organisations
Teams of scientists that test and give a seal of approval to gluten-free products and services so that you can have confidence buying them.

Association of European Coeliac Societies
www.aoecs.org/
Provides a link to coeliac organisations in Europe, coordinates the exchange of information, skills and knowledge amongst them and works towards consistent labelling and certification.

The Gluten-Free Certification Organization
https://gfco.org/
Helps manufacturers meet a strict 80-point standard, including that all starting ingredients and finished products test below the applicable gluten-free threshold of the country of sale, or 10 ppm (whichever is lower), and the prohibition of oats in countries where that is a requirement, such as Australia and New Zealand.

BRCGS
www.brcgs.com/our-standards/gluten-free-certification
The Brand Reputation through Compliance Global Standard, previously known as the British Retail Consortium sets standards globally for food safety, packaging, storage and distribution and is recognised by leading coeliac organisations around the world.